SOCIAL AND PSYCHOLOGICAL ASPECTS OF HIV/AIDS AND THEIR RAMIFICATIONS

Edited by **Gobopamang Letamo**

Social and Psychological Aspects of HIV/AIDS and Their Ramifications
Edited by Gobopamang Letamo

Published by InTech

Janeza Trdine 9, 51000 Rijeka, Croatia

Publishing Process Manager Alenka Urbancic

Technical Editor Teodora Smiljanic

Cover Designer InTech Design Team

Additional hard copies can be obtained from orders@intechopen.com

Social and Psychological Aspects of HIV/AIDS and Their Ramifications, Edited by Gobopamang Letamo
p. cm.
ISBN 978-953-307-640-9

For EU product safety concerns:
IN TECH d.o.o., Prolaz Marije Krucifikse Kozulić 3, 51000 Rijeka, Croatia,
info@intechopen.com or visit our website at intechopen.com.

Meet the editor

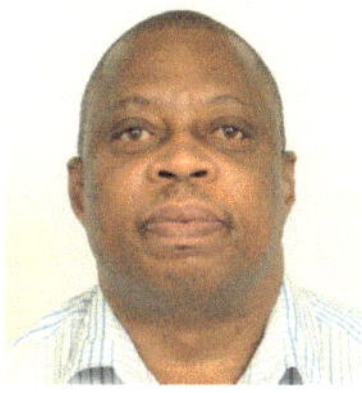

Professor Gobopamang Letamo is an Associate Professor in the Department of Population Studies at the University of Botswana. He has worked in the area of sexual and reproductive health, including HIV/AIDS, for 15 years and published extensively on the topic. He has also served as an External Examiner in Population Studies/ Demography at Makerere University in Uganda, North West University in South Africa and National University of Lesotho in Lesotho. In addition to working in academia, Professor Letamo has worked with United Nations Population Fund as an Assistant Representative in the Botswana country office where his responsibilities included programme monitoring and implementation for 2 years. Prof. Letamo has also served in various national committees and written peer-reviewed articles submitted for publication in journals of international reputation dealing with issues of HIV and AIDS.

Contents

Preface

Since the advent of HIV/AIDS, numerous publications have emerged on the subject, predominantly focussing on the biomedical aspects of the disease. In recent years, it has been recognized that HIV/AIDS is not just a medical condition, but also has political, social, psychological, economic and demographic ramifications that need to be dealt with. However, research addressing HIV/AIDS areas outside the biomedical side of research is limited.

This book was born out of desire among scholars researching in the field of HIV and AIDS to document the social and psychosocial aspects of HIV/AIDS epidemic, and the impact that these aspects have on HIV/AIDS-related behaviours. The book is titled "Social and Psychosocial Aspects of HIV/AIDS and their Ramifications" to reflect the multi-dimensionality of the HIV/AIDS epidemic. The book addresses key areas of HIV and AIDS, including, but not in any way limited to, care-seeking behaviour, adherence, access, psychosocial needs and support services, discrimination and the impact the epidemic has on various sectors of the economy. Researchers, students and other people interested in the HIV and AIDS in general will find this book informative and easy to read and understand. The book is an essential reading for academics, students and other people interested in the field of HIV and AIDS.

We are grateful for the helpful comments received from the various anonymous reviewers during the preparation of this book for publication. The facts and opinions expressed in this book are those of the authors/editors and do not necessarily reflect the views of the institutions they represent.

September 2011

Gobopamang Letamo

Department of Population Studies
University of Botswana

Part 1

Social Aspects of HIV / AIDS

1

The Experiences and Complexities of Care-Seeking Behavior of People Living with HIV/AIDS: A Qualitative Study in Nigeria

Ngozi C. Mbonu, Bart Van Den Borne and Nanne K. De Vries
School of Public Health and Primary Care (CAPHRI)
Faculty of Health Medicine and Life Sciences, Maastricht University
The Netherlands

1. Introduction

In 2009, approximately 2.98 million people in Nigeria were living with HIV/AIDS. More than 192,000 deaths were caused by AIDS and 2.175 million AIDS orphans are now living in Nigeria (UNAIDS, 2010). The availability of anti-retroviral therapy (ART) implies that people living with HIV/AIDS (PLWHA) should be able to carry out daily activities like the rest of society. However, there are a number of hindrances to the utilization of care, leading to suboptimal effectiveness of available treatment (Hilhorst et al., 2006; Morolake et al., 2009). One of the factors seems to be stigma; PLWHA and their care givers have to cope with negative reactions from the people directly around them as well as from the community (Mwinituo & Mill, 2006; Mitchell et al., 2007; Sabin et al., 2008; Adewuya et al., 2009; Hejoaka, 2009; Demmer, 2011). A study carried out among home based care givers in KwaZulu Natal South Africa showed that home based care givers experience high levels of burden and are targets of HIV-related prejudice and discrimination (Singh et al., 2011).

Not only does the discovery that one is infected with HIV lead to fear of progression into AIDS and fear of dying, it also creates an anticipation of negative social reactions among PLWHA. Sontag (1989) argues that it is not the suffering of the disease that is deeply feared, but the denigration that is suffered from having the disease that makes PLWHA vulnerable as individuals and within society. People in the community have a negative attitude towards PLWHA because they attribute the characteristic of promiscuity to those who are infected (Campbell et al., 2007). Societal norms and values in Nigeria are restrictive and secretive, while discussion about sex is often private for cultural and religious reasons (Ajuwon et al., 1998), making people who transgress these norms likely to be condemned because norms are very strong and strict.

Several studies around the world (Amirkhanian et al., 2003; Singh et al., 2009; Stevelink et al., 2011; Vlassoff & Ali, 2011) and in Africa indicate that PLWHA are still discriminated against (Muyinda et al., 1997; Duffy, 2005; Shisana et al., 2005; Muula & Mfutso-Bengo, 2005; Hilhorst et al., 2006; Liamputtong et al., 2009; Morolake et al., 2009; Amuri et al., 2011), making them resort to varied ways of coping with their problems (Mbonu et al., 2009). Despite these studies indicating the presence of stigma, literature have equally acknowledged that one of the positive noticeable interventions in the fight of HIV/AIDS and stigma is giving HIV/AIDS a human face (Fokolade et al., 2009; Morolake et al., 2009) but this implies that PLWHA who are active in public HIV/AIDS programmes may have to cope with additional problems. A UNAIDS summary of literature on HIV-related stigma and discrimination recognizes the strengthening of networks of PLWHA that take lead in addressing stigma and calls for more studies to evaluate stigma and discrimination programs (UNAIDS, 2009; UNAIDS, 2010). There is an urgent need for evidence-based research to meet the needs of those affected by HIV/AIDS (Doyal, 2009). Moreover, experiences of PLWHA who are members of an existing network will help in future HIV/AIDS policies that can be used in society and by health care institutions (Nyblade et al., 2009).

In this chapter, we aim to report results from a qualitative study that explores the stigmatization experiences, coping mechanisms and care-seeking choices of PLWHA who belong to an association network in Port Harcourt, Nigeria. We also explore the possible role of contextual factors related to these stigmatization experiences and the PLWHA's health care-seeking behavior as a consequence.

2. Theoretical framework

Following prior research on stigma in relation to HIV/AIDS (Mbonu, Van Den Borne & De Vries, 2009), using an inductive approach from an extensive literature review in Sub-Saharan Africa, we adapted the Precede portion of the Precede-Proceed model (Green & Kreuter, 1999) as an explanatory model. The PRECEDE-PROCEED model provides a systematic approach for assessing quality-of-life of health and for designing, implementing, and evaluating health education and health promotion programs. PRECEDE includes five phases. In phase 1, quality of life or social problems and needs of a population are identified. Phase 2 includes an epidemiological analysis in which the relevant health problems are identified. Phase 3 involves an analysis of the behavioral and environmental determinants of a key health problem. In the fourth phase, the factors that predispose (beliefs, knowledge, self-efficacy, social norms, etc.), reinforce (e.g. social support), and enable (facilities etc.) the health behavior, are identified. In phase 5, the focus is on the development of a health education or health promotion intervention that would encourage desired behavior change, changes in the environment, and changes in the determinants of behavior and environmental factors. PROCEED includes an implementation phase, an intervention process evaluation, impact evaluation of changes in behavior or environment, and an outcome evaluation in which the impact on health and quality of life is assessed (Green & Kreuter, 1999). Since models are constantly modified to fit the situation (Chiang et al., 2003), we specified the model to the health care-seeking behaviour among PLWHA and used it to analyse people's coping strategies in dealing with stigma-related problems (Mbonu et al., 2009). The model proposes that a complex health problem, such as care-seeking behaviour of PLWHA, is a function of various factors; and these factors have to be considered from a wider perspective of the social structural context.

The first component of the explanatory model is the analysis of the problem - that is, care-seeking behaviour of PLWHA and how stigma influences it (see [a] in Figure 1) and how it may have an impact on the socio-structural context within which PLWHA, society and healthcare professionals are embedded. The second component of the model involves identifying the predisposing, reinforcing and enabling factors. The predisposing factors are represented as variables such as beliefs, knowledge about HIV transmission and self-efficacy. Reinforcing and enabling factors are represented as moderating variables, such as poverty, gender, age, religion and policy and how stigma may impact on the variables that determine individuals' care-seeking behaviour. The model finally specifies different coping strategies (coping with self, coping directed at others and comparison with others, coping with solving the problems of HIV/AIDS) that can lead to various care-seeking choices, such as inappropriate self-care, inconsistent use of biochemical care or use of traditional healers and faith houses, which may result in non-utilisation of healthcare institutions. In our explanatory model, non-utilisation of healthcare institutions is the outcome variable (see [n] in Figure 1).

In this study, while the interview was left open for interviewees to express a variety of issues, thoughts and feelings with respect to stigma and other concepts, we use the explanatory model as a general framework for identifying relevant categories of variables.

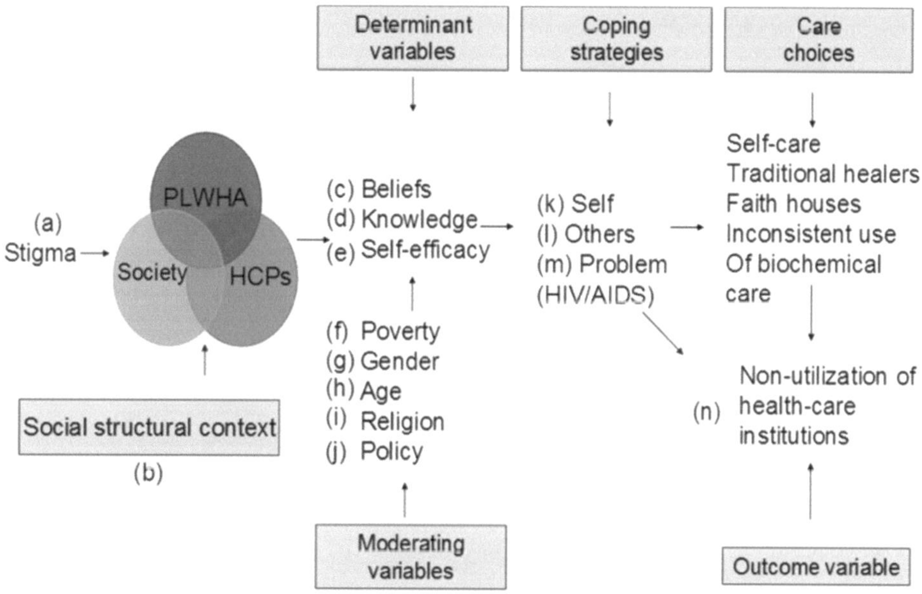

Fig. 1. Explanatory model of role of stigma in care-seeking behaviour.
Mbonu, Van den Borne, & De Vries, 2009

3. Methodology

We conducted in-depth semi-structured interviews with a purposive sample of 20 adults (12 females and 8 males) living with HIV/AIDS who were receiving care from a resource centre in Port Harcourt, Nigeria. Participants are members of network association of PLWHA and therefore were willing to be interviewed about their circumstances. All persons approached agreed to participate. Participants identified themselves as Christians and their ages ranged from 24 years to 48 years. In addition, ten of these participants (6 females and 4 males) participated in a focus group discussion which was conducted in the resource centre. The focus group discussion allowed the participants to exchange ideas and react to issues brought up by fellow participants. The resource centre was established to care for PLWHA and people with other sexually transmitted diseases. In addition, it provides pre and post HIV test counseling and nutritional advice for the PLWHA. Informed consent was obtained verbally from the persons who were interviewed and their anonymity was guaranteed. The aim of the study was explained to them before the interview took place. Interviews were conducted in the English language. Rivers State Agency for the control of AIDS approved the study.

The interviews were held in the resource centre or, in some cases, in people's residences (3 people). All the participants discussed freely the questions and issues covered in the study. The interviews were transcribed from audio tape and analyzed. The software package Nvivo 7 was used to analyze the data and identify major themes from Figure 1. Coding was done by the first author and subsequently validated by an independent researcher, who coded a random selection of data to look for new concepts. Emerging themes were compared by the independent researcher with the coding by the author. New entries and discrepancies were checked by re-reading the transcripts and fine-tuning interpretations until unambiguous categories and themes were agreed.

Table 1 shows information about the participants

Nr.	Gender	Status	Work	Reason for HIV test	Age	ART status
1	Female	Widow	Government Worker	went for test after the Husband was sick with HIV	40 years	On ART
2	Female	Widow	Government Worker	went for test after the Husband was sick with HIV	44 years	On ART
3	Female	Single	Office Worker in Company now unemployed	was sick and went for test afterwards	24 years	Not yet On ART because of lack of Money
4	Female	Single	Company Worker	was sick and was sent for testing	39 years	On ART
5	Female	Widow	Government Worker	went for test after the husband was dying From HIV	45 years	On ART
6	Male	Single	Private Office Worker	sent for test after being sick	35 years	Take herbs, Fruit, and Vegetable he stopped ART Reacts to ART
7	Female	Married	Housewife (husband lost job)	discovered HIV status during delivery of baby	29 years	On ART
8	Female	Married	Housewife	Discovered HIV status during delivery of baby	27 years	On ART
9	Female	Widow	Petty trader	went for test after husband died from HIV/AIDS	38 years	On ART

Nr.	Gender	Status	Work	Reason for HIV test	Age	ART status
10	Male	Separated	Government Worker	sent for test after sickness	41 years	On ART
11	Female	Married	Unemployed	went for test during delivery	29 years	On ART
12	Female	Widow	Government Worker	Pre-operative test screening	45 years	On ART
13	Female	Widow	Secretary (lost job)	Got sick and sent for test	40 years	On ART
14	Female	Married	Company worker	Got sick and sent for test	48 years	On ART
15	Male	Single	Banker	Got sick and sent for test	40 years	On ART
16	Male	Married	Government worker	Got sick and tested	38 years	On ART
17	Female	Widow	Petty trader	Husband was sick	47 years	On ART
18	Male	Single	Government worker	Was sick and went for test	28 years	On ART
19	Male	Single	Company worker (lost job)	Company screening	35 years	On ART
20	Male	Married	Unemployed	Was sick and tested	29 years	On ART

4. Results

The results of this study are organized according to the components of the explanatory model in Figure 1. Some basic distinguishing characteristics of participants are provided after the quote.

4.1 Stigma

Participants indicated that negative reactions towards them were the major problems they had, affecting the way they cope with HIV/AIDS and leading to non-utilization of health-care institutions. These negative reactions came from the community, including their close social networks, such as neighbors, family or their spouse. A participant explained the reaction of her neighbors when they discovered the positive status of her and her husband:
'My neighbors found out in the church that my husband and I are HIV positive, they now pursued [sic] (sent away) us from the compound. The landlord and the neighbors drove us away from the compound we are living in because they said HIV will affect them. We live in an uncompleted building now.' (Female, 29 years, housewife, participant 7, in-depth interview)
Some participants, even without revealing their HIV status to their partners, were abandoned because of suspicions of being HIV-infected. Others lived with their spouses although these spouses knew they were HIV-positive. But anticipated public reactions are apparently strong. A participant in the focus group discussion reported being abandoned by her partner when she went public with her positive status:
'I have lived with this man for five years. I have had HIV since then but he accepted it. He even was planning to marry me but then I went on a programme on the radio and his friends recognized my

voice. They immediately called him and after that he left me because he said he was ready to live with the knowledge of my HIV alone but not to share it with others. I find it stupid because he has lived with me all this long.' (Female, single, company worker, FGD)

This has implications for seeking care at health-care institutions if the participant needs her partner for financial support. Furthermore, some participants reported that health-care professionals (HCPs) also exhibit negative reactions towards PLWHA. The negative reactions from HCPs were enough to discourage them from going for treatment, leading to non-utilization of health-care institutions, as illustrated by these quotes:

'Some health care professionals are not friendly when they come to find out that someone is HIV-positive. They tend to discard [sic] someone. They will not attend to me in the clinic and ask me to wait by the corner while attending to others.' (Male, 41 years, separated, government worker, participant 10, in-depth interview)

'Before, I had a problem with health-care professionals in the hospital where I delivered my baby, they were not nice. It was there I found out my HIV status. They started running and avoiding me.' (Female, 29 years, housewife, participant 11, in-depth interview)

4.2 Determinant variables

The model also postulates that stigma has impact on three kinds of variables (beliefs, knowledge about HIV/AIDS, and self-efficacy) which are particularly important because of their impact on the coping strategies that PLWHA use and on the health-care choices they make leading to non-utilization of health care facilities.

4.2.1 Beliefs

Beliefs (see [c] in Figure 1) can either be general beliefs about HIV infection or about persons with HIV or AIDS, e.g the pathways of HIV infection. The following quotes illustrate this:

'I think HIV is a problem for everyone who has HIV because the society thinks you are loose [sic] promiscuous.' (Male, 35 years, single, company worker, participant 6, in-depth interview)

'People will blame me for having HIV because they will say I am a prostitute.' (Female, 24 years, single, unemployed, participant 3, in-depth interview)

The anticipation of reactions based on these popular beliefs makes PLWHA refrain from seeking care. It can also be beliefs about the reactions of others to the care-seeking behaviour of persons with HIV or AIDS, or specific beliefs about the feasibility of coping. This can lead to the non-utilization of health-care institutions and thereby make PLWHA unable to get the quality of care they need. Apparently, the expectation is that society will label every PLWHA as promiscuous and irresponsible. PLWHA are very aware of these societal beliefs. They expect to be blamed. As one participant said frankly to the interviewer:

'You should campaign more to people. You should tell people it is not only by sex that people have HIV, which is always the problem. When people change towards people with HIV then we can get better support and care at home and hospital.' (Female, 45 years, widow, government worker, participant 12, in-depth interview)

4.2.2 Knowledge

This can be knowledge about HIV and AIDS (see [d] in Figure 1), HIV status, HIV transmission and about effective treatment, which are important for the utilization of health-care institutions. In our study, all of the participants were aware of their HIV status and antiretroviral therapy (ART) because they belonged to an association network. In the general population, knowledge is expected to be limited. Furthermore, many of the participants felt that joining an association of people in the same situation helped them gain knowledge of HIV/AIDS and its care possibilities, for instance:

'Persons with HIV should join the association of people living with HIV and AIDS so they can get good information about the disease.' (Female, 40 years, widow, government worker, participant 1, in-depth interview)

4.2.3 Self-efficacy

Self-efficacy (see [e] in Figure 1) is the idea that one can carry out a task effectively and leads to problem-focused coping such as PLWHA finding the right health-care institution and the right treatment from health-care workers, going for HIV tests, or handling their condition and situation if others know about their HIV-positive status. Some of our participants had adequate self-efficacy in handling the situation when their HIV status was revealed to their relatives. For instance, a participant who is on ART described how he handled the situation with his brother when he disclosed his positive HIV status this way:

'My brother wanted to withdraw from me but when I talked to him, he understood ..I told him it can happen to even him, beside he has seen that I am not dying and I am still going on with my life.' (Male, 41 years, separated, government worker, participant 10, in-depth interview)

A few others had low self-efficacy in handling their situation when others heard about their HIV status. Some participants who looked at HIV/AIDS as a chronic illness felt more confident in handling their situation of being drug-compliant and going for treatment at hospitals. One participant explained that normally in society, one is expected not to talk about one's illness and HIV/AIDS is no different, so, based on this expectation she decided to keep it a secret from others that she was taking her ART medications:

'It is not only people with HIV that take drugs, hypertensive people take drugs, diabetes people take drugs and still these sicknesses do not go.' (Female, 40 years, widow, company worker, participant 13, in-depth interview)

By implication, the strong stigma around HIV inhibits high self-efficacy. PLWHA seem to regard HIV/AIDS as just another illness as a psychological means to increase their confidence in handling problems associated with HIV/AIDS and its care.

4.3 Moderating variables

The model also postulates that certain moderating variables (poverty, gender, age, religion and policy) have an impact on the coping and care-seeking behavior of PLWHA.

4.3.1 Poverty

Our participants reported that although many of them are aware of the benefits of ART, many are unable to utilize the health-care institutions and take ART because they do not have the money to procure it or pay for other medical and laboratory costs. Some, who do buy ART, are unable to routinely take their medication due to lack of money since many of them lost their jobs after HIV diagnosis. Participants were also concerned about how their financial problems affect the whole family. For instance, a participant explained her dilemma in going for treatment:

'I have not gone for treatment because I do not have money. I need money. I am broke. I have to feed myself. Right now, my husband is admitted in the ward. Even I have lab test to do but I have no money. I need money to buy food, drugs. My child is sick too with HIV.' (Female, 29 years, housewife, participant 7, in-depth interview)

Further discussion showed the difficulty with utilization of health-care institutions:

'In our organization, people living with HIV/AIDS are facing a lot of problems. Most of them are not working. Some of them were working before but because of their HIV status they were laid off from their work. Many of them are jobless that is why treatment is difficult. We lose our members often.' (Male, 41 years, separated, government worker, participant 10, in-depth interview)

4.3.2 Gender

Our study shows that due to stigma associated with HIV/AIDS, male PLWHA are not willing to disclose their positive HIV status to their wives causing delay in seeking care. There seems to be a clear difference in the timing of HIV/AIDS diagnosis between male and female participants. Women find out much later after being infected. There are a number of reasons for this. First, society expects women to be conservative and faithful to their partners; such cautiousness, however, does not protect women from HIV if their partners keep multiple partners and do not use protection during sexual intercourse. Moreover, even when women find out their HIV status, they have to disclose to their partners immediately if they want to secure financial aid for treatment. On the contrary, society tolerates men with multiple partners. Men who are HIV positive may still be angry when they find out and blame women for their HIV infection. In this study, married women, who contracted HIV from their partners, felt very bad and betrayed when they discovered their positive HIV status. Two of the female participants in particular (participant 1 and 5) expressed anger towards their partners because of assumed infidelity resulting in infection:

'The thing (HIV/AIDS) pains me (very angry). I married him as a virgin, I never played life. The thing pains me. You know if I played life as a young girl, I would feel better but I tell you, the thing pains me.' (Female, 45 years, widow, company worker, participant 5, in-depth interview)

Another said:

'I was very sad and confused. I now understand why my last three children died. When I was pregnant with them my pregnancy was not even up to nine months and they did not grow well like my first three children. They were always emaciated. They were premature and this man (her husband) knew he was HIV-positive and did not tell me. It is bad.' (Female, 40 years, widow, government worker, participant 1, in-depth interview)

Second, men take decisions in the family and are breadwinners while women are mostly dependent. These differences are shown at the diagnostic and during illness phases. At the diagnostic phase, some women in this study were diagnosed as part of routine blood tests at pregnancy. This led to women discovering their HIV status without being previously informed by their spouses. At the illness phase, some women in this study were ill but needed their partners' support and approval before seeking care. Women who are tested during pregnancy find out earlier in contrast to women who present themselves to the hospital for an HIV-related illness. Apparently, the male control and lack of support hinders women from making early effective care choices such as VCT. On the contrary, males cannot be diagnosed routinely because they are never pregnant. Male participants presented themselves with illness to the hospital before being sent for HIV test and did not need approval from their spouses before seeking care. An early diagnosis is important because when people find out their HIV status early, they are more likely to make an effective care choice especially for those who know about ART. Female participants emphasized their frustration at the lack of knowledge of their spouses' HIV status. This female participant put it this way:

'Imagine how my husband hid his HIV status from me so I now have HIV/AIDS from him. If I was a man, I would not be in this condition because I know myself.' (Female, 40 years, widow, government worker, participant 1, in-depth interview)

In summary, the gender issue is relevant in care seeking because it affects time of diagnosis, societal blame and necessity of disclosure to partner.

4.3.3 Age

Our study shows that young participants emphasized a strong interest in marrying and having children. This was particularly important for them to fulfill their societal role. The emphasis on reproduction was demonstrated by this participant:

'Infact this baby issue has given me a lot of stress. You know, I have to think of the uncertainties.' (Male, 35 years, single, company worker, participant 6, in-depth interview)

They believed that the ART will prevent their babies from being infected with HIV. This encouraged them to seek access to ART and care despite the costs involved in accessing care:

'I plan to have a baby because I do not have any. HIV will not affect my baby again provided I am taking my Anti retroviral therapy drugs.' (Female, 29 years, housewife, participant 11, in depth interview)

'I will like to have baby. I am looking forward to marriage. My unborn baby maybe infected but we are told in the hospital that if you take your drugs effectively the baby may not be infected.' (Male, 41 years, separated, Government worker, participant 10, in-depth interview)

On the contrary, due to fear of stigma young people may not want to go for HIV testing. This enhances the spread of HIV/AIDS and decreases prevention of vertical transmission. This participant who disclosed his positive HIV status to his girl friend found it difficult to convince her to go for HIV testing:

'I tried to encourage my girlfriend to go for HIV test but she did not agree to go for the HIV test. I gave her some money but she will turn and ask me whether she is sick? Why should she go for test? I told her it is important she goes for the test because I have the feeling that she has HIV because if she does not get it from me then she may get it from another person. She was angry with me that I am accusing her. At the end of the day she did not go for the test before we parted.' (Male, 28 years, single, government worker, participant 18, in-depth interview)

4.3.4 Religion

Our data show that some participants received spiritual and psychological support from the pastors in the church; however, the church congregation is not free from stigmatizing reactions. Since the church is made up of members of society, in further anticipation of gossip, this participant indicated a lack of trust in people at his church:

'In the church where I go, the moment they know my HIV status, they will start asking each other whether they have heard? It is even your closest friend that will give you out.' (Male, 48years, married, company worker, participant 14, in-depth interview)

Such anticipations of negative reactions of church members can discourage PLWHA from utilizing health-care institutions. This may also lead to not looking for and not getting support from relevant others.

4.3.5 Policy

Discussion with participants revealed that many of them wanted free anti-retroviral therapy and wanted the government to implement a policy for protected work and a financial policy for PLWHA such as provision of micro-credits, which would enable them to pay for health-care facilities. A participant said this:

'Government should come to our aid. They should give us work because many of us whose HIV status is known have lost their job. They should give us micro credit.' (Female, 40 years, widow, government worker, participant 1, in-depth interview)

At the time this study was carried, participants had access to subsidized ART, which means they still have to pay some expenses out of pocket which some of them could not afford. All the participants in this study went for HIV diagnosis with a clear reason. 5 women were tested after their husbands were sick or dying from HIV/AIDS, 3 women were tested during antenatal care, 4 women and 7 men were tested because of illness, and 1 man was tested at the behest of employers. Further discussion revealed that some employers send people for compulsory HIV testing without pre-informing them about the HIV test; afterwards they fire staff with a positive HIV diagnosis. A participant in the focus group discussion said this:

'What happens here is that immediately a company discovers one is HIV-positive, they will not terminate the appointment based on HIV. It will not be written in one's letter. They may say because of so much labor they want to downsize the company. I lost my job. The company had to go through HIV screening test. All the staff was involved. After discovering that some of us were HIV-positive, they had to lay us off. They did not call it HIV test, they called the test a different name because they know if they call it HIV test some people will not go for it. In the process some of us were affected and I am one of those people affected.' (FGD)

4.4 Coping mechanisms

In the following section, we report how PLWHA cope with HIV/AIDS and how different coping strategies affect PLWHA utilizing health-care institutions.

4.4.1 Coping with emotions because of HIV/AIDS

As shown in (k) of Figure 1, PLWHA may use different internal coping strategies directed at their own emotional problems. Some of our participants showed some fearful emotional reactions after diagnosis, such as thoughts of suicide and feelings that society would not show them sympathy if they knew about their positive status. A male participant reacted to the diagnosis like this:

'Initially, I felt very bad when I knew of my HIV status. I thought myself has finished in this world.' (Male, 41 years, separated, government worker, participant 10, in-depth interview)

A reaction from another participant was more extreme:

'I was scared when I was told I have HIV/AIDS. I felt like killing myself.' (Female, 24 years, single, unemployed, participant 3, in-depth interview)

The study's participants tried to cope with these emotional reactions through denial or by downplaying HIV/AIDS as a serious threat. They compared HIV/AIDS with other illnesses, denying that HIV/AIDS was any serious threat and that helped them to cope. Furthermore, they rather emphasized that HIV is not contracted from sex alone for example:

'HIV/AIDS is a normal sickness and anybody can have it, it can come by sex, sickness or even the Hausa people (some Northern people) that move around doing pedicure for people.' (Female, 40 years, widow, company worker, participant 13, in-depth interview)

4.4.2 Coping directed at others and comparison with others

Second, the coping strategy of PLWHA aimed at reducing the unfavorable reactions of others (see [l] in Figure 1) may include hiding tendencies, finding support from significant others or comparison with other people living with HIV/AIDS. This strategy may also involve trying to influence the meaning other people attach to HIV and AIDS (Goffman,

1963), such as attributing their HIV/AIDS to poison. Our study showed that the feasibility of hiding their HIV statuses depended on the stage of illness and use of ART. The concealment of their positive status enabled them to carry out their activities. In the focus group discussion, many participants explained why ART helped them cope with the physical features associated with HIV/AIDS. Many felt better with ART and did not have the look typical of AIDS patients, for instance:

'Since I started taking antiretroviral therapy, people do not know I have HIV/AIDS. They cannot suspect.' (Female, married, company worker, FGD)

Another way of coping reported by the participants was to withdraw from people who they thought may suspect or know their diagnosis. They resolved not to tell anybody, as illustrated by the following quotes:

'I have not told any other person. I did not tell my friends, If I tell them, na dey same thing [sic] (the same thing), they will run away from me.' (Female, 29 years, housewife, participant 7, in-depth interview)

'The society will not welcome me when they know my HIV status, so it is good keeping it to me instead of people running away from me. That alone can cause emotional stress to me. It can cause more problems to me when I am rejected.' (Male, 48 years, married, company worker, participant 14, in-depth interview)

Some of the participants chose to use selective disclosure. Selective disclosure was commonly made to people they trusted and who could support them:

'I told my girlfriend who is also HIV positive but we did not know before we met. I told my doctor and my God. I told my doctor because I need his advice. HIV is something between the person, his or her doctor and God.' (Male, 35 years, single, company worker, participant 6, in-depth interview)

'I told my husband, two of his sisters and one of my pastors. I told them because they are close to me.' (Female, 27 years, housewife, participant 8, in-depth interview)

Disclosure continues to be a huge problem. A few participants disclosed their status involuntarily out of necessity for financial support; while for some participants, people around them just ended up knowing. Some tried to deny it even when confronted. A participant, who discussed his positive HIV status on TV, still hides from his neighbors. He tries to deceive them into believing he is just working for an organization:

'I do not keep my HIV status quiet but I tend to keep it quiet within my vicinity; but outside my vicinity I expose it because they used to call me out for programme. My neighbors used to say they saw me on the television but I always tell them to confuse them that we have an organization or I belong to an organization that take care of people with HIV and AIDS.' (Male, 41 years, separated, government worker, participant 10, in-depth interview)

Others decided not to tell their colleagues because they did not want to lose their jobs. Concealment may be necessary for them to keep up with their financial obligations that would enable PLWHA utilize health-care facilities. This participant said the following when asked whether any of her colleagues knew about her positive status:

'Ah no… (Laughter). I have to tell you the truth, they [colleagues] will not mind to sum up one thing and that will be the reason for sending me out of the job. I will therefore tell nobody.' (Female, 40 years, widow, government worker, participant 1, in-depth interview)

Disclosing HIV status to children was particularly difficult due to what is widely believed to be the cause of HIV/AIDS and fear of losing role model status. Sometimes, PLWHA preferred to wait until they were actually sick with HIV. Another problem that PLWHA tried to cope with was with significant others such as their partners. Some of them had got married without informing their partners until pregnancy, while others hoped their ART would help when they get married. This has implications for the spread of the virus, as well as for the process of seeking appropriate care at an early stage. Many PLWHA felt it was difficult to give an explanation for being unfit to have children. On the contrary, a female participant who was already married and felt she had contracted HIV through a blood transfusion during childbirth received positive support from her spouse. PLWHA may also prefer to associate with other people with HIV/AIDS by joining association networks as a way of coping with their illness. Others simply ascribe HIV/AIDS to another, more acceptable cause, such as attributing HIV/AIDS to poison, which may encourage them to use traditional healers and prevent them from utilizing health-care institutions. For instance, the husband of this female participant who was HIV-positive said he was poisoned:

'This man (my husband) knew he was HIV-positive and did not tell me. It is bad. He told me his village people (his kindred) gave him juju (African charm/poison).' (Female, 40 years, widow, government worker, participant 1, in-depth interview)

4.4.3 Coping directed at problem solving

Third, to solve this problem related to HIV/AIDS, some participants reported strategies that excluded going to the hospital early and consistent use of ART (which are known to be effective). Instead, they preferred to try other options first rather than going to hospital for treatment with ART. Many of the participants mentioned using a combination of therapies; they went to faith houses, traditional healers, used herbs or combined them with attending a health-care institution. This strategy may affect consistent utilization of health-care institutions since some of them may abandon utilization of health care when they feel better and then use traditional healers and faith houses. Furthermore, we asked the participants their advice to other PLWHA. Their advice mostly was a reflection of what they practiced themselves:

'Persons with HIV should pray to God for a miracle.' (Female, 24 years, single, unemployed, participant 3, in-depth interview)

'My advice is that people with HIV should have hope in God.' (Female, 29 years, married, housewife, participant 7, in-depth interview)

'HIV people have to trust in God and God can always change things.' (Male, 48 years, married, company worker, participant 14, in-depth interview)

4.5 Care choices

Some participants made care choices, which made them refrain from treatment or stop their treatment after they had started. Others chose not to tell their pastors but went for prayers alone. Many of the participants believed God could cure them of HIV and combined it with going to hospital for ART. It was also common for them to resort to religion early to solve problems, hence it was not unusual that visiting faith houses such as churches were the early choices participants made when managing their sickness:

'I did not feel anything when I was told I had HIV because I know my God will heal me.' (Female, 47 years, widow, petty trader, participant 17, in-depth interview)

5. Discussion

Our study focused on factors associated with PLWHA making care choices. Our participants are different from other PLWHA because they have tested themselves and sought care however they still gave insight in the stigma related processes which affect utilization of health care institutions. Few participants in our study experienced positive support from their immediate family after disclosure of their positive HIV status and we found support for our main proposition that PLWHA still experience stigma in society including health care institutions, and in an effort to cope with stigma, utilized different care choices frequently which can affect utilization of health-care institutions. Our data revealed that poverty and religion were important in coping with HIV/AIDS as well as in making care choices, which affect utilization of health care institutions. Some PLWHA do not have money while others lost their jobs based on their positive HIV status, which has implications for them when deciding to seek care in health institutions especially since many people do not have health insurance or money to cover ART and care. The impact of stigma on PLWHA in Nigeria in the context of work constitutes an important barrier to seeking effective care and treatment. The right to work in Nigeria entails the rights of every person access to employment without any pre-condition except the necessary occupational qualifications (Iwuagwu et al., 2003). Moreover one of the guidelines in which Nigerian HIV/AIDS policy is based on is non-stigma and non-discrimination in recruitment, employment, admission and termination (National Agency for Control of AIDS (NACA), 2005) yet protection of PLWHA from dismissal from work poses some practical challenges. First, there is poor implementation of existing HIV/AIDS policies (National HIV/AIDS Policy Review Report, 2009) especially in private sectors that may cite other acceptable reasons (albeit non-HIV related reasons) for dismissal from work. Second, There is yet no legislation addressing HIV/AIDS related issues such as employment rights (Durojaye, 2003; National HIV/AIDS Policy Review Report, 2009) and the HIV/AIDS anti stigma bill is yet to be passed into law by the National Assembly of Nigeria. Oluduro and Ayankogbe (2003) noted that although there are treaties ratified by Nigerian government internationally including those concerning HIV/AIDS, some of them are yet to be domesticated (Oluduro & Ayankogbe, 2003). Furthermore treaties do not have force of law on their own and only treaties enacted into law by National Assembly of Nigeria can bind the Federal Republic of Nigeria (Oluduro & Ayankobe, 2003). Despite these challenges, Nigerian citizens have the fundamental rights enshrined in the constitution that guarantees every citizen freedom from stigma and discrimination and therefore can be applied to PLWHA (Azinge, 2003) to protect PLWHA legally while expectation of the eventual passage of the HIV/AIDS anti stigma law by the National Assembly. A different study carried out in Russia also reported job losses by PLWHA (Amirkhanian et al., 2003) making securing of a living and finances an integral part of coping and care-seeking in health-care institutions. Conversely, those participants who were still working and financially capable were able to cope and had less need to ask people for financial help, and hence, successfully hid their status while utilizing health care facilities and taking ART.

Many of the participants went for HIV testing with a clear reason. This has implications for early HIV diagnosis and the use of ART, due to the subsequent delay in visiting health-care institutions. In addition, early voluntary counseling and testing (VCT) will prepare, give people knowledge and the self-efficacy needed to cope with and manage HIV/AIDS. This finding is consistent with a study carried out in Thailand, which showed that the majority of the men underwent HIV testing for health reasons, while the majority of women were tested following family events, such as a spouse's passing away or pregnancy (Le Coeur et al., 2009). Fear of being identified as someone infected by HIV increases the likelihood of people avoiding VCT (Nyblade et al., 2009).

Our data showed that the discovery and disclosure of a positive HIV status may lead to family disharmony, generating a lot of suspicions. The findings show that concealment and disclosure remained an uphill task for PLWHA. The concealment affects their self-efficacy in seeking care in health institutions, which in turn can lead to non-utilization of health-care institutions because they will not want to be seen there. This study showed that some of the participants who disclosed, experienced negative consequences while others received support. Some of our participants had problems when they went on the radio programme as part of the PLWHA association activities because they revealed their positive HIV status and people who knew them recognized their voices. This shows the downside of PLWHA becoming active in HIV programs and has implication for support from their partners which is necessary to be able to utilize health care institutions. Furthermore, non-disclosure contributes to the spread of HIV/AIDS when people have unprotected sex.

Society can sometimes condemn PLWHA giving birth to children (Lekas et al., 2006; Valencia-Garcia et al., 2008), which affects their reproductive rights and self-efficacy of seeking early care. Our data shows that both unmarried and married participants did not plan to disclose their positive HIV status to their spouses but did want to have children. This is significant in Nigeria because high value is placed on children (Isiugo-Abanihe, 1994). Non-disclosure of positive HIV status to their spouses has implications for not seeking early treatment, as well as for the prevention of vertical transmission. Criminal prosecution for HIV transmission has already been applied in a few cases in the United Kingdom, where research showed that the majority of PLWHA in the study were against criminalization of reckless HIV transmission, while a few felt it might be justified if it changed the behavior of PLWHA (Dodds & Keogh, 2006). While the protection of individuals in society is important, the sexual rights, disclosure problems and further stigmatization of PLWHA remain a concern. Brown and colleagues noted that there are existing legislative tools to respond to actions that constitute criminally harmful behavior arguing that HIV-specific laws to punish PLWHA is unnecessary, counterproductive and jeopardizes the human rights of PLWHA (Brown et al., 2009). Furthermore, direct or indirect inclusion of criminalization of vertical transmission pose serious consequences for female PLWHA as well as undermine the success of vertical transmission programmes so far achieved (Csete et al., 2009).

The participants' coping strategies were highly determined by the anticipation of negative reactions from society and the link to non-monogamous heterosexual transmission. They utilized different coping strategies to hide their condition since they believed it would not be accepted in society. The ability to cope with HIV/AIDS further depended on their marital status. Discordant partners found it more challenging to cope, because some were abandoned by their partners due only to the suspicion of being HIV infected. Our data also showed that married people received support better. The route through which participants felt they contracted their HIV virus was related to their emotional reaction and the support they received. Literature has pointed out that many women living with HIV/AIDS consider themselves as innocent victims in order to escape moral judgment from society (Doyal, 2009).

Furthermore, our study showed that gender played a role in the knowledge of partner's HIV status, as some of the female participants did not know their partners were HIV-positive and could not seek care when they were infected with HIV/AIDS. Schur (1984), noted that the overall subordination of women can lead to a snowballing effect because of the difficulty for them to achieve desired goals, such as getting tested for HIV. Women are often dependent on their husbands for finances and decisionmaking in the family which are important when deciding to use the health-care institutions. Also, this has implications for prevention of vertical transmission for pregnant women with HIV/AIDS since they will not seek early treatment to initiate necessary ART. Studies have shown that husbands' refusal to disclose their status contributes to the spread of HIV infection (Neves & Gir, 2006; Chinkonde et al., 2009).

Our findings demonstrate the use and role of combined care choices in the care-seeking behavior of PLWHA such as visiting faith houses with taking ART from health care institutions. A combined care choice encourages opportunistic infections, ART drug resistance and complications that may result due to lack of drug adherence. This combination of treatments was also observed in health-seeking behavior for sexual concerns in Zimbabwe (Pearson & Makadzange, 2008), as well as in another study involving PLWHA in Ribeirao Preto, Brazil (Neves & Gir, 2006) corroborating findings obtained elsewhere.

6. Limitations

Although the findings from this study are informative, they must be interpreted in the context of some methodological limitations. First, this is a small exploratory, qualitative study. Second, the findings were organized within the explanatory model which was based on literature review of HIV-related stigma in Sub-Saharan Africa and so it is subject to the limitation of the search criteria used. Third, the findings cannot be generalized to the larger population. Fourth, the study was conducted with people who were open about their positive HIV status and belonged to a patient association. Finally, some of the participants were also on ART and enjoyed government, as well as social and company support.

7. Conclusion

In summary, the explanatory model applied in this study provided a framework for organizing the findings of this study. The model adapted from the Precede portion of the (Green & Kreuter, 1999) Precede-Proceed model was helpful in understanding HIV-stigma related problems, coping mechanisms and care-seeking behaviors of PLWHA which can affect utilization of health-care institutions (Mbonu et al., 2009). This study shows that certain determining and moderating variables are important for PLWHA, in order for them to cope with HIV/AIDS and to make care choices. These variables which are depicted in the model should be the target of context-specific interventions. The findings from this study can translate into practical issues if we understand how and why PLWHA seek care from health-care institutions. Societal reactions, whether anticipated or real, continue to play a vital role in the way PLWHA cope and seek care from health care institutions. It also makes people not to disclose their HIV status especially to their significant others such as their partners. This is because PLWHA believed that society blames them and perceives that it is only contracted through sex. Many PLWHA keep their HIV status information quiet but live with that burden to avoid societal judgment. PLWHA try also to compare HIV/AIDS in the way of route of transmission, lifetime medication and prognosis to other chronic illnesses as ways of coping even though they know in reality, HIV/AIDS is different medically and in terms of societal impressions, beliefs and reactions. Altering these coping methods, societal impressions and beliefs about HIV/AIDS is necessary in order for PLWHA to seek appropriate care. It is important that HIV patients are supported so that they are able to go for HIV test and get effective treatment. Proper counseling goes a long way to help PLWHA to accept their status and prepares them to live with HIV. Clearly, PLWHA need psychological, medical and material support. Access to antiretroviral drugs remains a very important step in the care of HIV patients because when people have access to drugs, their health greatly improves and they are less prone to complications so they can go to work, have normal relationships and interact fully with the people around them.

8. Recommendations

The government should, as suggested by some of the participants, support PLWHA whose positive HIV status is exposed through creating a protective work policy and providing them with free ART, as this will be a motivator for other people with positive HIV status to come forward for help. The government should help in providing micro credits for those trying to set-up a living and doing business. This is important for PLWHA who are poor and jobless to enable them pay their user fees, buy regular drugs, do laboratory investigations and take care of their families.

Government should continue with efforts to educate the population on HIV/AIDS-related stigma which, when reduced, will enable people to go for VCT and seek appropriate care in health-care institutions in an early stage. Furthermore, education of people about the options of ART and possibilities of care will increase the self-efficacy of PLWHA.

Government should continue to involve and commit stakeholders such as media, religious and community leaders in educating people about HIV/AIDS, stigma and HIV/AIDS care as that will help people in making appropriate care choices. Policymakers should also involve PLWHA at all levels of consultation to ensure that all their needs are well represented. Special attention should go to youths through special targeted HIV/AIDS programmes. In addition, effective gender-specific policies that protect women but include the role of men should be integrated into programmes to ensure full utilization and support such as protection of women who find out their positive HIV status in antenatal care. Finally, the national HIV strategies should involve and support the members of vulnerable groups such as the association networks of PLWHA which are important to continue efforts of reducing the broader stigma in society and health care institutions.

9. Acknowledgements

The authors wish to thank the participants that gave up their time for the interview and the staff of Resource Center, Port Harcourt, Rivers State Nigeria. Dr Anja Krumeich of Maastricht University The Netherlands is also thanked for her contribution in the designing of the questionnaire.

10. References

Adewuya, A.O., Afolabi, M.O., Ola, B.A., Ogundele, O.A., Ajibare, A.O., Oladipo, B.F., & Fakande, I. (2009). Post-traumatic stress disorder after stigma related events in HIV infected individuals in Nigeria, *Social Psychiatry and Psychiatric epidemiology,* 44 (9), 761-766.

Ajuwon, A.J., Oladepo, O., Adeniyi, J.D., & Brieger, W.R. (1998). Sexual practices that may favor the transmission of HIV in a rural community in Nigeria, In D. Buchanan and

G Cernada (eds) (pp 21-33), Progress in preventing AIDS? Dogma, Dissent and Innovation, Global perspectives, Amityville, New York: Baywood publishing Company, Inc.

Amirkhanian, Y.A., Kelly, J.A., & McAuliffe, T.L. (2003). Psychosocial needs, mental health and HIV transmission risk behavior among people living with HIV/AIDS in St Petersburg, Russia. *AIDS*, 17 (16), 2367-2374.

Amuri, M., Mitchell, S., Cockcroft, A., & Anderson, N (2011). Socio-economic status and HIV/AIDS stigma in Tanzania. AIDS Care, 23 (3): 378-382.

Azinge, E (2003), Challenges of applying International treaties on HIV/AIDS and human rights before Domestic courts, in HIV/AIDS: The role of judiciary, HIV/AIDS and human rights: The role of judiciary. Eds- Iwuagwu, S., Durojaye, E., Eziefule, B., Ekerete-Udofia, C., Nwanya, P., Nwanguma, B: Retrieved 16 May 2011 from http://www.aidslex.org/site_documents/G035E.pdf page 61 of 83Brown, W., Hanefeld, J., & Welsh, J. (2009). Criminalising HIV transmission: punishment without protection. *Reproductive Health Matters*, 17 (34), 119-126.

Campbell, C., Nair, Y., Maimane, S., & Nicholson, J. (2007). Dying twice: a multi-level model of the roots of AIDS stigma in two South African communities. *Journal of Health Psychology*, 12, 403-416.

Chiang, L.C., Huang, J.L., & Lu, C.M. (2003). Educational diagnosis of self management behaviors of patients with asthmatic children by triangulation based on Precede-Proceed model in Taiwan. *Patient Education and Counseling*, 49 (1), 19-25.

Chinkonde, J.R, Sundby, J., & Martinson, F. (2009). The prevention of mother-to-child HIV transmission programme in Lilongwe, Malawi: why do so many women drop out? *Reproductive Health Matters*, 17 (33), 143-155.

Csete, J., Pearshouse, R., & Symington, A. (2009). Vertical HIV transmission should be excluded from criminal prosecution. *Reproductive Health Matters*, 17 (34), 154-162.

Demmer, C. (2011). Experiences of families caring for an HIV-infected child in KwaZulu-Natal, South Africa: an exploratory study, PMID: 24400305.

Dodds, C., & Keogh, P. (2006). Criminal prosecution for HIV transmission: people living with HIV respond. *International Journal of STD and AIDS*, 17 (5), 315-318.

Doyal, L. (2009). Challenges in researching life with HIV/AIDS: an intersectional analysis of black African migrants in London. *Culture, Health and Sex*, 11 (2), 173-188.

Duffy, L. (2005). Suffering, shame and silence: The stigma of HIV/AIDS. *Journal of the Association of Nurses in AIDS Care*, 16(1), 13-20.

Durojaye, E. (2003). Nigeria launches New AIDS Policy. *Canadian HIV/AIDS Policy Law Review*, 8 (3), 41-42.Fakolade, R., Adebayo, S.B., Anyanti, J., & Ankomah, A. (2009). The impact of exposure to mass media campaigns and social support on levels and trends of HIV-related stigma and discrimination in Nigeria: Tools for enhancing effective HIV prevention programmes. *Journal of Biosocial Science*, 1-13 (PMID: 20018118).

Green, L.W., & Kreuter, M.W. (1999). Health-Promotion Planning. An Educational and Ecological Approach. California, United States of America: Mayfield Publishing Company.

Hejoaka, F. (2009). Care and secrecy: Being a mother of children living with HIV in Burkina Faso. *Social Science and Medicine,* 69 (6), 869-876.

Hilhorst, T., Van Liere, M.J., Ode, A.V., & de Koning, K. (2006). Impact of AIDS on rural livelihoods in Benue state, Nigeria. *Journal of Social Aspects of HIV/AIDS Research Alliance (SAHARA),* 3 (1), 382-393.

Isiugo-Abanihe, U.C. (1994). Reproductive motivation and family size preferences among Nigerian men. *Studies in Family Planning,* 25 (3), 149-161.

Iwuagwu, S., Durojaye, E., Oyebola, B., Oluduro, B., & Ayankogbe, O (2003). HIV/AIDS and Human Rights in Nigeria; Background paper for HIV/AIDS policy review in Nigeria: Retrieved 16 May 2011 from http://pdf.usaid.gov/pdf_docs/PNACX55.pdf.Le Coeur, S., Collins, J., Pannetier, J., & Lelievre, E. (2009). Gender and access to HIV testing and antiretroviral treatments in Thailand: Why women have more and earlier access? *Social Science and Medicine,* 69 (6), 846-853.

Lekas, H.M., Siegel, K., & Schrimshaw, E.W. (2006). Continuities and discontinuities in the experiences of felt and enacted stigma among women with HIV/AIDS. *Qualitative Health Research,* 16 (9), 1165-1190.

Liamputtong, P., Haritavorn, N., & Kiatying-Angsulee, N. (2009). HIV and AIDS, stigma and AIDS support groups: Perspectives from women living with HIV and AIDS in Central Thailand. *Social Science and Medicine,* 69 (6), 862-868.

The Joint United Nations Programme on HIV/AIDS (UNAIDS). Retrieved 11 May 2009 from UNAIDS website: www.unaids.org/en/countryresponses/countries/nigeria.asp.

The Joint United Nations Programme on HIV/AIDS (UNAIDS), (2009). HIV-related stigma and discrimination: A summary of recent literature (Prepared by: Macquarrie, K., Eckhaus, T., Nyblade, L. et al., 2009): Retrieved 27 January 2010 from UNAIDS website: http://data.UNAIDS.org/pub/report/2009/20091130_stigmasummary_en.pdf.

The Joint United Nations Programme on HIV/AIDS (UNAIDS), 2010 country progress report. Retrieved 17 March 2011 from UNAIDS website: http://www.unaids.org/en/dataanalysis/monitoringcountryprogress/2010progressreportssubmittedbycountries/nigeria_2010_country_progress_report_en.pdf.

Mitchell, S.K., Kelly, K.J.M., Potgieter, F.E., & Moon, M.W. (2007). Assessing social preparedness for antiretroviral therapy in a generalised AIDS epidemic: a diffusion of innovation approach. *AIDS and Behaviour,* 13 (1), 76-84.

Mbonu, N.C., Van Den Borne, B., & De Vries, N.K. (2009). A model for understanding the relationship between stigma and health care-seeking behaviour among people living with HIV/AIDS in Sub-Saharan Africa. *African Journal of AIDS Research (AJAR),* 8 (2), 201-212.

Morolake, O., Stephens, D., & Welbourn, A. (2009). Greater involvement of people living with HIV in health care. *Journal of International AIDS Society,* 12 (1), 4.

Muula, A. S., & Mfutso-Bengo, J. M. (2005). When is public disclosure of HIV seropositivity acceptable? *Nursing Ethics,* 12 (3), 288-295.

Muyinda, H., Seeley, J., Pickering, H., & Barton, T. (1997). Social aspects of AIDS- related stigma in rural Uganda. *Health and Place,* 3, 143-147.

Mwinituo, P.P., & Mill, J.E. (2006). Stigma associated with Ghanaian caregivers of AIDS patients. *Western Journal of Nursing Research,* 28(4), 369-382.

National Agency for Control of AIDS (NACA) 2005. The National Policy on HIV/AIDS for the education sector in Nigeria draft: Retrieved 17 May 2011 from http://www.naca.gov.ng/index2.php?option=com_docman&task=doc_view&gid=24&itemid=268.National HIV/AIDS Policy Review Report (2009): Retrieved 16 May 2011 from http://naca.gov.ng/index2.php?option=com_docman&task=doc_view&gid=67&itemid=268.

Neves, L.A., & Gir, E. (2006). HIV positive mothers' beliefs about mother-to-child transmission, *Revista Latino-Americana Enfermagem,* 14 (5), 781-788.

Nyblade, L., Stangl, A., Weiss, E., & Ashburn, K. (2009). Combating HIV stigma in health care setting: what works? *Journal of International AIDS Society,* 12(1), 15.

Oluduro, O & Ayankogbe, O (2003). Legal issues raised by HIV/AIDS in HIV/AIDS: The role of judiciary, HIV/AIDS and human rights: The role of judiciary. Eds- Iwuagwu, S., Durojaye, E., Eziefule, B., Ekerete-Udofia, C., Nwanya, P., Nwanguma, B. Retrieved 16 May 2011 from http://www.aidslex.org/site_documents/G035E.pdf page 18 of 83

Pearson, S., & Makadzange, P. (2008). Help-seeking behavior for sexual-health concerns: a qualitative study of men in Zimbabwe. *Culture Health and Sex,* 10 (4), 361-376.

Sabin, L.L., Desilva, M.B., Hamer, D.H., Keyi, X., Yue, Y., Wen, F., Tao, L., Heggenhougen, H.K., Seton, L., Wilson, I.B., & Gill, C.J. (2008). Barriers to adherence to antiretroviral medications among patients living with HIV in Southern China: a qualitative study. *AIDS Care,* 20 (10), 1242-1250.

Schur, E.M. (1984). Women and deviance: a social perspective, in: Labelling women deviant, gender, stigma, and social control. Philadelphia, USA: Temple university press.

Shisana, O., Rehle, T., Simbayi, L., Parker, W., Bhana, A., Zuma, K., et al. (2005). South African National HIV prevalence, incidence, behaviour and communication survey. Cape Town. Human sciences research council press.

Singh, M., Garg, S., Nath, A., & Gupta, V. (2009). An assessment of felt needs and expectations of people living with HIV/AIDS seeking treatment at NGOs in Delhi, India, *Asia Pacific Journal of Public Health,* PMID: 19443873.

Singh, D., Chaudoir, S.R., Escobar, M.C., & Kalichman, S. (2011). Stigma, burden, social support and willingness to care among caregivers of PLWHA in home-based care in South Africa. AIDS Care, PMID:21400316.

Sontag, S. (1989). Illness as metaphor and AIDS and its metaphors. New York: Doubleday publishers.

Stevelink, S.A., Van Brakel, W.H., Augustine, V. (2011). Stigma and social participation in Southern India: Differences and commonalities among persons affected by leprosy and persons living with HIV/AIDS, Psychology, Health and Medicine, PMID:21391136.

Valencia-Garcia, D., Starks, H., Strick, L., & Simoni, J. M. (2008). After the fall from grace: negotiation of new identities among HIV-positive women in Peru. *Culture, Health and Sex,* 10 (7), 739-52.

Vlassoff, C & Ali, F. (2011). HIV-related stigma among South Asians in Toronto, Ethnicity & Health, PMID: 21259140

2

Social Position as a Structural Determinant of Adherence to Treatment in Women Living with HIV/AIDS

Marcela Arrivillaga
Department of Public Health & Epidemiology
Pontificia Universidad Javeriana Cali
Colombia

1. Introduction

Adherence to treatment has been a matter of priority in the control of the HIV/AIDS epidemic. Due to the characteristics of the virus, adherence of at least 95% is necessary for the continuing suppression of the viral load, and to prevent the risk of AIDS progressing (Bangsberg et al., 2000). In view of the chronic nature of HIV/AIDS, and the benefits offered by antiretroviral therapy, a sufficient rate of adherence is essential for world public health.

There have been many efforts to control the behavior of people who suffer from HIV, in order to ensure that they follow their treatment instructions carefully. Nevertheless, in the conceptualization, research and intervention on the field of adherence, determinants of a general nature which could affect it have been seen as a minor issue.

Much of the research on HIV/AIDS adherence has been rooted in biomedical and behavioral approaches. Studied variables include age, gender, education (Carballo et al., 2004; Glass et al., 2006; Godin et al., 2005; Gordillo et al.,1999; Ickovics & Meade, 2002; Mocroft et al., 2001, Spire et al., 2002; Sternhell & Corr, 2002), health beliefs, coping styles, self-efficacy, control perception, stress, anxiety, depression (Chesney, 2000; Ingersoll, 2004; Turner-Cobb et al., 2002), pharmacological regimen, side effects, relationship with health care providers, geographical barriers, and social support (Burke et al., 2003; Chesney, Morin & Sherr, 2000).

Despite wide research on this topic, studies have not reach conceptual explanations about the relation between adherence to treatment in people diagnosed with HIV and structural determinants such as social position. Drawn from the current vision studying adherence, its definition has been limited to the degree that patients complete behaviors like following healthcare provider's instructions, taking antiretroviral medication and attending medical appointments. The gender perspective has also been restricted in spite of reports that compared to men, women face additional barriers including delays in medical attention, non-use of antiretroviral therapy, lack of financial support, poor quality of health care, and difficulties related to the doctor–patient relationship (Ickovics & Meade, 2002, Jia et al., 2004).

To complement the current biomedical and psychosocial view to the study of adherence in HIV cases, this chapter presents an approach from the social determinants of health focus. In particular, the social position category is analyzed as a structural determinant of adherence of women affected by the virus. This proposal emerges before the need to understand not only the role of social position in adherence but also gender determinants that can affect it. An integral comprehension of adherence could promote the application of more effective interventions to achieve hoped for results.

The chapter begins with a section titled *gender, social position and health,* where these concepts are defined, and the problem of gender equity and inequity is considered together with their impact in the field of public health. A continuation called an *overview of vulnerabilities for women affected by HIV/AIDS* is presented giving a description on how women must face up to a wide range of political, economic and cultural determinants. The chapter subsequently shows data derived from a study carried out between 2006 and 2009 with 352 Colombian women who had been diagnosed with HIV. The data is analyzed based on a review of the literature which describes the associations between adherent behaviors and different variables related to social position. According to these results, the following section offers a *conceptual proposal of the social determinants of adherence to treatment* in HIV/AIDS, applicable to women affected by the virus, as well as describing its components. Finally, the chapter presents conclusions which summarize the arguments made throughout this study for the recognition of social position as a structural determinant of adherence to treatment in HIV/AIDS. It observes that debate, conceptualization and research into adherence are still not enough, and it stresses the need to continue to progress in a direction which would include the probable influence of determinations in a macro social context, such as poverty, inequity, violence, health systems, work, and food security, among others. Readers are invited to understand adherence in an all-embracing sense, to carry out new forms of intervention, focused on social and gender-related equity.

2. Gender, social position and health

2.1 Gender equity and health

It is well known that the "gender" category has been redefined in terms of a social and cultural construction, and not as a condition which derives from biological pertinence to one sex or another. On the contrary, gender determines different roles in society, which are transformed into inequities in the access to financial resources and the power which is exercised over them. *Gender equity* means fairness and justice in the distribution of benefits, power, resources and responsibilities between women and men (Breilh, 1999; Gómez, 2002; Kottak, 1994). As a counterpart, *gender inequity* represents a group of inequities which are considered to be unnecessary, avoidable, and apart from that, unfair (Whitehead, 1990), and which are associated with systematic disadvantages at socioeconomic level between men and women.

In socioeconomic terms, according to the International Labor Organization, inclusion in economic and social life is determined by gender. Also, this organization acknowledges that although the situation of women who work has improved, progress continues to be slow. In several regions women often face stronger barriers in the labor market, and female unemployment rates exceeded those for males. For example, of all the people employed in the world, only 40% are women; the rate of unemployment is higher in women than in men; employed women tend to be engaged in less productive sectors of the economy, have fewer opportunities to access the social security system, and are frequently receive lower salaries than men. In Latin America, around a quarter of the women are employed in the informal sector, where their income can vary from day to day, and where the lack of social support systems makes them more vulnerable to market variations. In this region the percentage of women who do not have their own income is between 37 and 50 (International Labor Organization [ILO], 2010).

However, gender inequity is also expressed in socially and culturally constructed gender roles. Women who live in patriarchal societies come up against exposure to what has been called the "triple feminine load", which determines the roles they carry out (Breilh, 1999). The first load consists of conditions such as informal work, with discrimination in tasks and positions; the second refers to the double shift that many women have, as a result of domestic work with their families. This double shift also includes an unequal and sexist distribution of work in the home, where the women look after the children, the cleaning, cooking, shopping among other things. The third load refers to the biological demands made on women's bodies due to their reproductive activity related to menstruation, pregnancy and lactation (Breilh, 1999). These three loads produce physical deterioration and result in having a differential affect on women's health, in comparison with that of men.

Gender differences in health have been widely documented. There is sufficient evidence of this, and variations in life expectancy, the risk of morbidity and mortality, access to health services and treatment, the use of preventive health services and health behaviors have been found (Gómez, 2002; Payne, 2009). On a global level data shows that men experience higher mortality and a lower life expectancy than women, while women have a greater probability of higher morbidity and more years living with disability (Mathers et al, 2001; Payne, 2006). In the field of public health, for gender inequity to be reduced, what is required is the elimination of differences in the opportunities to enjoy good health, not to become ill, become disabled or die from preventable causes. In the case of women it is necessary to recognize that these differences are a reflection of: 1, different types of needs, 2, better use of health services, 3. differential patterns in the recognition of symptoms, perception of illness, and the way in which attention is sought, which are prevalent in different cultures, geographical regions, and socioeconomic status, and 4. the structural and institutional determinants of the health systems, which differentially facilitate or obstruct access to health services (Gómez, 2002; Weisman, 1998;). This situation is combined with roles as family caregivers, which obliges women, to a greater extent than men, to become familiar with symptoms of illness, and as a consequence, seek more medical attention.

The specific needs of women, their social position, the gender-based roles they assume in certain contexts, and the characteristics of the health systems to which they belong, highlight the importance of directing public policies with a gender mainstreaming approach, to promote their health and wellbeing. Health systems in particular have the commitment to promote gender equity and to reduce the gender gap in their daily operations as well as in the development of health policies.

2.2 Social position

Social position can be defined as the "place" or social stratum of a person in the society in which they live. It is derived from a specific context, which means that the classification of the social position varies between societies with different economic structures (Diderichsen, et al., 2001). Throughout history it has been seen that in every society the most valued resources are distributed are unevenly distributed between the different social positions, and that individuals and families with occupy the more favored positions are those who enjoy them more.

It is important to point out that the concepts of "socioeconomic level" and "socioeconomic status" are often used as synonyms for social position, but they have no explicit relationship with the economic and political forces which explain the lack of social and gender-based equity. Neither can social position be compared with the concept of "social class" in the style of Marx or Weber, since in its most classical sense this concept cannot but accept the transversal capacity that gender has as a category, not only in the differentiation of experiences between men and women, but also between women of different social positions. The relationship between social context and the manner in which people are distributed among certain social positions is a determinant of the health outcomes. At the same time, social position is influenced by other variables, such as the health network to which individuals have access, their academic level, and occupation or "earning a living".

In countries lacking complete universal access to health insurance or health services, people and families must absorb the direct costs of health care themselves (Dahlgren & Whitehead, 2007; Navarro, 1989). Although this phenomenon affects people of all social positions in the same way, their ability to deal with these costs is extremely varied, depending on the socioeconomic situation (Diderichsen, et al., 2001). In general, those who belong to the wealthier sectors are able to absorb more costs, often have private insurance policies, and will probably not get into serious debt in order to pay their health costs. For its part, the economic safety net of the poorest groups is smaller, these people are less likely to be able to pay for private health insurance and they are often obliged to find new sources of income produced by other members of the family, or become seriously indebted. Non-universal health systems may impose impoverishing charges on those who are able to use them, making the already existent inequities in their living conditions even worse (Borrell et al., 2007). Ill-health may commence an ascending spiral of excessive costs as a result of health care and the loss of income derived from work.

Women in particular are limited, as far as opportunities in the labor market are concerned; their ability to pay is less, but despite this they pay more than men for their medical costs. Health financing systems which require high out-of-pocket payments increase their outgoings, when added to their basic needs and use of services (Borrell et al., 2007). Access to health insurance is still more limited, because of the interruptions in their work, due to pregnancy and the raising of their children. Apart from this, the nature of "dependents" in insurance, places them at risk of being unprotected in the event of widowhood, abandonment, marital separation, changes in the employment situation of their partner, or changes in the regulations which govern the coverage of dependents. The fact that over 30% of homes in regions such as Latin America have women as heads of household (Pan American Health Organization [PAHO], 2009) serves as an indicator of their vulnerability.

Gender analysts have pointed out that health costs have a devastating effect on economies which are managed by women. When a woman becomes ill and at the same is head of the household, the family income which is destined for food, education and health care for children, is reduced (Payne, 2009). In the case of HIV/AIDS the effects have obviously been financially ruinous (International Community of Women Living with HIV/AIDS [ICW], 2005). It is thus accurate to conclude that the principle of gender-based equity in health, according to which the amount payable would be linked to the people's capacity to pay, is considerably threatened in the case of women, especially in the case of non-universal health systems, and are restricted to social security networks.

For its part, as far as *education* as a determinant associated to social position is concerned, there is sufficient data to show that each unit of increase in educational level or professional hierarchy is accompanied by a corresponding increase in the final health outcomes (Dahlgren & Whitehead, 1992); the probability of survival is greater in persons in social positions with higher educational levels. And with regard to *work/employment*, it has traditionally been suggested that the relationship between employment and health is based on whether people can earn sufficient income to support themselves, have access to resources and be productive (Benach & Muntaner, 2007; Raphael, 2004). The unemployed population presents higher mortality rates, while job security has an effect on life expectancy (Navarro, 2004; Raphael 2003).

In a global context, the growth in the number of women who work outside their homes in paid jobs has brought about qualitative changes in their political, legal, economic and social situation. In the private sphere, employment has an effect on the material conditions in which women live their lives on a day-to-day basis, their ability to negotiate in their marital and family relationships, the possibility of achieving economic independence and in their self-esteem as individuals. Nevertheless, social position as a category of analysis helps in the understanding of the connection which exists between one's place in the world of work, the social and cultural characteristics and the relationship of this position with gender inequities. The working world of women cannot be understood only as employment or unemployment from a traditional approach. This vision does not take into account different occupations and "ways of earning a living" that women have, such as informal and domestic work. The type of work done by women determines gender roles, and as Breilh (1999) has stated, has an impact on women's health with patterns of deterioration which are different from those of men.

3. Overview of vulnerabilities for women with HIV/AIDS

As has already been mentioned, conditions of gender inequity place women in positions of disadvantage in comparison with men, making them more vulnerable. The vulnerability approach has attracted attention with regard to the structural conditions which place women in a position of risk, beyond that of their "irresponsible" individual behavior in relation to HIV infection. Women must face a broad spectrum of political, economic and cultural determinants which affect the way in which they can protect themselves against infection, deal with the virus once they have been affected, or look after family members who are affected. In fact, a meta-analysis of research carried out in the field of social epidemiology in HIV/AIDS between 1981 and 2003 revealed that to be a woman is one of the determinants of structural violence and discrimination related with the infection (Poundstone et al., 2004).

Some of the conditions of vulnerability of women infected with HIV are described below.

Poverty. It is no secret that HIV has spread uncontrollably throughout the world, but not by chance; on the contrary it is intensified within the ranks of the poor and those who are powerless, such as women (Farmer, 2000). In this way, poverty has become a structural determinant which is clearly connected to the epidemic, and acts as a booster of the virus. Women in situations of poverty have few opportunities with respect to education, work, nutrition, and housing. They run a greater risk of infection and have limited care options at their disposal once they have been diagnosed with HIV. In this case inequity by social position is exacerbated by gender inequity.

On an individual level, research has revealed that women with HIV/AIDS, who are financially vulnerable have less chance of using a condom, terminate a possibly dangerous relationship, have access to information about sexual health care, and a greater possibility of relapsing into high-risk behavior to obtain financial resources (Marcovici, 2002). Women who have no work and are financially dependent on their partner are exposed to sexual relations in which the man takes the decision on whether to use a condom (ICW, 2005); those who are employed in the informal sector and have some income may be more empowered with regard to the taking of decisions about their sex life, have more flexibility but at the same time less stable opportunities of earning money, and when they become ill receive no financial assistance. In all cases, diagnosed women who live in poverty have less chance of being able to use health services, counseling or medication.

Ethnicity. HIV/AIDS-related inequities with ethnic connections have been reported in some literature (Poundstone et al., 2004). Going beyond individual behavior the ways in which the virus is concentrated in certain ethnic groups involves complex processes of economic and social deprivation, socialization patterns, socially inflicted trauma, ties with the illegal drugs trade, and limited access to health care and prevention services. An example of this can be found in the United States, where HIV/AIDS affects a disproportionate number of black women who are isolated and stigmatized by poverty, forming part of an ethnic minority, their association with the sub-culture of injectable drugs, or because they live in areas where the infection is prevalent. In this way contextual or structural determinants share a role in the socialization of patterns which contribute to ethnic inequities in HIV/AIDS. With regard to adherence, a small number of studies have revealed that this is lower in persons of African descent and that the data is not consistent (Glass et al., 2006). To the best of our knowledge, no studies have been found that relate specific ethnic characteristics to adherence among women.

Migration and wars. The migration of a population plays an important part in the spread of HIV through migration processes, human trafficking, and urbanization. Female migratory workers are vulnerable due to the pressures of poverty, the lack of information and access to services. The temporary nature of some of their couple relationships and long periods spent away from their families can lead to greater sexual activity of a commercial nature. Illegality can present a greater host of problems and generally, in these situations women do not have the necessary documentation to remain in the host country legally, and may encounter difficulties in receiving medical care, or can be reluctant to request these services for fear of being deported.

Studies of migration processes have revealed that human-trafficking[1] markets increase women's vulnerability to HIV/AIDS infection. In Latin American countries such as Colombia it has been estimated that about 35.000 women have left the country, to escape from the violence and inequitable conditions, and have been recruited for sexual work (Ward, 2002).

With regard to processes of urbanization, HIV/AIDS is a classic example of an urban health problem. Young women who move far away from their rural homes to seek work in factories in towns and cities become more vulnerable to infection. They become exposed to

[1] Understood as the capture, transportation, movement, acceptance or receiving of persons, resorting to threats or the use of force or other forms of coercion, abduction, fraud, trickery, the abuse of power, or a situation of vulnerability, or the payment of receiving of money or benefits to obtain the consent of a person who has authority over another, with the purpose of exploitation (UN, 2000).

the possibility of sexual exploitation in their work places and the loss of social support previously given by their families and communities. Internal conflicts, wars, the militarization of certain areas tend to increase migration, and are directly or indirectly related to HIV/AIDS. Wars break down social networks, destroy medical infrastructure and increase poverty and social instability (Hankins et al., 2002). Also, prostitution increases with the presence of military personnel in urban and rural areas.

Sexual, physical and psychological violence. Gender-related violence is understood as any act or threat of violence which results in detriment and/or suffering of physical, sexual or psychological health of women. Unfortunately the wielding of power by men over women leads to different forms of violence, which increases their degree of vulnerability.

Sexual violence increases the risk of HIV infection at the moment of abuse. Studies reveal that those who have been victims of physical ill-treatment or sexual abuse during childhood are more likely to present high-risk sexual behavior, and have difficulty in negotiating sexual relationships with their partners which involve adequate care (Marcovici, 2002). This type of violence can be perpetrated by partners or families; rape in marriage and in all forms of couple relationships is generalized and widespread. The political relationship of tenancy and property relationship in conjugality makes what happens in these relationships valid, in spite of the implicit health risks. Thus, it is probable that many women do not have safe sexual relations because their partners do not consider it necessary; in fact, is probable that a woman could have sexual contact against her wishes and as a consequence endure forced coitus. There are significantly high rates of infection by HIV among women who have been subjected to physical abuse or sexual aggression, or are dominated by their partners (Dunkle et al., 2004).

Stigma and discrimination. The stigma associated with HIV is a considered as a second epidemic because of the impact it has on the lives of people and societies. This occurs with anyone who is diagnosed with it, irrespective of age, gender or ethnicity. Discriminatory acts include the denial of education, denial of or destitution from employment, the obligation to take an HIV test as a condition of employment, travel or any other activity. Allied to this, there is a lack of confidentiality, detention, deportation, condemnation in the communication media, rejection by family, friends and community, and physical aggression, including murder (Foreman et al., 2003). Stigma has a negative impact on social interaction, emotional well-being and self-esteem.

Discriminatory actions on the part of institutions and health-care providers affect adherence, and can take the form of delayed treatment, the withholding of treatment, treatment given inadequately, the delay or withholding of care in other ways (eg. the presentation of food, hygiene etc.), premature discharge, objection to receiving a patient by the health-care center, inadequate attention to bedridden patients, or to those in outpatient centers, tests carried out without the patient's consent, the violation of confidentiality within and outside the health system, difficulty in giving a diagnosis, inappropriate comments and behavior, for example, shouting, foul language, etc. , and the use of excessive precautions among other things (Foreman et al., 2003). Any of these acts can have transcendental physiological or psychological consequences for the person being treated.

In a qualitative study it was found that the stigma caused by HIV/AIDS is as shocking as the diagnosis itself. In particular, women are not worried by the possible psychological changes, or by the death that the diagnosis implies, but by the attendant psychosocial consequences. This fear becomes a barrier to the adherence to treatment and to maintaining and improving their health (Carr & Gramling, 2004).

4. Social position and HIV/AIDS treatment adherence: The case of Colombian women living with HIV/AIDS

Research conducted between 2006 and 2009 by the author of this chapter, identified and analyzed the relationship between social position and adherence to treatment in a sample of 352 Colombian women living with HIV/AIDS in five major cities in that country (Cali, Bogotá, Medellín, Pasto and Villavicencio). The purpose of this study was to broaden the individual point of view of adherence in HIV/AIDS, and to advance towards the development of an alternative concept from a social determinant perspective. The research project was approved by the institutional review boards of the National University of Colombia (Universidad Nacional de Colombia, UN) and Javeriana University in Cali (Pontificia Universidad Javeriana Cali, PUJC). Written informed consent was obtained from all study participants.

A mixed method approach with a qualitative and quantitative cross-sectional design was applied. In the phase of formative research, semi-structured interviews (SSI) were conducted with 7 national experts in the field. The qualitative component of the study included 10 focus groups discussions (FGD) with a total of 83 women; in-depth interviews (IDI) were conducted with 14 of these participants. Another 269 women completed a sociodemographic and clinical questionnaire, an adherence to treatment questionnaire, and a social position survey designed according to the Colombian socioeconomic structure. Content analyses were applied to analyze the qualitative data and logistic regressions used to analyze the quantitative data. The general results show significant statistical associations and qualitative patterns between adherence and social position. Women in a medium and high social position were more likely to present higher adherence behaviors than women in low social position (See table 1).

	Regression coefficient (b)	Wald test statistic	DF[a]	p-value	OR (95% CI[b])
Constant (b_0)	-1.7427	18.0960	1	<0.0001	NA[c]
Low social position (b_1)	1.7319	15.8323	1	<0.0001	5.651 (2.408-13.262)

[a] DF = degrees of freedom. [b] CI = confidence interval. [c] NA = not applicable.

Table 1. Univariate logistic regression analysis of the association between low adherence to treatment and low social position (versus medium and high social position) among 269 HIV-positive women in five Colombian cities

The findings of the study show the importance of social determinants in adherence, and make clear that the way in which women with HIV occupy a place in the social hierarchy and in a specific context, is linked to critical processes which advance or obstruct adherence to treatment. The social position was determined by a group of characteristics which occur jointly in the Colombian context and define it. These characteristics were: place of residence (urban or rural), official socioeconomic stratum in Colombia[2], educational level, type of affiliation to a health system or type of access to health services [3], labor profile or "way of

[2] The official socioeconomic stratification classifies Colombian citizens in six levels: 1-2 (Low), 3-4 (Middle) and 5-6 (High).

[3] The General Colombian Health System has two main types of health care coverage: Contributive and Subsidized. In addition, a special category called "*Vinculados*" (meaning "Attached") exists for

earning a living"[4] (referring to considerations of gender, income level, access to property, and access to credit with banks).
Described below are the characteristics of adherence to treatment in the women who took part in the study, broken down into three levels, according to their social position. The information shown is taken mainly from the qualitative phase of the study.

4.1 Low social position and HIV/AIDS treatment adherence

"Having AIDS is horrible and being a woman alone and with children is worse!
There is never enough money.
Besides food, it is difficult to pay transportation to go to the doctor"
(HIV-positive women, age 29, FGD)

The findings of the study showed that the lives of Colombian women with HIV/AIDS of low social position or in poverty conditions are compromised by limited access to economic and financial resources. Women placed in the lowest social level were women with no formal education, or had some degree of primary schooling, had limited access to subsidized health services, had an occupational profile which included being housewives, in some cases heads of family, with principal financial responsibility for the home, were manual workers, factory workers, self-employed or farm workers. They had incomes of less than US $200, did not own their own home and had no access to credit. The precarious nature of their lives was related to the difficulty they experienced in adhering to treatment once they had been diagnosed with HIV.
The conditions of poverty were reflected in the unsatisfactory response to these women's basic needs. In nutritional terms, they reported serious limitations, with negative consequences for their adherence. These were women whose incomes were insufficient to provide adequate nutrition - many of them ate one meal per day and apart from this shared their small rations of food with their families and in particular with their children. Some women chose not to take their antiretroviral medication in order to avoid gastrointestinal disorders, and to literally have an "empty stomach".
One of the greatest difficulties mentioned by these women belonging to a low social position was in obtaining money for transport to medical centers and to pay the excessive administration fees of the health insurance companies. Out-of-pocket expenses increased when they had to make a number or "trips" to attend medical appointments, collect

---

economically disadvantaged people who are not formally recognized by the two main coverage types. The Subsidized and the "*Vinculados*" systems include the poorest sector of the population in Colombia.
[4] Three profiles of female work were analyzed in the case of Colombian women: Profile A, made up of workers, factory workers or manual workers in companies not of their ownership, farmers, self-employed workers (e.g. car watcher (guard), street salesperson, cook, washerwoman and maid). Profile B, includes owners of small businesses, or small traders, (e.g. bakeries, butchers, dressmakers, hairdressers, store, etc.), semi-salaried with regular income from commissions from sales (e.g. cosmetics or underwear salesperson, working from a catalogue), women who work in public or private companies with operational functions with employment contracts, (e.g. secretary, receptionist, office assistant), and independent professional with an undergraduate degrees. Profile C, made up of company owners and managers with their own business, independent workers with postgraduate degrees, and women working for public or private companies with administrative, technical duties, or those involving control and supervision with employment contracts (e.g. manager, director, head of department).

medication, or go for tests. Added to this was the cost of travelling from urban or rural areas far from their homes. Every journey meant more expense, which affected the family finances, more so when the women were heads of family who in many cases had to pay for food, housing, services and their children's education.

Conditions such as poverty, unemployment, exposure to violence, the lack of education and the difficulty in satisfying basic financial needs for food, clothing, housing and access to public services, were explanations of why some women in a low social position decided to sell their antiretroviral medications once they had obtained them from the health system, just to satisfy their basic needs. There were also cases where their partners forced them to sell these medications.

The low educational level of these women affected their understanding of HIV/AIDS, its treatment, and the consequences of not taking medication, or taking it incorrectly. All of these living conditions resulted in tendencies towards low adherence, resistance to medication, exposure to opportunistic infections, and the risk of mortality.

By way of a summary, Figure 1 shows the living conditions and adherence behavior in this group of women.

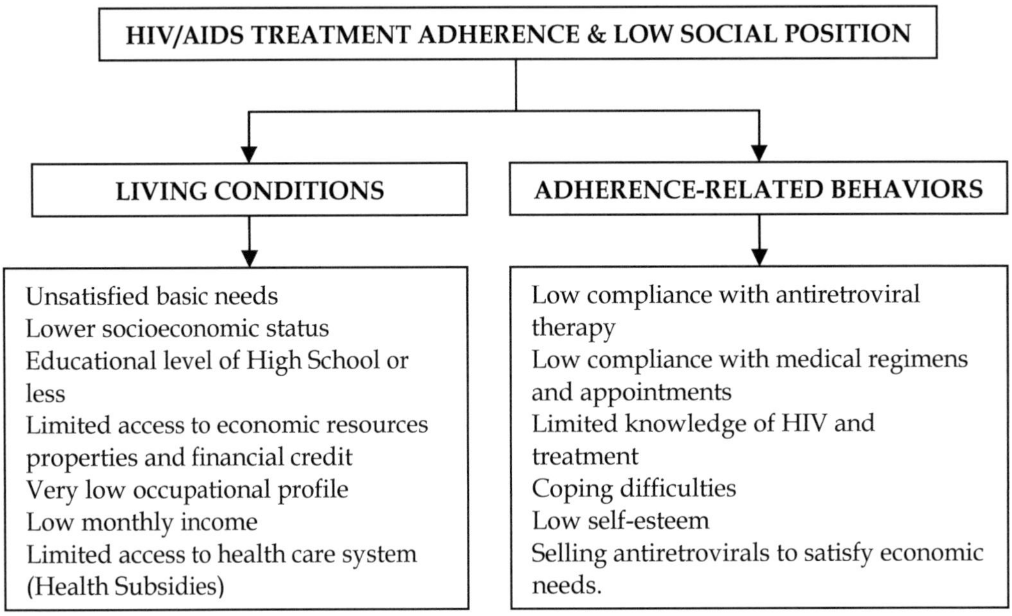

Fig. 1. HIV/AIDS Treatment Adherence & Low Social Position. HIV-Positive Women. Colombia - South America. 2007-2010.

4.2 Medium social position and HIV/AIDS treatment adherence

"In general, women from a medium social position adhere to treatment more easily than poor women and even better than women from a high economic status. They have characteristics such as a degree of economic independence which does not imply they are rich women living on their money but they work and become good patients who adhere well"
(HIV/AIDS National Expert -Physician-. SSI)

For women belonging to the medium social position, the results of the study indicate that they share similar living conditions and socioeconomic characteristics. Some were financially independent and were heads of household, while others produced income from their jobs to contribute to the upkeep of the family. On receiving the diagnosis, the initial effect on these women was one of dismay, anger and sadness, but these were also women who showed a positive attitude in coping with the illness and the treatment. In contrast with the women of a low social position, these women were more aware of the benefits of adherence to treatment. In other words we were dealing with women with complete or partial financial independence, who maintained an active role in the upkeep of their homes after their diagnosis, and they took responsibility for the new situation regarding their health. The *"economic/financial power"* that working women with their own income are supposed to have places them in a relational sphere of exercising their autonomy, and of recognizing themselves as persons who are capable of dealing with a diagnosis such as that of HIV.

The social position of this group of women has given them access to formal education and the ability to understand the complexity of antiretroviral treatment, and the benefits of following it correctly. Activities aimed at seeking information about HIV/AIDS -once this had been diagnosed- were highlighted in this group. They stated that they usually began to read, carefully selecting what they read, became skilled at choosing reliable information, attended workshops and conferences, and those who had access to it, consulted Internet. In all cases, explanations offered by these women about HIV/AIDS and its treatment, were more detailed, complex, and in the most outstanding cases, analytical and critical in comparison with women from low social positions. Thanks to the quality of life enjoyed as a consequence their social position, these practices which benefited their adherence may be added to *"the power of accumulated knowledge"*.

The knowledge of HIV and antiretroviral therapy in this group of women resulted in their being more able to negotiate the type of therapy with their doctor, and discuss any recommended changes with health-care personnel. These women were familiar with the antiretroviral medication, the corresponding doses, and their possible adverse effects. They knew how to interpret the results of the tests, relating them to their compliance with the therapy.

The *empowerment* evident in these women of medium social position manifested itself in their defense of their rights as users of the health system. In fact, of the three groups of women, it was this group of medium social position who most exercised their health rights in this regard, even taking into account the fear and stigma associated with HIV. They went as far as to initiate legal action to be able to ensure opportune and continuous access to treatment, direct and active communication with their doctors and health-care personnel, and compliance with their appointments, without fear of being identified as HIV carriers. The defense of these rights was linked to the knowledge they had of how the health system worked, and for this reason they were able to have medical attention, and access to medication in a relatively stable and uninterrupted manner.

Based on the above, we can affirm that the "place" in Colombian society of women belonging to the medium social position, puts them in a situation of being well able to consider themselves privileged when they have to accept HIV diagnosis. This is a social group in which the pattern of an *empowered woman* converges with conditions of economic and financial possibilities, which, although not the best situation, is very favorable for adherence on the part of this sample in the study.

Figure 2 summarizes living conditions as well as adherence conduct in women of a medium social position who took part in the study.

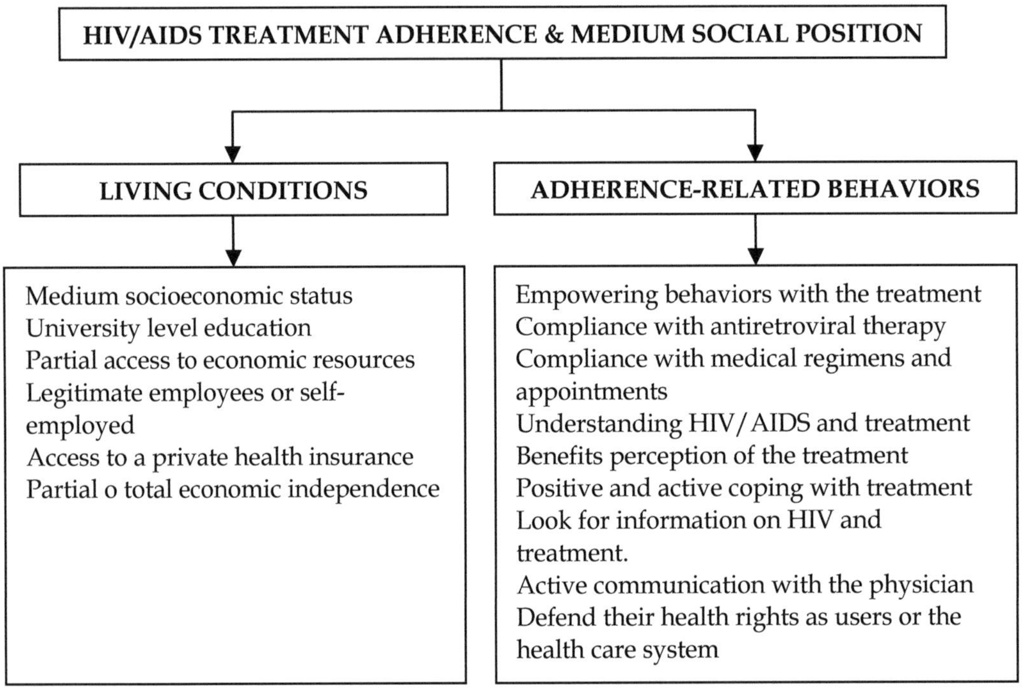

Fig. 2. HIV/AIDS Treatment Adherence & Medium Social Position. HIV-Positive Women. Colombia - South America. 2007-2010

4.3 High social position and HIV/AIDS treatment adherence

"I do even the impossible and pay what is necessary to hide my diagnosis. Nobody must know! It would end my career. I take my medication religiously to not get sick and that no one notices that I have HIV"
(HIV-positive women, age 36, IDI)

Women from a high social position with HIV/AIDS who took part in the study had no financial difficulties and therefore enjoyed a satisfactory life style. These were women with university education up to postgraduate level, with property, access to credit with banks, and with professional profiles of company owners and management positions in different companies. These conditions favored adherence when beginning antiretroviral therapy.

In spite of this, significant findings from the study show how these women lived with HIV, the social role they tried to maintain after being diagnosed, and how difficult it was for them to accept being HIV-positive, in comparison to the experience of women from the lower social positions. They presented chronic stress as a result of the diagnosis, which in itself represented a threat to their health.

In the first place, it is important to mention that women who occupy a high social position are generally affiliated to private health insurance companies as well as having complementary health plans. Nevertheless, some of these women reported that they would prefer to pay for their HIV treatment themselves, so that their HIV-positive status would not be registered in the health system. They even went as far as to invest money in visits to private consultations with specialists in other Colombian cities. Women from a high social position felt that they would not be seen consulting certain doctors, whose medical experience may associate them with HIV treatment, and at the same time reducing the threat to the confidentiality of their diagnosis. In all of this the financial cost involved was unimportant; what was important for them was the need to maintain secrecy.

In comparison with women of low and medium social positions, women belonging to a high social position thought of HIV/AIDS as more of an "illness" of which they should be ashamed; they considered that for society it is not the same to talk about another illness, however fatal this may be, as to talk about HIV/AIDS. Also, for them, to become "ill" means to depend, be helped and attended to, which goes against their personal and professional model of an independent woman. At the same time they had strong convictions about the possible discrimination, rejection, and pity associated with the diagnosis; some women even said that they would move away from the city in the event of their state of health being revealed. They were extremely afraid that their families would find out about the HIV diagnosis; also that the image formed around them would be destroyed, and moreover that their sexual practices could be questioned. For this group of women the emotional cost of the diagnosis caused them suffering which at times was exhausting.

To maintain secrecy about their diagnosis, these women limited the number of people who knew about it to a minimum, preferring to deal only with their own physician, and avoiding contact with the other health-care providers. When in the waiting room of the clinic they resort to strategies in order not to be identified by their name, and carefully plan ways of covering up HIV/AIDS in the event of illness, hospitalization or death. Under no circumstances do they take part in support groups or become involved with organizations which help HIV-positive people. Although they limit their possibilities of receiving comprehensive health care, the secret of their diagnosis - their closest ally - would not interfere with adherence to their treatment.

Conserving their physical appearance, image and personal aesthetic formed an essential part of the secret and was a motivating determinant in adherence. This is a case of women who were aware of the need to protect their bodies and take care of their health to hide HIV from their family and from society. Their self-care behavior included a healthy and balanced diet with vitamins, practicing yoga and taking natural remedies.

In spite of all this, women in a high social position in our study, who had many advantages bestowed by their status in Colombian society, developed a profound conviction about the importance and benefits of adherence. Although they came up against stigma-related threats, they marshalled all of their personal and material resources to care for their health.

Figure 3 shows the living conditions and adherence behavior among women of a high social position.

4.4 Discussing the results of the study in Colombia – South America

In the first place, the general trend found in the study was that HIV-positive women and in antiretroviral treatment belonging to the highest social position were more likely to present higher adherence, and the conditions of poverty or low social position in women served to increase -up to five times- the probability of non-adherence.

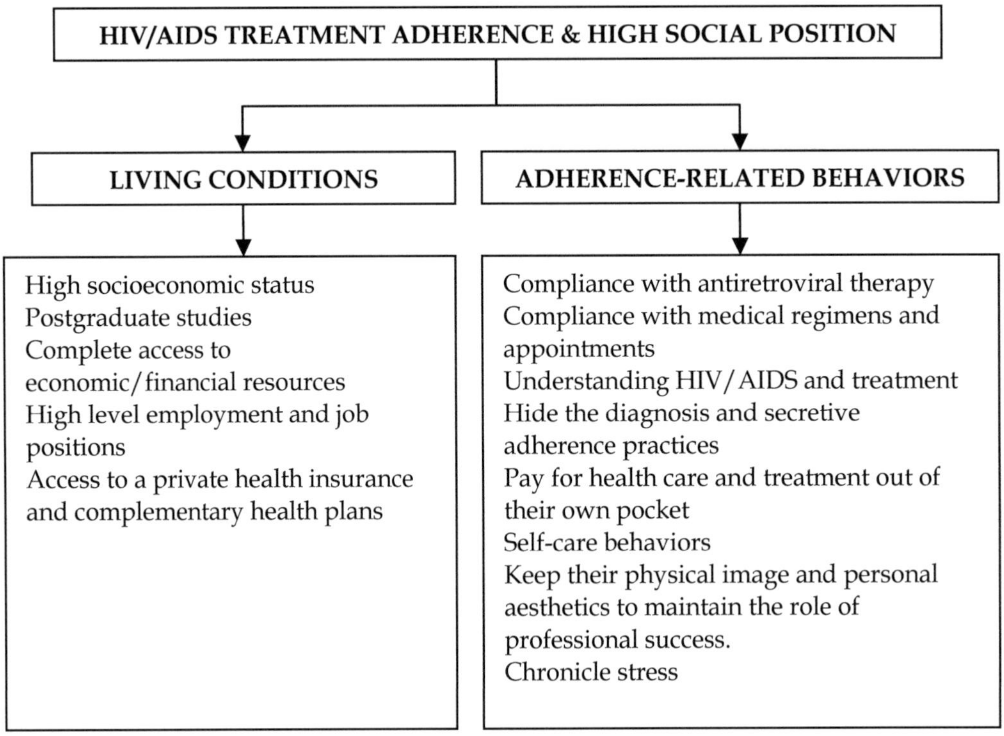

Fig. 3. HIV/AIDS Treatment Adherence & High Social Position. HIV-Positive Women. Colombia. 2007-2010

The relationship between socioeconomic status and adherence in HIV/AIDS-related cases is a subject which has been covered in different ways and with diverse results in scientific literature. In their sociodemographic descriptions, the majority of authors include variable income levels as the closest variable to social position. In general, socioeconomic variables are measured as independent factors, and as was the case in this study similar reports measuring *social position as a group of conditions which act together to determine the place of HIV-positive women in Colombian society* have not been found. Neither has the link between social position and the specific features which characterize adherence in the different groups been clear.

Although the relationship between the poverty of women and HIV/AIDS has been recognized as an essential determinant of the dynamics of the epidemic (Farmer, 1996; Herrera & Campero, 2002; Rao, 2004; Wingood & Diclemente, 2000), adherence among this population is a topic on which there has been little research and the results are not consistent. A systematic literature review of 116 studies presents the conclusion that even though there is a positive trend in relation to adherence in various chronic illnesses and some areas of socioeconomic status, for example income, education and occupation, there is insufficient evidence about statistically significant associations between socioeconomic status and adherence among patients with HIV/AIDS (Falagas, 2008). On the contrary, other studies carried out with men and women reveal associations between a deficient financial situation and non-adherence (Carballo et al., 2004; Castro, 2005; Chesney, 2000;

Chesney et al., 2000; Gifford et al., 2000; Glass, et al., 2006; Gordillo, 1999; Ickovics & Meade, 2002; Kleeberger et al., 2001).

The truth is that poverty accounts for a higher probability of social disadvantages associated with risks to adherence. In this study the relationship between the conditions of women of a low social position and low adherence was clearly seen. As far back as 1996 it had been reported that poor women with HIV/AIDS undergoing antiretroviral therapy, by comparison with samples of men with the virus, are more exposed to delays in being diagnosed, access to the health system and the corresponding care, which contributes to a bad prognosis and evolution of HIV (Daily et al., 1996). The problem of the lack of access to economic/financial resources due to their low social position, reduces their ability to obtain and continue with treatment (Amaro et al., 2001; Rao, 2004), or to satisfactorily maintain any type of therapy.

Some of the afore-mentioned variables have been analyzed independently by other authors, who have presented similar findings to those of this study. There is data on academic income and unemployment-related levels.

Regarding levels of education and adherence, as is the case with this study, some authors (Goldman & Smith, 2002; Golin et al., 2002; Kalichman et al., 1999; Kleeberger et al., 2004) have demonstrated significant associations. Results of research also illustrate the way in which adherence of women of higher social positions benefit from access to formal education and the cultural baggage accumulated in these social groups. High levels of education contribute to the ability to deal with the HIV diagnosis, serve in the taking of decisions, facilitate the search for information on access to health-related resources, and are advantageous in understanding HIV and its treatment. On the other hand, low levels of education, as with women of a low social position, produce patterns of vulnerability associated with low adherence. Allied to the other conditions which are typical of the lives of poor HIV-positive women, low education level can trigger a bad prognosis and the high risk of death from AIDS.

With respect to income level, some authors have suggested that there are associations with adherence (Carballo et al., 2004; Ickovics & Meade, 2002), and propose that it would be reasonable to argue that attention to basic needs is more beneficial than direct attention to adherence. In particular, women of a low social position could receive social support for the satisfaction of their basic needs.

This is also especially important in the case of unemployed women. Some authors contend that unemployment could contribute to reduced intention or capacity to continue taking antiretroviral medication, in keeping with the doses and times prescribed (Adler & Newman 2002; Fong et al., 2003). Bearing in mind that work is a central category of social position, it is necessary to develop new studies that will show the possible effects on adherence of employment/unemployment and the working/occupational situation of HIV-positive people. In the case of women, gender considerations should be taken into account with regard to the particular characteristics of women's work, and according to their social position.

The findings of the Colombian study also showed that in women of medium social position a pattern of empowered behavior converges, which favors adherence. In this regard, new approaches to the problem of HIV have referred to the importance of the "empowerment" category, identifying six sources of fundamental power for the support women with HIV: information and education, skills, access to services and prevention technologies, access to financial resources, social capital and the opportunity to be heard in the taking of decisions at all levels (Gupta, 2000). These proposals coincide with the characteristics of the group of women of medium social position who took part in the study.

Other authors have dealt with the topic of the empowerment of HIV- positive women, from interventions based on microfinance to reduce violence against women, social exclusion, obtain access to health services, and promote mental health (Kim et al., 2007; Mohindra et al., 2008). The authors estimate that providing women with financial benefits such as access to credit services would contribute to their empowerment, increase their self-esteem, self confidence, their ability to resolve conflicts and take decisions. In any event, it would be well worthwhile to investigate more deeply the relationship between empowerment and adherence with future studies which would conserve the social nature of the concepts, since, as has been pointed out, empowerment means a change in unequal relationships between genders on a social level; strengthening prevention networks, the promotion and defense of social, economical, cultural, sexual and reproductive rights; change those life styles which place women at the risk of HIV infection, and fight against the stigma associated with the diagnosis (Herrera & Campero, 2002).

And it is precisely the social stigma which is the main characteristic associated with women of high social position in the study. Some authors relate HIV stigma and discrimination with socioeconomic and gender-related inequities (Altman, 2007); others have focused on the psychosocial consequences it produces (Arregui, 2007; Carr & Gramling, 2004; Pecheny et al., 2007; Ruiz-Torres et al., 2007). It has been said that women are the population most subjected to rejection and discrimination when diagnosed with HIV, also that they suffer from more discrimination than men (Arregui, 2007). In this study it was found that the perception of social stigma on the part of women of a high social position indirectly contributes to adherence. Although this is paradoxical, these women have adherence-related practices which with the purpose of conserving their appearance and in this way hide HIV from their families, their immediate social circle, and society in general. This self-care conduct has the result of favoring adherent practices.

This does not mean to say that the experience of stigma is a positive one for HIV- positive Colombian women of a high social position; for them, the moment of diagnosis is crucial in their biography since HIV is not only a medical diagnosis but on the contrary, begins to define their personal identity (Altman, 2007; Carr & Gramling, 2004; Pecheny et al., 2007). The first personal dimension to be affected by the HIV/AIDS-associated stigma is that of self-image; the woman first reflects every prejudice and rejection learned in society in herself. She is invaded by rational and irrational fears, and silence can take control of her life (Arregui, 2007). Thus, the main challenge of the women of high social position who took part in the study was to keep their diagnosis a secret at all costs. As previously mentioned by other authors (Pecheny et al., 2007), among the reasons for not revealing their diagnosis are avoiding embarrassment and shame, being able to keep to their daily routine, avoiding potentially discriminating situations, the fear of being treated differently and rejected, being the object of ridicule, suspicion and ill-intentioned comments in their social environment. According to reports in literature and the findings of the study, among the consequences of this perceived stigma are the deterioration of interpersonal relationships, negative emotions such as anxiety, depression and guilt, a low level of social support, isolation, difficulties with family relationships, and the deterioration of relationships with health-care providers (Ruiz-Torres et al., 2007).

5. The social determinants of adherence to treatment of HIV/AIDS

Based on the evidence presented, adherence to treatment can be considered as a dynamic process, which moves in a continuum between critical processes related to general determinants and critical processes related to individual determinants.

The critical processes related to general determinants are illustrated in Figure 4 and include consideration of the *social position* as a structural determinant of adherence. In every society and socioeconomic context value must be placed on the characteristics which jointly make up and define the "place" or social stratum of the person living with HIV/AIDS. In the level of the *health system*, the health right to continuous and opportune treatment and comprehensive care by qualified health care providers are necessary conditions for adherence on the part of those who suffer from the virus. For its part, the "*mode of living*" (Almeida-Filho, 2000; Breilh 2003), represents a bonding category between general determinants and the complex behavior of treatment adherence. This category can be considered as a related group of practices connected especially with adherence, influenced by people's living conditions, socio historical processes, the dynamics of gender pertinence, and the influence of social position.

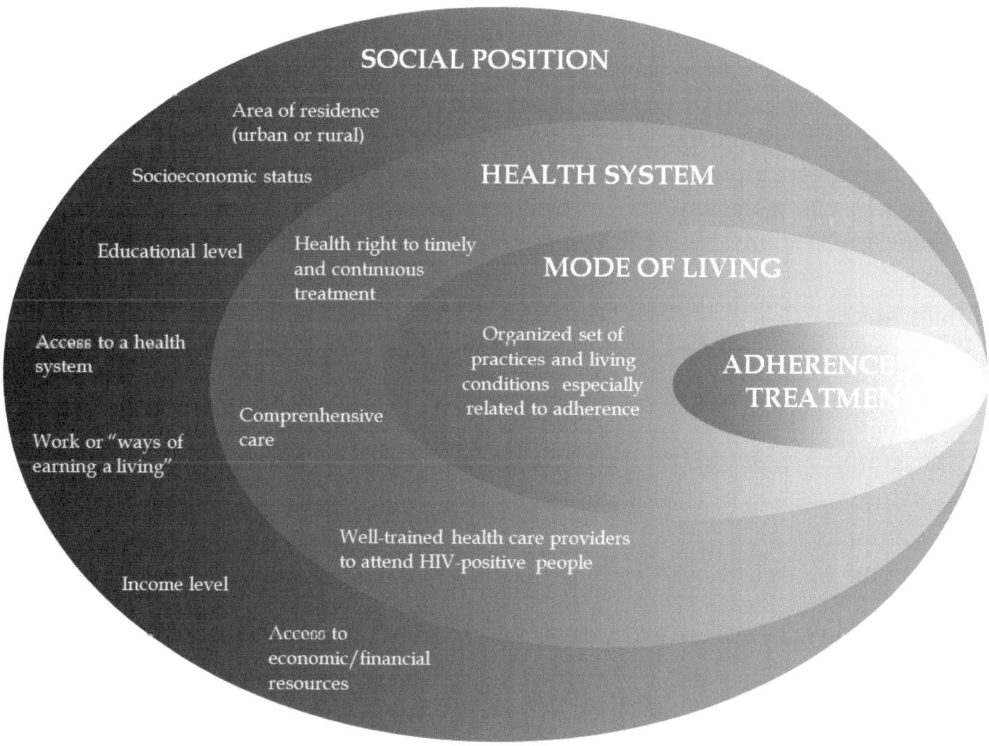

Fig. 4. Critical processes related to social determinants of treatment adherence in people living with HIV/AIDS.

The critical processes related to individual determinants of adherence cannot be understood isolated from the general determinants described above, but rather, subsumed in them. The life course trajectories taken through life lead to different forms of facing up to HIV/AIDS and its treatment, and also, gender roles and their impact on adherence must be taken into account.

Contrary to biomedical and individualistic traditions, and from an approach of the social determinants of health, which offers a framework of theoretical, epistemological and praxiological comprehension on the health-related processes of social life (Breilh, 2003), adherence to treatment can be considered as a *complex behavior promoting adaptation, psychological adjustment, appropriate health care, and quality of life during the HIV/AIDS infection process, determined by mode of living, social position, and the health care system.* With this concept of adherence it is possible to broaden the vision, and attend to the specific matters which are imposed by the general determinants such as individual influences. The critical processes described here, not only when conceptualizing but also when investigating and intervening adherence to HIV/AIDS treatment.

6. Conclusions

The limited understanding of adherence to HIV/AIDS treatment, which is traditionally defined in an individual, biomedical and psychosocial context, and the evidence of the rates of low adherence which still occur in some populations affected by the virus, indicate that an approximation of adherence in relation to other categories of social analysis, and integrated with individual categories, could be useful to advance in the arguments of the negative effects of non-adherence. It is probable that if this concept is understood from the point of view of social determinants of health, new interventions could be proposed and better policies and plans for attention could be developed, with strategies aimed at social and gender-based equity.

7. References

Adler, N.E. & Newman, K. (2002). Socioeconomic disparities in health: pathways and policies. *Health Affairs,* Vol.21, No. 2, (March 2002), pp. 60-76, ISSN 0278-2715

Almeida-Filho, N. (2000). *La ciencia tímida. Ensayos de deconstrucción de la Epidemiología,* Lugar Editorial, ISBN 950- 892-095-5, Buenos Aires, Argentina.

Altice, F.L, Mostashari, F. & Friedland, G.H. (2001). Trust and acceptance of and adherence to antiretroviral therapy. *Journal of acquired immune deficiency syndromes,* Vol. 28, No. 1. pp. 47-58, ISSN 1525-4135

Altman, D. (2007). Rights Matter: Structural interventions and vulnerable communities. *Interamerican Journal of Psychology,* Vol. 41, No. 1, (n.d 2007), pp. 87-92, ISSN 0034-9690

Amaro, H., Raj, A. & Reed, E. (2001). Women's Sexual Health: The need for feminist analyses in Public Health in The Decade of Behavior. *Psychology of Women Quarterly,* Vol. 25, (March 2001), pp. 324-334, ISSN 0361-6843

Amigo, I. (1998). *Manual de psicología de la salud,* Pirámide, ISBN 9788436823400, Madrid, Spain.

Arregui, M. (2007). Living with HIV in the Dominican Republic. *Interamerican Journal of Psychology,* Vol. 41, No. 1, (n.d 2007), pp. 31-40, ISSN 0034-9690

Bangsberg, D.R. et. al. (2000). Adherence to protease inhibitors, HIV-1 viral load, and development of drug resistance in an indigent population. *AIDS,* Vol. 14, No. 4 (March, 2000), pp. 357-366, ISSN 0269-9370

Barfod, T., Gerstoft, J., Rodkjaer, L., Pedersen, C., Nielsen, H., Moller, A., et. al. (2005). Patients´ answers to simple questions about treatment satisfaction and adherence and depression are associated with failure of HAART: A cross-sectional survey. *AIDS Care,* Vol. 19, No.5, pp. 317-328, ISSN 0954-0121

Bayes, R. (1998). El problema de la adhesión en la terapéutica de la infección por el virus de inmunodeficiencia humana (VIH). *Intervención Psicosocial, Revista sobre igualdad y calidad de vida,* Vol.7, No. 2, pp. 229-237, ISSN 1132-0559.

Bedell, S.E. et. al. (2000). Discrepancies in the use of medications: Their extent and predictors in an outpatient practice. *Archives of Internal Medicine,* Vol. 160, (July 2000), pp. 2129-2134, ISSN 0003-9926.

Benach, J. & Muntaner, C. (2007). Precarious employment and health: developing a research agenda *Journal of Epidemiology and Community Health,* Vol. 61, (September 2007), pp 276-277, ISSN 0143-005X

Berg, K., Demas, P., Howard, A., Schoenbaum, E., Gourevitch, M. & Arnsten, J. (2004). Gender differences in factors associated with adherence to antiretroviral therapy. *Journal of General Internal Medicine,* Vol.19, No.11, pp. 1111-1117, ISSN 0884-8734

Borrell, C., Espelt, A., Rodríguez-Sanz, M. & Navarro, V. (2007). Relationship between politics and health - Editorial: Politics and health. *Journal of Epidemiology and Community Health,* Vol. 61, (September 2007), pp. 658-659, ISSN 0143-005X

Breilh J. (2003). *Epidemiología Crítica: Ciencia emancipadora e interculturalidad,* Lugar Editorial, ISBN 950-892-147-1, Buenos Aires, Argentina.

Breilh, J. (1999). El género entre fuegos de inequidad y esperanza, In : *Antología latinoamericana y del caribe: mujer y género,* I. Bermúdez, W. Dierckxsens & L. Guzmán, (Eds.), 57-62, Universidad Centroamericana [UCA], ISBN 99924-36-02-6, Managua, Nicaragua.

Burke, J.K., Cook, M., Cohen, T., Wilson, K., Anastos, M., Young, H., et. al. (2003). Dissatisfaction with medical care among women with VIH: dimensions and associated factors. *AIDS Care,* Vol.15, No.4, (August 2003), pp. 451-462, ISSN 0954-0121

Carballo, E. & Cadarso-Suárez, C., Carrera, I., Fraga, J., De la Fuente, J., Ocampo, A., et. al. (2004). Assessing relationships between health-related quality of life and adherence to antiretroviral therapy. *Quality of Life Research,* Vol.13, No.3, (April 2004), pp. 587-599, ISSN 0962-9343

Carr, R. & Gramling, L. (2004). A health barrier for women with HIV/aids. *Journal of the association of nurses in AIDS care,* Vol.15, No.5, (September 2004), pp. 30-39, ISSN 1055-3290

Castro, A. (2005). Adherence to antiretroviral therapy: Merging the clinical and social course of AIDS. *PLoS Medicine,* Vol.2, No.12, (October 2005), pp. e338, ISSN 1549-1277

Catz, S.L., Kelly, J.A., Bogart, L.M., Benotsch, E.G., & McAuliffe, T.L. (2000). Patterns, correlates, and barriers to medication adherence among persons prescribe new treatments for HIV disease. *Health Psychology,* Vol.19, No.2, (March 2000), pp. 124-133, ISSN 1020-4989

Catz, S.L., McClure, J. B., Jones, G.N., & Brantley, P.J. (1999). Predictors of outpatient medical appointment attendance among persons with IHV. *AIDS Care,* Vol.11, No.3 (June 1999), pp. 361-373, ISSN 0954-0121

Chesney M.A. & Morin, M., Sherr, L. (2000). Adherence to HIV combination therapy. *Social Science & Medicine,* Vol.50, No.11, (June 2000), pp. 1599–1605, ISSN 0277-9536

Chesney, M.A. (2000). Factors affecting adherence to antiretroviral therapy. *Clinical Infectious Diseases,* Vol.30, No.2, (June 2000), pp. S171–176, ISSN 1058-4838

Dahlgren, G. & Whitehead, M. (1992). *Policies and strategies to promote equity in health.* WHO, Regional Office for Europe, ISBN 978-91-85619-18-4, Copenhagen

Dahlgren, G. & Whitehead, M. (2007). Framework for assessing health systems from the public's perspective: the ALPS approach. *International Journal of Health Services,* Vol. 37, No. 2, pp. 363–378, ISSN 0020-7314

Daily, J., Farmer, P., Rhatigan, J., Katz, J. & Furin, J. (1996). Women and HIV infection: A different disease? In : *Women, Poverty, and AIDS,* P. Farmer, M. Connors & J. Simmons. (Eds.), 125-144, Common Courage Press, ISBN 978-1567510744, Monroe, Maine.

De la Cruz, J.J. & Gordillo, M.V. (2003). Adherencia y fallo terapéutico en el seguimiento de una muestra de sujetos VIH+: Algunas hipótesis desde la Psicología. *Psicothema,* Vol.15, No.2, (November 2003), pp. 227-233, ISSN 0214-9915

Diderichsen, F., Evans, T. & Whitehead, M. (2001). The social basis of disparities in health. In: *Challenging Inequities in Health: From Ethics to Action,* T. Evans, M. Whitehead, F. Diderichsen, A. Bhuiya & M. Wirt. (Eds.), 13-23, Oxford University Press, ISBN-13: 978-0195137408, New York, United States.

DiMatteo, M.R. (2004). Variations in Patients' Adherence to Medical. Recommendations. A Quantitative Review of 50 Years of Research. *Medical Care,* Vol.42, No.3, (March 2004), pp. 200-209, ISSN: 0025-7079

Dunkle, K.L., Jewkes, R.K. & Brown, H.C. (2004). Gender-based violence, relationship power, and risk of HIV infection among women attending antenatal clinics in South Africa. *The Lancet,* Vol.363, No. 9419 (May 2004), pp. 1415–1421, ISSN 0140-6736

Eldred, L.J., Wu, A.W., Chaisson, R. & Moore, R. (1998). Adherence to antiretroviral and pneumocystis prophylaxis in HIV disease. *Journal of Acquired Immune Deficiency Syndromes,* Vol.18, No.2, (June 1998), pp. 117–125, ISSN 1077-9450

Falagas, M.E., Zarkadoulia, E.A., Pliatsika, P.A. & Panos, G. (2008). Socioeconomic status (SES) as a determinant of adherence to treatment in HIV infected patients: A systematic review of the literature. *Retrovirology,* Vol.5, No.13, (Frebruary 2008), ISSN 1742-4690.

Farmer, P. (1996). Poverty, and AIDS, Sex, drug and structural violence. In: *Women, Poverty, and AIDS,* P. Farmer, M. Connors y J. Simmons, (Eds.), 3-38, Common Courage Press, ISBN: 978-1567510744, Monroe, Maine.

Farmer, P. (2000). Desigualdades sociales y enfermedades infecciosas emergentes. *Papeles de Población*, Vol.23, No. 2, (Marzo 2000), pp. 181-201, ISSN 1405-7425

Fong, O.W., Ho, C.F., Fung, L.Y., Lee, F.K., Tse, W.H., Yuen, C.Y., et. al. (2003). Determinants of adherence to highly active antiretroviral therapy (HAART) in Chinese HIV/AIDS patients. *HIV Medicine*, Vol.4, No.2, (April 2003), pp. 133-138, ISSN : 1464-2662

Foreman, M., Lyra, P. & Breinbauer, C. (2003). *Comprensión y respuesta al estigma y a la discriminación por el VIH/SIDA en el sector salud*, OPS, ISBN 9275324719, Washington, United States.

Friedman, H.S. & Di Matteo, M.R. (1989). Adherence and practitioner patient relationship. In: Health Psychology, H.S. Friedman & M.R. Di Matteo (Eds.), 68-100, Prentice Hall, ISBN-13: 978-0133848922, New York, United States.

Gao, X., Nua, D.P., Rosenbluth, S.A., Scott, V. & Woodward, C. (2000). The relationship of disease severity, health beliefs and medication adherence among HIV patients. *AIDS Care*, Vol.12, No.4, (August 2000), pp. 387–398, ISSN 0954-0121.

Gifford, A., Bormann, J., Shively, M., Wright, B., Richman, D. & Bozzette, S. (2000). Predictors of self-reported adherence and plasma HIV concentrations in patients on multidrug antiretroviral regimens. *Journal of Acquired Immune De sciency Syndrome*, Vol.23, No.5, (April 2000), pp. 386–395, ISSN 1525-4135.

Ginarte, Y. (2001). La Adherencia Terapéutica. *Revista Cubana de Medicina General Integral*, Vol.17, No.5, (n.d 2001), pp. 502-505, ISSN 0864-2125

Glass, T.R., Geest, S.G., Weber, R., Vernazza, P.L., Rickenbach, M., Furrer, H., et. al. (2006). Correlates of self-reported nonadherence to Antiretroviral Therapy in HIV-Infected patients. *The Swiss HIV Cohort Study. Journal of Acquired Immune Deficiency Syndromes*, Vol.41, No.3, (March 2006), pp. 385-392, ISSN 1525-4135

Godin, G., Co^Té, J., Naccache, H., Lambert. L.D. & Trottier, S. (2005). Prediction of adherence to antiretroviral therapy: a one-year longitudinal study. AIDS Care, 17(4), 493-504

Goldman, D.P. & Smith, J.P. (2002). Can patient self-management help explain the SES health gradient? *Proceedings of the National Academy of Sciences of USA*, Vol.99, No.16, (February 2002), pp. 10929-34, ISSN 1525-4135

Golin, E.C., Liu, H., Hays, R.D., Miller, L.G., Beck, C.K., Ickovics, J., et al. (2002). A prospective study of predictors of adherence to combination antiretroviral medication. *Journal of General Internal Medicine*, Vol.17, No.10, (October 2002), pp. 756-65, ISSN 0884-8734

Gómez, E. (2002). Género, equidad y acceso a los servicios de salud: una aproximación empírica. *Revista Panamericana de Salud Pública*, Vol.11, No.5, (September 2002), pp. 327-334, ISSN 1020-4989

González, J.S., Penedo, F.J., Antoni, M.H., Durán R.E., Fernández, M.I., McPherson-Baker, S., et al. (2004). Social support, positive states of mind, and HIV treatment adherence in men and women living with HIV/AIDS. *Health Psychology*, Vol.23, No.4, (July 2004), pp. 413–418, ISSN 1020-4989

Gordillo, V., Del Amo, J., Soriano, V. & Gonzalez, J. (1999). Sociodemographic and psychological variables influencing adherente to antiretroviral therapy. *AIDS*, Vol.13, No.13, (September 1999), pp. 1763-69, ISSN 0269-9370

Gupta, G. (2000). Approaches for empowering women in the HIV/AIDS Pandemic: A gender perspective. In: *Expert Groups Meeting on "The HIV/AIDS Pandemic and its Gender Implications*, 17.02.2009, Available from http://www.un.org/womenwatch/daw/csw/hivaids/Gupta.html

Halkitis, P., Parsons, J., Wolitski, R., & Remien, R. (2003). Characteristics of HIV antiretroviral treatments, access and adherence in an ethnically diverse sample of men who have sex with men. *AIDS Care*, Vol.15, No.1, (February 2003), pp. 89-102, ISSN 0954-0121

Hankins, C., Friedman, S., Zafar, T. & Strathdee, S. (2002). Transmission and prevention of HIV and sexually transmitted infections in war settings: implications for current and future armed conflicts. *AIDS*, Vol.16, No.17, (November 2002), pp. 2245-2252, ISSN 0269-9370

Herrera, C. & Campero, L. (2002). La vulnerabilidad e invisibilidad de las mujeres ante el VIH/SIDA: constantes y cambios en el tema. *Salud Pública de México*, Vol.44, No.6, (Septiembre 2002), pp. 554-564, ISSN 0036-3634

Holzemer, W., Corless, I., Nokes, K., Turner, J., Brown, M., Powell-Cope, et. al. (1999). Predictors of self-reported adherence in persons living with HIV-disease. *AIDS Patient Care and STDS*, Vol.13, No.3, (March 1999), pp. 185-197, ISSN 1087-2914

Ickovics, J. R. & Meade, C. S. (2002). Adherence to HAART among patients with HIV: breakthroughs and barriers. *AIDS Care*, Vol.14, No.3, (June 2002), pp. 309–318, ISSN 0954-0121

Ingersoll, K. (2004).The Impact of Psychiatric Symptoms, Drug Use, and Medication Regimen on Nonadherence to HIV Treatment. *AIDS Care*, Vol.16, No.2, (February 2004), pp. 199-211, ISSN 0954-0121

International Community of Women Living with HIV/AIDS [ICW]. (2005). La visión de ICW3: mujeres seropositivas, pobreza y desigualdad de género. In : *ICW*, 10.09.2005. October 2007, Available from http://www.icwlatina.org/icw/imagenes/biblioteca/cuad.3.pdf

International Labour Office [ILO]. (2010). *Global Employment Trends*, ILO, ISBN 978-92-2-123256-8, Geneva, Switzerland

Jia, H., Uphold, C., Wu, S., Reid, K., Findley, K. & Duncan, P. (2004). Health-Related Quality of Life among men with HIV Infection: effects of social support, coping, and depression. *AIDS Patient Care STDS*, Vol.18, No.10, (October 2004), pp.584-603, ISSN 1087-2914

Kalichman, S.C., Ramacandran, B. & Catz, S. (1999). Adherence to combination antiretroviral therapies in HIV patients of low health literacy. *Journal of General Internal Medicine*, Vol.14, No.5, (May 1999), pp. 267-73, ISSN 0884-8734

Kim, J.C., Watts, C., Hargreaves, J.R., Ndhlovu, L.X., Phetla, G., Morison, L.A., et. al. (2007). Understanding the impact of a Microfinance-Based Intervention on women´s empowerment and the reduction of intimate partner violence in South Africa.

American Journal of Public Health, Vol.97, No.10, (October 2007), pp. 1794 - 1802, ISSN 00900036

Kleeberger, C., Phair, J., Strathdee, S., Detels, R., Kingsley, L. & Jacobson, L. (2001). Determinants of heterogenous adherence to HIV-antiretroviral therapies in the multicenter AIDS cohort study. *Journal of acquired immune deficiency syndromes*, Vol.26, No.1, (June 2001), pp. 82-92, ISSN 0213-9111

Koopman, C., Gore-Felton, C., Marouf, F., Butler, L., Field, N., Gill, M., et. al. (2000). Relationships of perceived stress to coping, attachment, and social support among HIV-positive persons. *AIDS Care*, Vol.12, No.5, (July 2000), pp. 663-672, ISSN 0954-0121

Kottak, C.P. (1994). *Antropología: Una exploración de la diversidad humana con temas de la cultura hispana*, Mc Graw Hill, ISBN: 8448118049, Madrid, España

Landero R. & González M. (2003). Autoeficacia y escolaridad como predictores de la información sobre VIH-SIDA en Mujeres. *Revista de Psicología Social*, Vol.18, No.1, (June 2003), pp. 61-70, ISSN 0213-4748

Marcovici, K. (2002). *El UNGASS, género y la vulnerabilidad de la mujer al VIH/SIDA en América Latina y el Caribe*, OPS, Available from http://www.paho.org/spanish/hdp/hdw/GenderandHIVSpanish.pdf

Martín, L. & Grau, J.A. (2004). La investigación de la adherencia terapéutica como un problema de la psicología de la salud. *Psicologia y Salud*, Vol.4, No.1, (Junio 2004), pp. 89-99, ISSN 1405-1109

Martin, L. (2004). Acerca del concepto de adherencia terapéutica. *Revista Cubana de Salud Pública*, Vol.30, No.4, (n.d. 2004), pp. 350-352, ISSN 0864-3466

Mathers C.R., et al. (2001). Healthy life expectancy in 191 countries, 1999. *The Lancet*, Vol.357, No.9269, (May 2001), pp. 1685–1691, ISSN 0140-6736

Max, B., & Sherer, R. (2000). Management of the adverse effects of antiretroviral therapy and medication adherence. *Clinical Infectious Diseases*, Vol.30, No.2, (June 2000), pp. S96–S116, ISSN 1058-4838

Meichenbaum, D. & Turk, D. (1991). *Cómo facilitar el seguimiento de los tratamientos terapéutico*, Desclée de Brouwer, ISBN 84-330-0877-3, Spain.

Millar, L. (2003). Factores asociados a la adherencia a tratamiento en pacientes enfermos de SIDA de la Región del Bío Bío. *Psykhe*. Vol.12, No.1, (Agosto 2003), pp. 145-160, ISSN 1058-4838.

Mocroft, A., Youle, M., Moore, A., Sabin, C., Madge, S., Lepri, A., et al. (2001). Reasons for modification and discontinuation of antiretro-virals: Results from a single treatment centre. *AIDS*, Vol.15, No.2, (January 2001), pp. 185-194, ISSN 0269-9370

Mohindra, K.S., Haddad, S. & Narayana, D. (2008). Can microcredit help improve the health of poor women? Some findings from a cross-sectional study in Kerala, India. *International Journal for Equity in Health*, Vol.7, No.2, (January 2008), ISSN 1475-9276

Morrison, M., Petitto, J., Ten Have, T., Gettes, D., Chiappini, M.S., Weber, A.L., et. al. (2002). Depressive and anxiety disorders in women with HIV infection. *The American Journal of Psychiatry*, Vol.159, No.5, (May 2002), pp. 789-796, ISSN 0002-953X

Murphy, D., Wilson, C., Durako, S., Muenz, L., & Belzer, M. (2001). Antiretroviral medication adherence among the reach HIV-infected adolescent cohort in the USA. *AIDS Care*, Vol.13, No.1, (February 2001), pp. 27-40, ISSN 0954-0121

Navarro V. (1989). Why some countries have national health insurance, others have national health services, and the United States has neither. *International Journal of Health Services*, Vol. 19 (n.d 1989), 383–404, ISSN 0020-7314

Navarro, V., et al. (2004). The importance of the political and the social in explaining mortality differentials among the countries of the OECD, 1950–1998, In: *The Political and Social Contexts of Health*, V. Navarro (Ed), 11-86, Baywood, ISBN 0-89503-299-6, Amityville, NY, United States

Pan American Health Organization [PAHO], United Nations Population Fund [UNFPA] & United Nations Development Fund for Women [UNIFEM], (2009). *Gender, Health, and Development in the Americas Basic Indicators 2009*, WHO.

Paredes, N. (2003). *Derecho a la Salud: su situación en Colombia*, CINEP-GTZ, ISBN 9586440818, Bogotá, Colombia.

Paterson, D.L., Swindells, S., Mohr, J., Brester, M., Vergis, E.N., Squier, C., et al. (2000). Adherence to protease inhibitor therapy and outcomes in patients with HIV infection. *Annals of Internal Medicine*, Vol.133, No.1, (July 2000), pp. 21–30, ISSN 0003-4819

Payne, S. (2006). *The health of men and women*, Polity, ISBN 9780745634531, Cambridge, England.

Payne, S. (2009). How can gender equity be addressed through health systems? *Health Systems and Policy Analysis*, Vol.12, (n.d 2009), pp. 1-45, ISSN 1997-8073

Pecheny, M., Manzelly, H.M. & Jones, D.E. (2007). The experience of Stigma: People living with HIV/AIDS and Hepatitis C in Argentina. *Interamerican Journal of Psychology*, Vol.41, No.1, (April 2007), pp. 17-30, ISSN 0034-9690

Poundstone, K.E., Strathdee, S.A. & Celentano, D.D. (2004). The social epidemiology of Human Immunodeficiency Virus/Acquired Immunodeficiency Syndrome. *Epidemiologic Reviews*, Vol.26, No.1, (February 2004), pp. 22-35, ISSN 0193-936X

Rao, G. (2004). Globalization, Women and the HIV/AIDS Epidemic. *Peace Review*, Vol.16, No.1, (March 2004), pp. 79–83, ISSN 1040-2659

Raphael, D. (2003). A society in decline: The social, economic, and political determinants of health inequalities in the USA, In: *Health and Social Justice: A Reader on Politics, Ideology, and Inequity in the Distribution of Disease*, R. Hofrichter (Ed.), 59-88, Jossey Bass, ISBN 0-7879-6733-5, San Francisco, United States

Raphael, D. (ed.). (2004). *Social Determinants of Health: Canadian Perspectives*. Canadian Scholars' Press, ISBN 1551302373, Toronto

Remor, E.A. (2002). Valoración de la adhesión de al tratamiento antirretroviral en pacientes VIH +. *Psicothema*, Vol.4, No.2, (November 2002), pp. 262 - 267, ISSN 0214-9915

Roberts, K. & Mann, T. (2000). Barriers to antiretroviral medication adherence in HIV-infected women. *AIDS Care*, Vol.12, No.4, (August 2000), pp. 377–386, ISSN 0954-0121

Rodríguez-Marín, J. (1995). Efectos de la interacción entre el profesional sanitario y el paciente. Satisfacción del paciente. Cumplimiento de las prescripciones terapéuticas. In: *Psicología social de la salud,* J. Rodríguez-Marín (Ed.), 151-160, Síntesis, ISBN 8477382891, Madrid, España.

Ruiz-Torres, Y., Cintrón-Bou, F. & Varas-Diaz, N. (2007). AIDS-related stigma and health professionals in Puerto Rico. *Interamerican Journal of Psychology,* Vol.41, No.1, (April 2007), pp. 49-56, ISSN 0034-9690

Singh, N., Berman, S.M., Swindells, S., Justis, J.C., Mohr, J.A., Squier, C., et. al. (1999). Adherence of human immunodeficiency virus infected patients to antiretroviral therapy. *Clinical Infectious Diseases,* Vol.29, No.4, (October 1999), pp. 824-30, ISSN 1537-6591

Spire, B., Duran, S., Souville, M., Leport, C., Raffi, F., Moatti, J.P. et al. (2002). Adherence to highly active antiretroviral therapies (HAART) in HIV-infected patients: from a predictive to a dynamic approach. Social Science & Medicine, 54, 1481-1496

Stein, M., Rich, J. D., Maksad, J., Chen, M. H., Hu, P., Sobota, M., et. al. (2000). Adherence to antiretroviral therapy among HIV-infected methadone patients: effects of ongoing illicit drug use. *American Journal of Drug and Alcohol Abuse,* Vol.26, No.2, (May 2000), pp. 195–205, ISSN 0095-2990

Sternhell, P.S. & Corr, M.J. (2002). Psychiatric morbidity and adherence to antiretroviral medication in patients with HIV/AIDS. Australian and New Zealand Journal of Psychiatry, 36, 528-533

Stone, V., Clarke, J., Lovell, J., Steger, K., Hirschhorn, L., Boswell, S., et al. (1998). HIV/AIDS patients' perspectives on adhering to regimens containing protease inhibitors. *Journal of General Internal Medicine,* Vol.13, No.9, (September 1998), pp. 586–593, ISSN 0884-8734

Turner-Cobb, J., Gore-Felton, C., Maroua, F., Koopman, C., Kim, P., Israelski, D., et. al. (2002). Coping, social support, and attachment style as psychosocial correlates of adjustment in men and women with HIV/AIDS. *Journal of Behavioral Medicine,* Vol.25, No.4, (April 2002), pp. 337-354, ISSN 0160-7715

Ward, J. (2002). *If not now. When? Addressing gender-based violence in refugee internally displaced and post-conflict setting,* Reproductive Health for Refugees Consortium, ISBN 1-58030-017-0, Washington, United States

Weidle, P., Ganea, C., Irwin, K., Mcgowan, J., Ernst, J., Olivio, N., et. al. (1999). Adherence to antiretroviral medications in an inner-city population. *Journal of AIDS,* Vol.22, No.5, (December 1999), pp. 498–502, ISSN 1525-4135

Weisman, C. S. (1998). *Women´s health care,* The Johns Hopkins University Press, ISBN 0801858267, Baltimore, United States

Weiss, S.M. et al. (2011). Enhancing the health of women living with HIV: the SMART/EST Women's Project. *International Journal of Women's Health,* Vol. 2011, No.3, (February 2011), pp. 63-77, ISSN 1179-1411

Whitehead, M. (1990). The concepts and principles of equity and health, In: World Health Organization Office for Europe, March 2006, Available from:
http://salud.ciee.flacso.org.ar/flacso/optativas/equity_and_health.pdf

Wingood, G. & Diclemente, R. (2000). Application of the Theory of Gender and Power to examine HIV-related exposures, risks factors and effective interventions for women. *Health Education & Behavior*, Vol.27, No.5, (October 2000), pp. 539-565, ISSN 1090-1981

World Health Organization [WHO]. (2003). *Adherence to long-term therapies: Evidence for action*. WHO, ISBN 92 4 154599 2, Switzerland

3

Intergenerational Sexual Relationship in Nigeria: Implications for Negotiating Safe Sexual Practices

Oyediran, K.A., Odutolu, O. and Atobatele, A.O.
MEASURE Evaluation/JSI, World Bank/Nigeria and USAID/Nigeria
Nigeria

1. Introduction

In Nigeria, young people aged 15-24 years old contribute significant number to the new HIV infections with the majority of those infections occurring in young women and girls. From NARHS 2007, HIV prevalence rate among young women is approximately 2.5 times that of young men within the age group. This disproportionate rate of HIV infection in young women is similarly found in many other countries in sub-Saharan Africa. For instance, data show that in general young women age 15-24 in sub-Saharan Africa are three times more likely to be infected with HIV than young men of the same age (UNAIDS, 2006). In Zambia and Zimbabwe, young women are four and five times respectively more likely to have HIV infection compared to their male counterparts (UNAIDS 2004). While biological factors may account for women's greater susceptibility to HIV; the difference is marked and cannot be explained on the basis of biology alone. It therefore raises the question of differences in sexual behaviour among the group within the context of cultures; lifestyle; and structural and environmental factors. As a result of this alarming HIV infection, the sexual behavior of this population is of great public health concern.

Within this premise and in order to understand the sexual behaviour of young women, intergenerational sex has been widely explored in literature. There is clear empirical evidence that age-mixing between young women and older men plays an important role in the differences in the observed epidemiological pattern (Gregson et al., 2002). Studies indicate that relationships between young women and older men are common in many parts of sub-Saharan Africa and are significantly related with unsafe sexual behaviour and increased vulnerability to HIV infection (Glynn et al., 2001; Kelly et al., 2003; Longfield et al., 2004). For instance, Langeni (2007) in the study of 800 men in Botswana found that for every year's increase in the age difference between partners there was a 28 percent increase in the odds of having unprotected sex. Similar studies reveal that such relationships are largely premised upon material gains, the greater the economic asymmetries between partners and the greater the value of a gift, service, or money exchanged for sex, the less likely the practice of safer sex (Luke, 2003; Wojciki, 2005). In this regard, intergenerational sex is similar to transactional sex because sex is exchanged for money and other materials, but the concept of intergenerational sex is clearly differentiated from commercial sex or prostitution. The former is based on material support mainly through relationships with 'sugar daddy or sugar mummy' (Moore & Biddlecom, 2006).

2. Intergenerational sex

Intergenerational sex is similarly referred to as cross-generational sex or age-mixing or age-disparate relationships in literature. It is a pattern of sexual behaviour between young women and older men within or outside of marriage. The term suggests wide variation in the ages of the partners with the men being commonly the older partner. The phenomenon is observed also between young men and older women; but this is less common, less overt and has not been linked with high HIV prevalence among the young men. Intergenerational sex has been more clearly defined, within both the UNAIDS general population survey and the Demographic and Health Surveys (DHS) AIDS modules, as *'Young women ages 15 to 19 who "have had non-marital sex in the last 12 months with men who are 10 or more years older than themselves."* But the definition is being expanded to include sexual relationships in which the age difference between the partners is only five years by other researchers. This revision is based on the observation that having sexual relations with a man only five years older has been clearly associated with increased risk of HIV in girls.

The practice of intergeneration sex is pervasive and is inherent in many cultures and traditions. Although, intergenerational sex is not limited to sub-Saharan Africa, the high prevalence of HIV infection in the region, especially among young adults, has led to studying behaviours that are associated with increased incidence thus making most available data on the practice to be in the region as it is associated with a higher risk of HIV infection. Furthermore, relationships between young women and older men are considered to be the norm in some cultural contexts. However, women in sexual relationships with older male partners have been found to have poor reproductive outcomes, including increased risk for HIV infection (Kelly, et. al., 2003; Gregson, et. al., 2002; Jewkes, et. al., 2002). Dissassortive sexual age mixing patterns can provide entryway for HIV and STIs into the younger generation (Jewkes, et. al., 2002). In the context of poverty and gender inequality, intergenerational sex often involves sex in exchange for money or goods and characterised by less condom use and greater sexual coercion (Gregson, et. al., 2002; Luke, 2005; Longfield, et. al., 2004). The risks associated with intergenerational sex may be, in part, due to the power imbalances between the partners (Blanc, 2001; Mensch and Lloyd, 1998). Particularly if a young woman is dependent on an older man for financial support, she may have little power to negotiate safe sex (Luke and Kurz, 2002). Furthermore, in instances where a young woman does assert herself, she may face sexual and physical violence (Kaufman and Stavrou, 2002; Wood, Maforah and Jewkes, 1998).

Several factors have been identified within age-mixing relationships that increase the risk of sexually transmitted infections (STIs) and HIV infection. Firstly, for both partners *risk perception* is often very low. According to Longfield et al. (2004), men in Kenya often report a preference for young sexual partners, basically because they are adjudged more likely to be free from HIV infection. While in South Africa, young women viewed older men in much the same way; as 'safe' partners because they appear to be less risk-taking, more stable and more responsible (Leclerc-Madlala, 2003). Young women are also found to be more concerned about the risk of becoming pregnant or of being 'found out' in their relationships with older men, than of STI or HIV (Silberschmidt and Rasch, 2000; Jones, 2006; Nkosana and Rosenthal, 2007). Secondly, in this relationship of unequal partners, young women's power to negotiate condom use is often compromised by age disparities and economic dependence. Young women have reported that they often cannot insist on safe sex practices, and doing so would jeopardize their economic goals in the relationships (Glynn, et. al., 2001; Luke, 2005; Longfield, et. al., 2004). According to a 17 year old out of school Ugandan young woman who was 15 years younger than her partner:

'He would pick me from home secretly and take me for film shows in town. I would always lie to my mother that I had gone to my Auntie's place and would spend nights with him. At the end of it all he asked me to show him that I loved him by having sex with him and I complied. I could not refuse because I was ashamed of all the things he had done for me.' (Moore and Biddlecom 2007)

The young women oblige to have sex within the relationship more out of a feeling of 'pay back' or appreciation of what the man has done or being in a position to meet his needs, more or else taking responsibility to please him. Men are also known to threaten to abandon the young women for another. The next section explores these and other reasons why the practice has continued to thrive despite the risk of STI and HIV infection.

2.1 Reasons for engaging in intergenerational sex

Several qualitative and few small-scale quantitative studies have explored factors luring young girls to engaging in intergenerational sexual relations in sub-Saharan Africa. Studies from Cameron, Kenya, Nigeria, Tanzania, Ghana, Swaziland and Uganda among others find that young women engage in sexual relationship with older partners for economic survival; funds to cover education-related expenses; enhanced status and connections in social networks; improved life opportunities and options; security; love and probably the option of marriage(Calves et al., 1996; Weiss et. al., 1996; Komba_Malekela and Lijestorm, 1994; Nyanzi, et. al., 2000; Akuffo, 1987; Stavrou and Kaufman, 2000; Gage, 1998; Orubuloye, et. al., 1992; Meekers and Calves, 1997). Scholars have documented that girls are motivated to engage in sexual relations with older partners due to their perceived view that older men are marriageable types and more likely to marry or support them in case of unintended pregnancy (Weiss, et. al., 1996; Komba-Malekela and Liljestrom, 1994; Nyanzi, et. al., 2000; Gorgen, et. al., 1998). Also of significant importance is the fact that parents often pressurize girls to form relationships with older, established partners that may lead to marriage - or at least where the partner can support their daughter if she becomes pregnant unintentionally (Gage, 1998). As shown by other studies, parents could indirectly encourage the relationship by warning their daughters not to bear a poor boy's child (Gorgen, et. al., 1998; Gorgen, et. al., 1993). On the other hand, parents disapprove of girls' relationship with older men when observed that the man is not interested in marriage (McLean, 1995).

A study conducted in Swaziland among girls 14 years and older reported that 20 percent of the girls reported being sexually active because of financial reasons (McLean, 1995). Another study in rural Tanzania found that 52 percent of female primary school students and 10 percent of female secondary school students reported that the reason for having sex was for money or presents (Matasha, et. al., 1998). In addition, in a study in rural Ghana, the majority of both in-school and drop-out girls admitted that the most important reason for having boyfriends was financial, and a further one-third said the reason was for the purchase of clothing and other goods (Akuffo, 1987). With respect to economic survival, evidence from several studies indicates that many girls need resources from older men for basic needs or in times of economic crisis (MacPhail and Campbell, 2001; Stavrou and Kaufman, 2000; Feldman et. al., 1997). For instance, scholars reported that parents may directly pressurize their daughters to enter into relationships with older, well-off men because they demand assistance from their children, including the money given to girls by their older partners (Gage, 1998; Komba-Malekela and Liljestrom, 1994). Furthermore, numerous studies point to adolescent girls' motivations to secure life opportunities and enhance long-term goals of higher economic status and security through their involvement with older partners. Stavrou and Kaufman (2000) and Abang (1996) reported that some young women engage in relations with older partners to help pay for tuition, living expenses, university housing, clothes and food. Scholars further observed that older partners of young women help them to meet prestigious people and establish themselves in an occupation or career (Gage, 1998; Meekers and Calves, 1997a, 1997b; Orubuloye, et. al., 1992).

Evidence from a few relatively small-scale quantitative studies indicated that socio-demographic attributes could be used to explain the context of cross-generational sex. In Lesotho, an important finding is that there is a strong relationship between wealth index and urban-rural residence and the likelihood of engaging in intergenerational sexual partnerships: women in lower wealth quintiles and in rural areas are more likely than others to engage in cross-generational partnerships (ORC, Macro, 2007).

2.2 Intergenerational sex and HIV infection

Evidence from the literature clearly links intergeneration sex with high HIV infection in young women. Young women who engage in sexual relationship with older men are more likely to have HIV infection compared to their male counterparts who do not. A study in rural Rakai, Uganda (Kelly, et. al., 2001) analyzed the relationship between HIV prevalence and the age of adolescent girls' primary sexual partner, whether marital or non-marital. In a multivariate analysis, among girls aged 15 -19, the adjusted relative risk of HIV infection doubled among those reporting a most recent sexual partner 10 or more years older, compared to those with partner 0-4 years older. Among young women 20 - 24, the adjusted relative risk of HIV infection was 24 percent greater, and among young women aged 25 - 29, it was 9 percent lower. Additional results suggest that 12.4 percent of the HIV prevalence in girls aged 15 - 19, and 5.1 percent in young women aged 20-24, can be attributed to relationships with men 10 or more years older, largely within marital relationships. Another study in rural Zimbabwe (Gregson, et. al., 2002) also finds a significant positive effect of age difference, with most recent marital or non marital partner; on HIV infection for all adolescents aged 17 - 24. In a multivariate analysis, the authors conclude that a one-year increase in age difference between partners is associated with a 4 percent increase in the risk of HIV infection. In a related analysis of the effect of age difference between partners in town urban cities in Africa: Kisumu, Kenya and Ndola, Zambia, Glynn et. al. (2001) find a significant positive association between larger age difference with husband and HIV infection. The authors reported that for girls with less than a four-years age difference with their husbands, none are infected with HIV, whereas 38 percent in Kisumu and 34 percent in Ndola are infected if the age difference with their husbands is four years or greater.

In the Nigerian context, there are empirical evidences of intergenerational sexual relationships; the 2003 DHS reported that the prevalence of intergenerational sex among girls aged 15-17 years is 21.3% percent. This represents the highest prevalence among the countries shown in a table 1 below. Significantly there is the practice of early marriage in the northern part of the country and more often than not the young women are married to men who are much older than themselves. In general terms the practice is cultural; so also is polygamy. Could it be a situation of double jeopardy? Unfortunately, the subject has not been well researched as to its implication on STI and HIV infection.

RECENT DHS SURVEYS ON INTERGENERATIONAL SEX

Country, Year of DHS	Percentage of sexually active women aged 15-17 with partner at least 10 years older in the past year	Percentage of sexually active women aged 18-19 with partner at least 10 years older in the past year
Ghana 2003	1.7	7.9
Nigeria 2003	21.3	4.2
Malawi 2004	0.9	2.4
Tanzania 2004	4.9	7.8
Lesotho 2004	7.5	7
Uganda 2004-2005	9.4	9.9

Source: DHS Reports ORC MACRO

Table 1. Recent DHS Surveys on intergenerational sex

Consequently, there is a knowledge gap on the spread of the practice; factors promoting the practice; the ability of the young women to negotiate safe sex and HIV infection in the age group. Hence, understanding the underlying factors and prevalence of the intergenerational sex is a priority study for Nigeria. The main thrust of this paper is to examine the prevalence of, and factors associated with intergenerational sexual relationship among young women aged 15 - 24 years and examine the implications of the practice on safe sex and HIV infection. The study will analyze the 2008 Nigeria Demographic and Health Survey (NDHS) to explore the relationship between young women's individual socio-demographic attributes and behaviour. Lastly, the paper will proffer programmatic and policy recommendations.

3. Methods

This study used data from the 2008 Nigeria Demographic and Health Survey (NDHS), which was carried out by ORC Macro and the National Population Commission. The sample was selected using a stratified 2-stage cluster design consisting of 888 clusters taken from a list of enumeration areas developed for the 2006 Population Census. A nationally representative probability sample of 36,800 households was then selected from the clusters, with a minimum target of 950 completed interviews per state, in which all women aged 15 to 49 years were eligible to be interviewed. The men's questionnaire was administered to all men aged 15 to 59 years in a sub-sample of half of the households. The survey collected information between June and October 2008. The data are intended to furnish program managers and policy makers with detailed information on the levels and trends in fertility; nuptiality; sexual activity; fertility preferences; awareness and use of family planning methods; infants and young children feeding practices; nutritional status of mothers and young children; early childhood mortality and maternal mortality; maternal and child health; and awareness and behavior regarding HIV/AIDS and other sexually transmitted infections. The data also provided information on malaria prevention and treatment; neglected tropical diseases; domestic violence; fistulae and female genital cutting.

Since the main thrust of this paper is to examine the prevalence of, and factors associated with intergenerational sexual relationship among young women aged 15 - 24 years; we examined the relevant questions within the survey to provide information on the indicators. Specifically, young women age 15 -24 who had sex with a non-marital, non-cohabiting partners in the 12 months prior to the survey were asked whether the man was younger, about the same age, or older than they were. If older, they were asked if they thought he was less than ten years older or ten or more years older. The analysis was restricted to those who had sexual relationship with a man who was 10 or more years older than them.

The dependent variable was binary and defined as the occurrence of the young women aged 15 - 24 years reporting having had sex with non-marital and non cohabitating male partners in the past 12 months who are at least 10 years older and those who did not. Possible confounders and other independent variables identified through the literature and theoretic reasoning fell into two (2) main groups: socio-economic and behavioural variables. In the first group were length of time away from home, place of residence (urban/rural), religion, ethnicity, regions, age, and educational attainment. While variables such as age at sexual debut, age difference between respondent and her first sexual partner and frequency of media exposure were considered in second group. Demographic, socio-economic and behavioural variables were included in the analysis to identify factors for possible intervention and to act as control variables in the analytical models.

The data analysis employed both descriptive and analytical techniques. Both descriptive and analytical analyses were conducted to ascertain the association and net effect of the respondents' background characteristics and identified confounders on the dependent variable (intergenerational sex) when controls for the selected background characteristics were introduced. The statistical analyses were undertaken in two phases. The descriptive statistics show the distribution of respondents by the key variables, and in the bivariate analysis, the relationship between each explanatory variable and the dependent variable was examined. Finally, multivariate logistic regression analysis was utilized to examine the net effects of the variables on the likelihood of having an intergenerational sexual relationship. First, socio-demographic characteristics and behavioural factors thought to be related to the intergenerational sexual relationships were examined using a Pearson x^2 test.

Multivariate logistic regression analyses were performed to calculate the adjusted odds ratios (ORs) and 95% confidence intervals (CIs) for predictors of women reporting high-risk sex within the last 12 months with older men of at least 10 years and older. Four structured regression models were estimated to describe the likelihood that a young woman would have had intergenerational sex when the different categories of the covariates are statistically controlled. Model 1 treats the likelihood of intergenerational sex as a function of the basic socio-economic variables (age, education, wealth index). Model 2 adds measures of socio-cultural influences (place of residence and ethnicity). The third model adds measures of attitudes and behavioural factors (age at sexual debut and age difference between respondent and her first sexual partner). Finally, model 4 adds a measure of media exposure (frequency of watching television) and socio-cultural influence (region). This analytical procedure provides an opportunity to examine how each set of explanatory factors is associated with young women's engagement in intergenerational sex.

Logistic regression was used in determining the effects of predictor variables on the outcome variable (intergenerational sexual relationship). The logistic regression model also offers ease of interpretation through the use of odds ratios. The logistic regression function has the form In $(p/q) = B_0 + B_1X_1 + \ldots + B_kX_k$, where p is the probability that a respondent who engaged in higher risk sexual relationship with a man 10 years or more older; q (or 1-p) is the probability that the respondent did not have sex with a man 10 years or more older in the past 12 month prior to their interview. B_0, B_1, … B_k are regression coefficients, and X_1, X_2, … X_k are factors. The exponential of the regression coefficients of the parameter estimated gives the odds ratios in the logistic regression models, which is interpreted as the likelihood of intergenerational sex under the given scenario

3.1 Variable definition and relations

As earlier stated, the 2008 NDHS questionnaire elicited information on sexual activity with non-marital partners and in the 12-months preceding the survey and whether the male sexual partner is 10 years older. The dependent variable, intergenerational sex, - defined as relationships between younger women and older men who are 10 or more years older in the last 12-months. The operational variables include age, ethnicity, place of residence, wealth index (poverty proxy), education, region, age difference between respondent and her first sexual partner and age at sexual debut. The socio-cultural and demographic variables were transformed either into categorical or dichotomous variables and entered as dummy variables in the multivariate analysis.

It is hypothesized that intergenerational sexual experience will decrease with age. Because the younger the girl experiencing sex, the older her partners will be and presumably by age 18, many of the girls would be ceasing the relationship with the much older partner and have taken a sexual partner closer to their own age which may likely be their permanent suitor. Current age of respondents is grouped into four categories (15 - 17; 18- 21 and 22 - 24) and the likelihood of having intergenerational sexual relationship is expected to decrease with age. Age at sexual debut is included as an explanatory variable because it has been found to be significantly associated high risk sexual behavior (Gomez, et. al., 2008). It is therefore necessary to explore whether this association holds among Nigerian girls. Age at first sexual encounter is sub-divided into four categories: below 15, 15 - 17, 18 years and older.

Religion is believed to have a profound impact on the behaviour and viewpoint of individuals. Even in the face of modernization and its consequences on cultural practices, religion still seems to hold a firm grip on moral values relating to sexual practices and behaviour. Therefore, girls who are more religious are more likely to hold strong, rigid, and fundamentalist religious beliefs that may discourage their sexual escapades before marriage in order to remain virgin. However, the relationship between religious affiliation and sexual practices, particularly intergenerational sex, is likely to be mediated by social and demographic factors, such as education of the respondent and region of residence. The religious affiliation sub-groups used are Catholic, Other Christians and Islam.

Ethnicity is an important proxy of cultural factors affecting sexual behaviour since it encompasses values and norms that govern the behavioural and psychological aspects of social interaction between men and women in a particular socio-cultural space. It may also reflect the level of openness to influences of and/or adherence to other cultures due to interactions with different areas and/or regions. With more than 389 ethnic groups in Nigeria, ethnic differences are critical in explaining cultural differences and behavioural patterns, including sexual relations and practices. Also the heterogeneity of ethnic groups in Nigeria implies that social changes takes place at different paces and in a non-uniform manner since some ethnic groups may be more receptive to change than others. For this paper, ethnic affiliation is categorized into five sub-groups based on their numerical strength and affinity. The ethnic sub-divisions used are Igbo, Yoruba, northern minorities, southern minorities and others due to small number of cases for Hausa/Fulani ethnic group. The northern and southern minorities comprise numerous smaller ethnic groups in the north and south respectively while other ethnic group consist mainly small tribe with less than 2 percent of the country population, whose sample sizes were too small to stand alone in the analysis. This analytical convenience, however, does not suggest that each of the two broad ethnic groupings is homogeneous in their socio-cultural environment or behaviour.

In view of the paucity of research on regional differential in intergenerational sex, it is significant in this paper to explore the phenomenon within the 2008 NDHS data that contain comparable and representative regional information. Apart from underscoring the structural patterns within the Nigerian community, region represents differences in the socio-economic and cultural influence on respondent sexual practices, particularly intergenerational sexuality. It is important also to note that regions constitute a proxy for social change or development. In this paper, Nigeria is sub-divided into two distinct geo-political regions namely; Northern and Southern region. Place of residence is also included to capture the influence of urban and rural residence on the likelihood of intergenerational sex.

It is hypothesized that younger women at lower wealth quintile are more likely to engage in intergenerational relations than those at higher wealth quintiles. However, this relationship depends on the interplay of several other confounding factors such as age of the respondent, educational attainment, and place of residence. Since studies have reported a key motivational factor while young girls engage in sexual activity with older men is because of their economic status (Gage, 1998; Orubuloye, et. al., 1992; Meekers and Calves, 1997) it is important to see whether wealth index as constructed in the NDHS could help shed light on the interplay of poverty with intergenerational sexual relationships. Wealth index was constructed from the household facilities and ownership of a certain consumer items such as television, radio, bicycle, car, as well as dwelling characteristics such as source of drinking water, power supply, type of sanitation facilities, and type of material used in flooring and roofing the dwelling units. Each household was assigned a score for each asset, and the scores were summed up; individuals were ranked according to the total score of the household in which they resided. The aggregate scores were then divided into quintiles, from one to five, corresponding to the poorest and the wealthiest groups.

Educational attainment was categorized as less than secondary education, secondary education and post-secondary education. Residence and region were included based on the method of sampling used by the NDHS. Although original sampling was performed using the 37 states, the analysis included regions because of the relatively few number of cases in some states and risk of non-convergence in the multivariate statistical methods. Finally, media exposure was categorized according to self-reported frequency of watching, listening to, or reading the television, radio, or newspapers/magazines.

3.2 Respondents' profile

A total of 12, 649 young females, aged 15-24 years were interviewed during the 2008 NDHS and 2,029 of these young women who engaged in higher-risk sexual intercourse in the past 12 months were analyzed in this study. The basic-demographic characteristics of the study population are provided in Table 2. About 44 percent of them were 15-19 years of age while the remaining 56.5 percent were aged 20-24 years. The median age of the respondents was 20.0 years. The survey indicated that 6 out of 10 of the respondents resided in rural areas and regional spatial distribution of the study population shows that 74.1 percent of them resided in the southern regions of South-east, south-south and south-west, while the remaining 25.9 percent resided in the three-regions in the northern part of the country. The distribution of respondents by ethnic affiliation shows that 12.9 percent are Igbo, 13.0 percent are Yoruba; 1.1 percent are Hausa/Fulani; minority ethnic groups constitute 26.5 percent. Of the minority ethnic groups, the northern minorities constitute 5.0 percent of the respondents, while southern minorities constitute 21.5.0 percent. Other ethnic groups in Nigeria with population less than 1 percent of the country population constitute 33.1 percent Majority (73.4 percent) of the young women under study had secondary education. While about 15 per cent of them had post-secondary education, 9.7 percent and 2.1 percent had primary education and no formal education respectively. Christians constituted a majority of the sampled population with about nine out of ten young females being Christians. Muslims constituted 12.4 per cent. Another important background characteristic considered in the analysis was the wealth quintile. Wealth quintile constructed from the household facilities is used as a proxy for economic status. The level of wealth quintile ranges from the first to the fifth quintile, corresponding to the least and most well off respectively. The Wealth quintile revealed that about one out of four young women were from households classified in the fifth quintile.

Table 2 reveals a high level of exposure to electronic media. Three out of ten of the respondents listened to the radio at least once in a while and about 32.6 percent of young women who engaged in higher-risk sexual intercourse in the past 12 months reported listening to the radio every day. About a quarter (22.7 percent) had never watched television; while 37.7 percent watched television every day. The reading of newspaper or magazine is low among the study population. Over half 56.3 percent had never read newspaper or magazine while 4.5 percent read newspaper or magazine every day. The results indicate widespread access to media.

Table 2 further compared the characteristics of sexually experienced young women and those among them that engaged in higher-risk sexual intercourse in the preceding 12 months before the survey. The result reveals that there is no major difference between those who are sexually experienced and those among them engaged in higher-risk sexual relationship with men ten years or more years older than them. For instance, 43.5 percent of those who had intergenerational sexual relationships are 15 - 19 as compared with 37.9 percent of the counterparts that are sexually experienced. The median age for both subgroups was 20.0 years. Furthermore, those young women who engaged in higher-risk sexual intercourse are likely to reside more in urban areas; reside more in southern regions, more educated, come from more affluence households, belong to Christian religious especially those who are protestants or Pentecostals and have more access to the media than sexually experienced young women age 15 - 24 interviewed during the 2008 NDHS.

Characteristics	Number (N=7,979)	Percentage of women age 15 - 24 who had had sexual experience	Percentage of women age 15 - 24 who had high-risk sexual intercourse in the past 12 months (N = 2,029)
Age group			
15-19	3,021	37.9	43.5
20-24	4,958	62.1(20.0)	56.5(20.0)
Place of residence			
Urban	2,137	26.8	40.3
Rural	5,842	73.2	59.7
Region of residence			
Northern	5,016	63.6	25.9
Southern	2,903	36.4	74.1
Ethnicity			
Hausa/Fulani	2,834	35.7	1.1
Igbo	793	10.0	18.3
Yoruba	886	11.1	21.0
Southern minority	725	9.1	21.5
Northern minority	611	7.6	5.0
Others	2,101	26.4	33.1
Educational level			
No education	3,280	41.1	2.1
Primary	1,220	15.3	9.7
Secondary	3,030	38.0	73.4
Tertiary	449	5.6	14.8
Religious affiliation			
Catholic	767	9.7	16.5
Other Christians	2,939	37.0	70.3
Islam	4,108	51.8	12.4
Traditional/Others	121	1.5	0.4
Wealth quintile			
First	2,032	25.3	7.7
Second	1,745	21..9	13.5
Third	1,547	19.4	21.1
Fourth	1,583	19.8	31.2
Fifth	1,072	13.4	26.5
Frequency of watching television			
Never	4,403	55.4	22.7
Less than once a week	867	10.9	16.5
At least once a week	1,068	13.4	23.1
Almost everyday	1,603	20.2	37.7
Frequency of listening to radio			
Never	2,848	35.8	19.3
Less than once a week	1,222	15.4	17.4
At least once a week	1,820	22.9	30.8
Almost everyday	2,059	25.9	32.6

Note:-Median age of respondent are indicated in the bracket

Table 2. Percentage distribution of young women (aged 15-24 years) sexually experienced and those who had high-risk by selected socio-demographic characteristics (NDHS 2008)

3.3 Prevalence of intergenerational sex in Nigeria

Nearly one in six (2,029 of 12, 694) of the young women included in the survey reported having higher-risk in the preceding 12 months before their interview during the 2008 NDHS. The results presented in Table 3 show that among women age 15 - 24 who had higher-risk sexual intercourse in the 12 months preceding the survey, 14.6 percent had higher-risk sex with a man ten or more years older than them. The median age of sexual debut among the young women who had engaged in higher-risk sexual intercourse in the past year was 17 years. The analysis reveals that the proportions of respondents who had intergenerational sex in the past 12 months before the survey interview decreased with age. For instance, 16.5 percent of young women age 15-17 years, 15.2 percent of those age 18 - 21 years and 12.6 percent of their older peers aged 22-24 years had engaged in higher-risk sexual behaviour in the 12 months with a man 10 years or more years older.

Characteristics	Number of women age 15 - 24 who had high-risk sexual intercourse in the past 12 months	Percentage of young women age 15-24 who had high risk sexual intercourse with a man 10+ years
Age group*		
15 - 17	407	16.5
18 - 21	950	15.2
22 - 24	672	12.6
Place of residence**		
Urban	818	12.5
Rural	1,211	16.0
Region***		
Northern	526	24.1
Southern	1,503	11.2
Ethnic affiliation***		
Igbo	370	17.0
Yoruba	426	7.0
Northern Minority[1]	124	20.2
Southern Minority	435	10.3
Others	671	19.8
Educational attainment***		
Less than secondary education	239	23.8
Secondary education	1,489	13.4
Post-secondary education	301	13.3
Religious affiliation		
Catholic	334	15.3
Other Christians	1,422	14.1
Islam	258	16.7
Wealth quintile***		
First	157	21.0
Second	274	16.4
Third	428	18.5
Fourth	633	12.8
Fifth	537	10.8

[1] Include few cases of Hausa and Fulani who are predominantly resident in the northern part of Nigeria

Characteristics	Number of women age 15 - 24 who had high-risk sexual intercourse in the past 12 months	Percentage of young women age 15-24 who had high risk sexual intercourse with a man 10+ years
Age at sexual debut* **		
Less than 15 years	298	19.1
15 - 17 years	904	15.3
18 years and above	810	11.6
Age difference between respondent and first sexual partner* **		
Less than 5 years	1,165	4.1
5 - 9 years	316	11.1
10 years and above	69	85.5
Frequency of reading newspaper or magazine **		
Never	1,134	16.5
Less than once a week	430	11.9
At least once a week	364	12.6
Almost everyday	91	12.1
Frequency of listening to radio* **		
Never	390	18.5
Less than once a week	351	16.0
At least once a week	622	14.1
Almost everyday	659	12.1
Frequency of watching television* **		
Never	460	20.7
Less than once a week	335	16.7
At least once a week	468	13.0
Almost everyday	763	11.0
Total 15 - 24	2,029	14.6

Note:- *p<.05; **p<.01; ***p<.001

Table 3. Percentage of young women age 15 - 24 who had high-risk sexual intercourse in the past 12 months with a man who was 10 or more years older than them by selected socio-demographic characteristics

The analysis reveals that an intergenerational sexual relationship is more common among rural dwellers than young women who reside in urban areas (16.0% vs. 12.5%). There is a large variation in the prevalence of intergenerational sex by region: about four out of 10 young women in the northern region had intergenerational sex, compared with 11.2 percent of young women in the southern region. Ethnic affiliation of respondent reveals similar result with region of residence. Intergenerational sexual relationship is most prevalent among northern minority young women (20.2 percent) and least among the Yoruba young women (7.0 percent). Intergenerational sexual relationship is more prevalent among young women with less than secondary education (23.8 percent) and least prevalent among young women with secondary education (13.4 percent) and post-secondary education (13.3. percent).

It is evident from the table 3 that young women who had their sexual debut with a first partner that was 10 or more years older than them are more likely to engage in cross generational sex. Wealth index is negatively associated with intergenerational sexual behaviour - young Nigeria women from poorer households are more likely to engage in high-risk sexual relationships affairs than their wealthier counterparts. For instance, 21.0 percent of young women age 15 - 24 reported having sexual intercourse with a man 10 years or more their own age as compared with 10.8 percent of their counterparts from the most wealthier households. The prevalence of intergenerational sex declines from 19.1 percent among young women who had their sexual debut before age 15, to 11.6 percent among those who had their first sexual relation at 18 years and older. Intergenerational sexual relationships are more common among young women who are Muslim, ever married, and those who had never read newspapers or magazine, listened to radio or watched television.

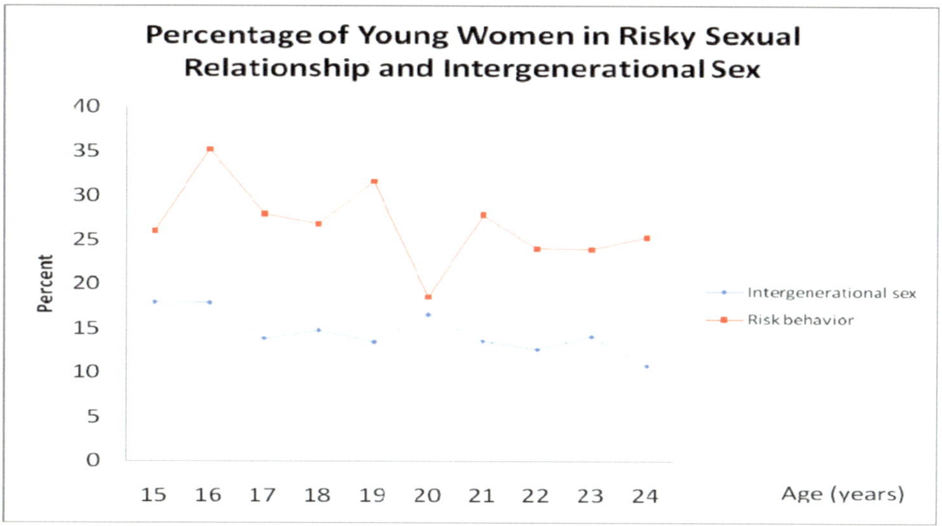

Fig. 1. Percentage of young women in risky sexual relationship and intergenerational sex

3.4 Multivariate analysis

Table 4 presents odds ratio for four equations that model the effects of the explanatory variables on the likelihood that Nigerian women (15 - 24 years) would engage in higher-risk sexual relationships with a man 10 years or older. In the first logistic regression model, only education and wealth index were significantly related to young women's engagement in cross generational sexual activities. Young women with secondary school education and those with post-secondary education were less likely than those with less secondary education to have had high-risk sex with a man 10 years or older in the past 12 months (odds ratio of less than 1). For instance, young women with secondary school education and post-secondary school education are 43 percent and 25 percent less likely to engage in intergenerational sex respectively than those with less than secondary education. The finding is statistically significant for the secondary school education. The regression model reveals that young women in the second to fifth quintile of the wealth index are less likely to have engaged in the intergenerational sex as compared with their counterparts in the first quintile of the wealth index. The result was statistically significant for those within the fifth quintile wealth and marginally for those in the fourth quintile wealth index. The other personal attributes added as covariates in the regression equation - individual age - was not significantly associated with intergenerational sex.

Background Characteristics	Model 1	Model 2	Model 3	Model 4
Age Group				
15 - 17 years (ref.)	1.00	1.00	1.00	1.00
18 – 21 years	0.94	0.96	2.06**	2.02**
22 – 24 years	0.79	0.75	2.57**	2.46**
Educational Attainment				
Les than secondary education (ref.)	1.00	1.00	1.00	1.00
Secondary education	0.57***	0.60***	0.61	0.68
Post-secondary education	0.75	0.87	1.29	1.53
Wealth Index				
First quintile (ref.)	1.00	1.00	1.00	1.00
Second quintile	0.74	0.91	0.85	0.89
Third quintile	0.94	1.11	0.58	0.70
Fourth quintile	0.65*	0.77	0.86	1.16
Fifth quintile	0.53**	0.64	0.69	1.07
Place of residence				
Urban		1.00	1.00	1.00
Rural		0.96	1.36	1.30
Ethnic Affiliation				
Northern Minority		1.00	1.00	1.00
Igbo		0.95	0.73	1.10
Yoruba		0.34***	0.35**	0.51
Southern Minority		0.50**	0.42*	0.71
Others		1.06	0.71	0.83
Age at sexual debut				
Less than 14 years			1.00	1.00
15 – 17 years			0.60	0.60
18 years and above			0.30***	0.30***
Age diff. b/t her 1st sexual partner				
<= 4 years			1.00	1.00
5 – 9 years			3.41***	3.21***
10 years and above			175.25***	159.89***
Region				
Northern				1.00
Southern				0.63
Frequency of watching television				
Not at all				0.78
Less than once a week				0.75
At least once a week				0.54*
Almost everyday				1.00
-2Log-likelihood (df)	-813.53	- 792.14	- 311.56	- 308.70

*p<.05; **p<.01; ***p<.001; +p<.10. 1.00=reference group

Table 4. Odds ratios from logistic regression analyses examining associations between selected characteristics and young women engaging in higher-risk sexual relationship with a man 10 years and older (NDHS, 2008)

While the significant association between wealth index and intergenerational sex disappears on adding place of residence (urban or rural) and ethnicity to the equation in Model 2 the significant relationship between secondary school education and intergenerational sex remains. The analysis shows that place of residence on its own does not significantly influence intergenerational sexual behavior in Nigeria. Ethnicity is significantly associated with intergenerational sex on controlling other variables. The results support the assumption that sexual behavior is guided by the cultural values and norms of the various ethnic groups. Young Yoruba women are 66 percent less likely to have engaged in cross generational sex than those from northern minority ethnic groups. Furthermore, young women from the southern ethnic minorities are significantly less likely to engage in intergenerational sex (odds ratio of 0.50) than those of northern minority ethnic groups. The odds of involvement in intergenerational sexual relationship are lower among young women residing in urban areas; the difference is not statistically significant.

In the third model, the significant association between education and intergenerational sex disappears on adding age at sexual debut and age difference between respondent and her first sexual partner while the association for the age becomes statistically significant to the equation in Model 2. In the logistic regression model 3, young women aged 18 - 21 years were (2.06 times) more likely than those 15-17 years to have had higher risk sexual relationship with a man 10 years or older in the past 12 months prior to the interview. Similarly, young women aged 22 -24 years are 2.57 times more likely than those 15 -17 years to have had intergenerational sex in the past 12 months compared with those young women aged 15-17. The results are statistically significant. The odds of engaging in intergenerational sex were lower among Yoruba and southern minority ethnic groups as compared with their northern minority ethnic group. The odds of engaging in higher risk sexual relationship with a man 10 years or older was significantly lower for young women who had first sexual experience 18 years or more as compared with those who started sexual experience before age 15. Furthermore, young women who reported having a partner 5 to 9 years and 10 years or more older at first sex were more likely (OR: 3.41 and 175.25 respectively) to report involvement in risky intergenerational sex, compared to young women whose first sexual partners was younger or less than 5 years older. These differences were statistically significant.

The third model (Table 4) shows that the odds of engaging in intergenerational sex were higher among urban (1.36) young women than their rural counterparts, a finding that is statistically significant. Young women from households classified into second quintile, third quintile, fourth quintile and fifth quintile were less likely to have had intergenerational sex as compared with those from household rank in first quintile. . For instance, young women in the fifth quintile wealth index are 31 percent less likely to have had intergenerational sex compared with those in the first quintile of the wealth index. The differences were not statistically significant.

In the final model, age at sexual debut and age differences between respondent and her first sexual partner remains statistically significantly associated with intergenerational sexual relationships when media exposure variable (frequency of watching television) and region of residence were included into the third equation. The results show that young women aged 18 - 21 years were (2.02 times) more likely than those 15-17 years to have had cross generational sexual relationship in the past 12 months prior to the interview. Similarly, young women aged 22 -24 years are 2.46 times more likely than those 15 -17 years to have had high-risk sexual relationship with a man 10 years or older in the past 12 months before their interview compared with those young women aged 15-17. The difference remains statistically significant. Other variables statistically significantly associated with intergenerational sex are age at sexual debut, age difference between respondent and their first sexual partner. As can be seen from table under model 4, young women who reported starting sexual intercourse by age 18 and above are less likely to have had intergenerational sex compared with those who reported starting before age 15. For instance, those who reported their sexual debut age to be 18 years and above are 7-times less likely to have had intergenerational sex as compared with those who reported their sexual debut age at less than 15 years. The difference was statistically significant. The statistical significant association between age difference of the respondent and their first sexual partner and intergenerational sex remains after controlling for all the variables.

Table 4, model 4 shows that young women who reported having a partner 5 to 9 years and 10 years or more older at first sex were more likely (OR: 3.21 and 159.89 respectively) to have had high risk sexual relationship with a man 10 or more years older compared with young women whose first sexual partners was younger or less than 5 years older. These differences were statistically significant. Other factor statistically significantly associated with intergenerational sex is watching television at least once a week as compared to those who reported to "not at all." The results show that young women residing in the southern region are less likely to engage in intergenerational sexual relationship than those living in the northern region. The statistical significance of the ethnicity disappears when variable on exposure to media (television) was introduced. Wealth index remain non-significant from model 2 to 4 while place of residence (urban vs. rural) remain non-significant since it has been introduced into the equation in model 2.

4. Discussion

The growing interest in intergenerational sex is borne out of the concern for the sexual and reproductive health and rights of young women particularly in sub Saharan Africa where the population bears the highest toll of the HIV/AIDS epidemic. From the several iterations of Demographic and Health Surveys and other studies, intergenerational sex is pervasive and this study based on the 2008 Nigeria Demographic and Health Survey confirms the prevalence of the phenomenon in Nigeria. Clearly, from the 2008 NDHS data a sizeable number of young women age 15 - 24 years engage in risky sexual behavior that may contribute to the spread of HIV/AIDS. In this study, one-quarter of young women in Nigeria reported having sex with a non-cohabitating and non-marital partners in the last 12 months while 14.6 percent of young women engaged in high risk sexual relationship with a man 10 or more years older than themselves, demonstrating the prevalence of intergenerational sex in the young Nigerian women population and thus the risk of HIV transmission. This estimate seems to be consistent with findings from other studies (Glynn et al., 2001; Kelly et al., 2003; Longfield et al., 2004; NDHS 2003). From this study 16.5 percent of young women aged 15-17 years engaged in intergenerational sex which is almost five-point lower than for women of similar age in the 2003 NDHS. It is too early however to say that the rate is falling. Broadly, this study reveals that the likelihood of engaging in intergenerational sexual relationship varies according to the personal attributes of respondents as well as cultural, attitudinal and behavioral factors.

This study paid particular attention to age of the respondents with regard to sexual risk. The practice of intergenerational sex decreases with age. The study revealed that 16.5 percent of young women age 15-17 years, 15.2 percent of those age 18 - 21 years and 12.6 percent of their older peers aged 22-24 years had engaged in higher-risk sexual behaviour in the 12 months with a man 10 years or more years older. The fact that the practice is commonest among 15-17 years is suggestive that the young women are vulnerable to inducements or coercion and those older girls bear the pressure for sex from the older men better. Basically, the younger girls may have little or no knowledge of the implications of their actions; cannot effectively assess the risk involved in the sexual relationship neither do they have the skill to negotiate safer sex. Most girls in this age group are preys and the predators have not spared them. The implications are multiple but essentially speak to the need for the commencement of reproductive health education and life skills programme for young girls early enough so that they are better placed to protect themselves. This is especially important for out - of - school girls as it is assumed that in some of our schools family life education is taught to young people. It is similarly essential to pay particular attention to young girls in the rural areas as intergenerational sexual relationship is **more** common among rural dwellers than young women who reside in urban areas. Another major approach would be to work directly with men to challenge the socio-cultural norms and perceptions that allows for and sanction engagement in intergenerational sex (Leclerc - Madlala 2002, 2003).

The expected result from the two recommended approaches above is to help young girls to increase the age at sexual debut significantly so that they can make informed decision about sex and how to protect themselves. As this study also shows that the odds of engaging in higher risk sexual relationship with a man 10 years or older was significantly lower for young women who had first sexual experience 18 years or more as compared with those who started sexual experience before age 15. The likelihood of having intergenerational sex tends to increase with intergenerational first sexual experience which has been reported to be linked with poor reproductive health outcomes. For instance, examining a longitudinal, representative sample of adolescents in the United States, Ryan and others found that women who initiated sex before age 16 with an older partner had a greater likelihood of testing positive for an STI in young adulthood. It is evident from the paper that intergenerational sexual relation varies according to personal, cultural and behavioral attributes of the respondents. These attributes should be considered when designing programs to promote safe and healthy sexuality and effective HIV/AIDS/STIs prevention,. In addition, the study suggests that several young Nigerians are vulnerable to HIV infection through high risk sexual behaviour and relatively low levels of condom use. HIV-prevention efforts should target the entire young population, rather than attempting to identify and focus attention only on high risk groups.

Another significant finding from this study is educational attainment. This is particularly important as we look at environment and structural factors that predispose to poor health outcomes importantly in our case the risk of HIV infection. The study shows that young women with secondary school education and those with post-secondary education were less likely than those with less secondary education to have had high-risk sex with a man 10 or more years older in the past 12 months. The implication is that the more educated the girl child is the higher the likelihood of better health outcomes. Nigeria has Universal Basic Education (UBE) programme which ensures at least nine (9) years of formal education, it is free and compulsory - compelled by law but in practice not enforced. In effect, Nigeria can greatly reduce the prevalence of intergenerational sex by enforcing the law that established Universal Basic Education.

In another age and educated related finding, the result reveals that age has a positive relationship with intergenerational sex particularly in models three and four, the result indicate that older young women who engage in high-risk sexual relationship may be the higher education students. Although the relationship between education and intergenerational sex become non-significant at multivariate analyses in equation 3 and 4, the higher prevalence of intergenerational sex among those in post-secondary schools may be due to the fact that young women exchange sex to get funds to cover education-related expenses and gain connections in social networks (Barker and Rich, 1992; Kaufman et. al., 2001; Meekers and Calves, 1997). This is a converse relationship when compared with young women in intergenerational sex. The older women are not 'victims' in the relationship, as they actively search for and establish such relationships to their advantage; studies reveal 'that many play active roles in seeking and exploiting relationships with older men and do not perceive themselves as victims' (Silberschmidt & Rasch 2000, Leclerc-Madlala 2003, Nkosana 2006)

The practice is consistent within the context of growing economic inequalities and cultural expectations for men to give and women to receive a compensation for sex, paves way for young women to gain materially, affirm self-worth, achieve social/educational goals, increase longer-term life chances, or otherwise add value and enjoyment to life.

It is important to mention it for affirmation, that poverty plays an important role in intergenerational sex such as in commercial sex work. The study reveals, from the regression model, that young women in the second to fifth quintile of the wealth index are less likely to engage in the intergenerational sex as compared with their counterparts in the first quintile of the wealth index. This confirms the link between poverty and risky sexual behavior - such as intergenerational sex, survival sex and prostitution. Young women's vulnerability to HIV is fueled by financial dependence and economic stress makes them susceptible to involvement in intergenerational relationship. As earlier mentioned access to education is a major route out of ongoing poverty and dependence. (Leclerc-Madlala 2003) Greater opportunity should also be given to women empowerment programmes (Odutolu et al 2003).

Broad categories of Northern and Southern regions rather than six geo-political regions and states were included in the models, because the number of cases was too low to allow for either region or state specific analyses. Future in-depth studies should therefore be carried out within region and states because of the heterogeneity of the country. Further evidence of Nigeria heterogeneity exists even within ethnic groups, such as the Yoruba who are made up of sub-ethnic groups with distinctive cultures; therefore, it is important to use caution when making generalizations about Nigerian populations. Although this study examined risk factors on a national level in Nigeria, some of the non-significant associations may have been a result of these intraregional differences, leading to a null association. Quantitative and qualitative state or region-specific studies should be carried out to probe the association between intergenerational sex, individual attributes, behavior and cultural factors so as to help programme implementers and policy makers targeting high risk groups.

The regional patterns of intergenerational sexual relationships found in this study suggest ethnicity may be an important factor to be considered when studying adolescents or young people's sexuality and sexual behavior. Ethnicity is significantly associated with intergenerational sex on controlling other variables. The results support the assumption that sexual behavior is guided by the cultural values and norms of the various ethnic groups. Young Yoruba women are 66 percent less likely to have engaged in cross generational sex than those from northern minority ethnic groups. However, this influence of cultural norms may be changing due to globalization and education, especially in the cities where people are more likely to abandon traditions because of the heterogeneity of populations. Still for many Nigerians, ethnic affiliation, which is usually a regional element, means shared language and norms governing behaviour and sexuality issues. The results of this study support the view that intergenerational sexual relationships is a function of varied socio-cultural factors including religion, level of exposure to formal education, urban-rural residence among others. Based on the notion that intergenerational sex predisposes to HIV infection, it is important for government and other programme planners to factor ethnic differences to HIV prevention programmes and make them more specific to the needs of the various ethnic groups and regions. The bane of HIV programming in Nigeria has always been one size fits all concepts and interventions. It is time that the interventions are evidence based and appropriately targeted.

The study results shed further light as regards the challenges facing programmes aimed at improving the reproductive health situation of adolescents and young adults in Nigeria, as well as opportunities for intervention. One major challenge is the sizeable number and diverse nature of factors that appeared to influence young women high risk behaviour. Some of these were particular characteristics of the environment in which they are reared. Therefore, a single, easy-to-implement intervention is unlikely to provide a solution to the risky behavior being engaged upon and its attendant consequences of vulnerability to STI and HIV/AIDS transmission in Nigeria. This is consistent with conclusion that when in a given setting and a multitude of correlates exists, each having a small impact on sexual behaviour, rather than a few correlates, each having a large impact, a single "magic bullet" is unlikely to be found to change adolescent sexual behaviour significantly.

These results have important policy implications. Because factors associated with intergenerational sexual behaviour among Nigerian young women vary according to education, ethnic affiliation, age, age at sexual debut, age difference between respondent and her first sexual partner, exposure to media and wealth quintile, programs may need to position intervention differently for different target populations. The study established that there is a relatively high risk sexual activity thus making the sampled population vulnerable to HIV infection. In addition, unwanted pregnancy could lead to termination of education especially the sexual partner refuses to claim the pregnancy; as a result, young women could face a bleak economic and social future. Therefore, behavioural change communication activities should be strengthened with extensive education on safe-sexual behaviour through culturally appropriate messages, as is currently undertaken by various NGOs in the country. In particular, more effort should be made to reach the young women from poor household and rural areas, who typically had earlier sexual debut and also tended to be more engaged in cross-generational sex, with adequate information on behavioural change, prevention of unwanted pregnancy and protection from sexually transmitted infections, including HIV/AIDS.

Although this research does not focus on the relationships between intergenerational sex and STI/HIV/AIDS situation in Nigeria, it highlights the importance of intergenerational sexuality in contributing to the spread of STI/HIV/AIDS especially in cultures where women are subjugated to male social hegemony. Furthermore, the ethnic differences in intergenerational sex observed in this study are consistently found in other studies on sexual and reproductive behavior in Africa. Since little is known on how cultural norms and

values affect intergenerational sexual behaviors in Nigeria, more research is required to explore these relationships.
The quality of self-reported information particularly the dependent variable may be unreliable. If anything, however, such sexual behavior as high risk sex, ever paid for sex, condom use at last sex and history of STDs would be underreported, biasing the association towards the null. Therefore, any significant association found may be an attenuated one.

5. Conclusion

This study confirms the prevalence of intergenerational sex in Nigeria and identifies associated factors. It assuages that the practice may promote the spread of HIV infection among Nigeria's teeming youth population leading to HIV infected young women bearing the burden of the disease. The messages are clear that delayed onset of sexual debut; education; women economic empowerment, increased life options for women and working with men to challenge the socio-cultural norms and perceptions that allows for and sanction engagement in intergenerational sex would go a long way to reduce the practice and lead to improvement in the health outcomes of the young women including reduction in HIV infection in the group. The authors have suggested several policy options but policies need to be put in context within the different regions of Nigeria and the health and sustainable development objectives of the country. Importantly, more qualitative studies should be carried out to identify other social factors promoting the practice in Nigeria and studies directed at intergenerational sex and HIV infection would definitely be very instructive.
There is need to make concerted efforts with programmatic responses to counter power imbalances from gender, age and economic or materials differences between young women and their older male partners. As programmatic responses are mounted, it is important that they are accompanied by intervention research to test their feasibility and ultimately, their impact on reducing intergenerational sex or the inherent power imbalances therein, that facilitate vulnerability of the young women particularly HIV transmission and unwanted pregnancy. Furthermore, the authors suggested a number of policy issues, any process to garner policy support must also be accompanied by policy research to document and analyze the most salient elements of the resulting social change process.

6. Acknowledgement

The authors acknowledge the helpful comments of Dr. Gbenga Ishola of Jhpiego in the preparation of this article. Dr. Dayo Adeyemi of the MEASURE Evaluation/JSI contributed immensely during the multivariate analysis. The contribution of Adrienne Cox and Noureddine Abderrahim both of ICF Macro in the construction of the outcome variable added value to the in-depth knowledge of analysis in the use of NDHS data. Finally, we thank the ICF Macro and National Population Commission, Nigeria for making the data of the Nigeria Demographic and Health Survey (NDHS) available for use. The opinions expressed in this article are solely those of the authors and do not represent the views of their institutions.

7. References

Abang, Mkpe (1996). Promoting HIV/AIDS prevention on Nigerian campuses: Students take the lead AIDScaptions 111(3).

Akuffo, FO (1987). Teenage pregnancies and school drop-outs: The relevance of family life education and vocation training to girls' employment opportunities. In Christine Oppong, ed. *Sex roles, population and development in West Africa*. Portsmouth, NH. Heinemann

Allison P. (1984). Event History Analysis: Regression for Longitudinal Data. Sage. pp 23-34

Barker, Gary Knaul and Susan Rich. 1992. "Influences on Adolescent Sexuality in Nigeria and Kenya: Findings from Recent Focus-Group Discussions." *Studies in Family Planning* 23: 199–210.

Blanc AK (2001): The effect of power in sexual relationships on sexual and reproductive health: an examination of the evidence. *Studies in Family Planning*, 32 (10):189-213.

Calves, Anne Emmanuele, Gretchen T. Cornwell, and Parfait Eloundou Enyegue. (1996). *Adolescent Sexual Activity in Sub-Saharan Africa: Do Men Have the Same Strategies and Motivations as Women?* University Park, PA: Population Research Institute.

Federal Ministry of Health (2009) National HIV/AIDS and Reproductive Health Survey (NARHS 2007), Abuja Nigeria

Feldman, Douglas A., Peggy O'Hara, K.S., Baboo, Ndashi W. Chitalu, and Ying Lu. (1997): HIV prevention among Zambian adolescents: Developing a value utilization/norm change model. *Social Science and Medicine*, 44(4): 455-468

Gage, AJ. (1998). Sexual activity and contraceptive use: The components of the decision making process. *Studies in Family Planning*, 29(2): 154-166

Glynn, J.R, Carael, M., Auvert, B., Kahindo, M., Chege J., Musonda, R., Kaona, F., and Buve, A.(2001). Why do young women have a much higher prevalence of HIV than young men? A study in Kisumu, Kenya, and Ndola, Zambia. *AIDS*, 15 (Supplement 4): 51-60.

Gomez, Anu Manchikanti, Ilene S. Speizer, Heidi Reynolds, Nancy Murray and Harry Beauvals (2008). "Age difference at sexual debut and subsequent reproductive health: Is there a link" ? Reproductive Health, 2008 5:8 doi.10. 1186/712 1755 5 8

Gorgen, Regina, Mohamed Yansane, Michael Marx, and Dominique Millimonunou. (1998). "Sexual Behaviour and Attitudes Among Unmarried Urban Youths in Guinea. *International Family Planning Prespectives*, 24(2): 65–71.

Gregson S, Nyamukapa CA, Garnett GP, Mason PR, Zhuwau T, Carael M, Chandiwana SK, and Anderson RM (2002): Sexual mixing patterns and sex-differentials in teenage exposure to HIV infection in rural Zimbabwe. *Lancet*, 359:1896-1903. (5)

Gregson, Simon, Constance A. Nyamukapa, Geoffrey P. Garnett, Peter R. Mason, Ton Zhuwau, Michel Carael, Stephen K. Chandiwana, and Roy M. Anderson. (2002). "Sexual Mixing Patterns and Sex- Differentials in Teenage Exposure to HIV Infection in Rural Zimbabwe." *The Lancet* 359: 1896–1903.

Jewkes R, Levin J, Mbananga N, and Bradshaw D (2002): Rape of girls in South Africa. *Lancet*, 359 (6):319-320.

Jones, L. (2006). Sexual decision-making by urban youth in AIDS-afflicted Swaziland. *African Journal of AIDS Research*, 5(2): 145-157.

Kaufman CE, Stavrou SE (2002): "Bus Fare, Please": The Economics of Sex and Gifts Among Adolescents in Urban South Africa. In *Policy Research Division Working Papers*. New York: Population Council; (12)

Kelly, R., Gray, R., Sewankambo, N., Serwadda, D., Wabwire-Mangen, F., Lutalo, T. & Wawer, M. (2003). Age differences in sexual partners and risk of HIV-1 infection in rural Uganda. *Journal of Acquired Immune Deficiency Syndrome,* 32(4): 441-451.

Kirby Douglas (1999). Antecents of Adolescents Sexual Risk Taking, Pregnancy and childbearing: Implications for Research and Programs. Washington, DC: National Campaign to Prevent Teen Pregnancy.

Komba-Malekela, Betty and Rita Liljestorm (1994). Looking for men. In Zubeida Tumbo-Masabo and Rita Liljestorm, eds, Chelewa, chelewa. The dilemma of teenage girls. The Scaninavian Institute of African studies

Langeni, T. (2007). Contextual factors associated with treatment-seeking and higher-risk sexual behaviour in Botswana among men with symptoms of sexually transmitted infections. African Journal of AIDS Research 6(3): 261-269.

Leclerc-Madlala, S. (2002). On the virgin cleansing myth: gendered bodies, AIDS and ethnomedicine. *African Journal of AIDS Research,* 1: 87-95.

Leclerc-Madlala, S. (2003). Transactional sex and the pursuit of modernity. *Social Dynamics,* 29(2): 213-233.

Longfield, K., Glick, A., Waithaka, and Berman, J. (2004) Relationships between older men and younger women: Implications for STIs/HIV in Kenya. *Studies in Family Planning,* 35(2): 125-134.

Luke, N. (2003). "Age and economic asymmetries in the sexual relationships of adolescent girls in sub-Saharan Africa." *Studies in Family Planning,* 34(2): 67-86.

Luke N (2005): Confronting the 'sugar daddy' stereotype: age and economic asymmetries and risky sexual behavior in urban Kenya. *International Family Planning Perspective,* 31 (7):6-14.

Luke N, and Kurz KM (2002): *Cross-generational and Transactional Sexual Relations in Sub-Saharan Africa: Prevalence of Behavior and Implications for Negotiating Safer Sexual Practices.* Washington, D.C.: Population Services International; (8)

Machel, J. (2001). Unsafe sexual behaviour among schoolgirls in Mozambique: a matter of gender and class. *Reproductive Health Matters* 9(17): 82-90.

MacPhail C, Campbell C. 'I think condoms are good but, aai, I hate those things': condom use among adolescents and young people in a Southern African township. Social Science and Medicine 2001; 52 (11): 1613 - 1627

Matasha, E., T. Ntembelea, W. Saidi, J. Todd, B. Mujaya and L., Tendo-Wambua (1998). Sexual and reproductive health among primary and secondary school pupils in Mwanza, Tanzania.: Need for Intervention. *AIDS Care,* 10(5): 572-582

Mclean, Polly (1995). Sexual behaviours and attitudes of high school students in the Kingdom of Swaziland. *Journal of Adolescent Research,* 10(3): 400-420

Meekers, Dominique and Anne-Emmanuele Calves. (1997a). "'Main' Girlfriends, Girlfriends, Marriage, and Money: The Social Context of HIV Risk Behaviour in Sub-Saharan Africa." *Health Transition Review* 7(Supplement): 316–375.

Meekers, Dominique and Anne-Emmanuele Calves. (1997b). Gender differentials in adolescent sexual activity and reproductive health risks in Cameroon Washington, Dc. PSI Research Division Working Paper No. 4.

Mensch BS, Lloyd CB (1998): Gender differences in the schooling experiences of adolescents in low-income countries: the case of Kenya. *Studies in Family Planning*, 29:167-184. (11)

Moore, AM and Biddlecom, A. (2007). Transactional sex among Adolescents in Sub-Saharan Africa amid the HIV Epidemic. Paper presented at the Annual Meetings of the Population Association of America, New York, March 29 - 31.

National Population Commission (NPC) [Nigeria] and ICF Macro. 2009. Nigeria Demographic and Health Survey 2008. Abuja, Nigeria: National Population Commission and ICF Macro

Nkosana, J. (2006). Intergenerational relationships in urban Botswana. *Unpublished PhD thesis,*Department of Public Health, University of Melbourne.

Nkosana, J. and Rosenthal, D. (2007). The dynamics of intergenerational sexual relationships: the experience of schoolgirls in Botswana. *Sexual Health*, 4(3): 181-187.

Nyanzi S, Pool R, and Kinsman J (2000). The negotiation of sexual relationships among school pupils in south-westernUganda, *AIDS Care*; 13(1): 83-98

Nyanzi and Kinsman 2001

Odutolu Oluwole, Adebola Adedimeji, Omobola Odutolu, Olatunde Baruwa and Funmilayo Olatidoye. (2003) Economic Empowerment and Reproductive Behaviour of Young Women in Osun State. *Nigeria African Journal of Reproductive Health*, 7 (3): 92-100

Orubuloye I, Caldwell J, and Caldwell P. (1992). Diffusion and focus in sexual networking: identifying partners and partners' partners. *Studies in Family Planning*, 23(6) :343-351

Poulin, M. (2007). "Sex, money, and premarital partnerships in southern Malawi." *Social Science and Medicine*, 65: 2383-2393.

Ryan, S.; Franzetta, K.; Manlove, JS. and Schealer, E (2008): "Older Sexual Partners during adolescence: links to reproductive health outcomes in young adulthood. Perspect Sex Reproductive Health, 40: 17 - 26.

Silberschmidt, M., & Rasch, V. (2000) Adolescent girls, illegal abortion and 'sugar daddies' in Dares Salaam: Vulnerable victims and active social agents. *Social Science and Medicine* 52: 1815-1826.

Stavrou, SE and Kaufman, CE (2000). „Bus fare please" The economics of sex, gifts and violence among adolescents in urban South Africa. Paper presented at the Annual Meetings of the Population Association of America, Los Angeles, March 23 -25.

UNAIDS (2004), *Facing the Future Together: Report of the Secretary Generals' Task Force on Women, Girls, and HIV/AIDS in Southern Africa.* Joint United Nations Programme on HIV/AIDS (Geneva: UNAIDS, 2004).

UNAIDS (2006), Report on the Global AIDS Epidemic (Geneva: UNAIDS, 2006)

Weiss, Ellen, Daniel Whelan and Geeta Rao Gupta (1996). Vulnerability and opportunity. Adolescents and HIV/AIDS in the developing world. Washington, Dc: International centre for Research on Women.

Wojciki, JM. (2005). Socioeconomic status as a risk factor for HIV infection in women in East, Central and Southern Africa: a systematic review. *Journal of Biosocial Science*, 37:1-36.

Wood K, Maforah F, and Jewkes R (1998): "He forced me to love him": putting violence on adolescent sexual health agendas. *Social Science Medicine*, 47 (13):233-242 (13)

4

HIV Infection and Schooling Experiences of Adolescents in Uganda

Harriet Birungi[1], Francis Obare[1], Anne Katahoire[2] and David Kibenge[3]
[1]*Population Council, Nairobi*
[2]*Makerere University, Kampala*
[3]*Ministry of Education and Sports*
[1]*Kenya*
[2,3]*Uganda*

1. Introduction

The increased availability of anti-retroviral treatment (ART) for HIV in parts of sub-Saharan Africa (SSA) has enabled many children who were perinatally infected to survive to school-going age and even longer. For instance, a study conducted in 2007 in Uganda among adolescents aged 15-19 years who were perinatally infected with HIV found that about 70% of them were attending school at the time of the survey and many desired to be in school to avoid social isolation (Birungi et al., 2008). With an increasing number of HIV-positive young people attending school, most governments in SSA have begun to recognize the challenges this situation presents to the education sector (Kelly, 2003). Many governments have formulated Education Sector Policies on HIV/AIDS that encompass all learners, employees, managers and administrators in all learning institutions at all levels of the education system (for example, Ministry of Education and Sports- Uganda, 2006; Ministry of Education- Kenya, 2004). The policies predominantly revolve around a legal framework that recognizes and upholds the rights of all people with a special focus on marginalized and vulnerable groups and those with special needs. They also recognize the need for universal access to HIV/AIDS information, access to treatment and care, protection from discrimination and stigma, and care for orphans and vulnerable in-school young people.

In spite of the recognition of school-going HIV-positive young people as a vulnerable group, education sector responses to HIV/AIDS in the SSA region are predominantly curriculum-based. The focus is almost entirely on developing the capacity of learners in the areas of better knowledge about the diseases, skills that enhance the ability to protect oneself against infection, and approaches that acknowledge the rights and dignities of those infected and affected (Bennell et al., 2002; Cohen, 2004; Kelly, 2000; Rugalema & Khanye, 2004). Insufficient attention has been paid to ways of supporting in-school HIV-positive young people partly because their needs in school are still largely unknown given that this is an emerging issue in the region. It could also be due to the dilemma of how to tackle the issue of HIV in schools based on fears that having specific programs targeting in-school HIV-positive young people could reinforce stigma and discrimination against them.

Whatever the reason for the lack of appropriate education sector responses in this area, a key issue that emerges is the need for evidence on in-school experiences of HIV-positive young people in the region. This should in turn inform appropriate interventions aimed at ensuring an inclusive education system that adequately responds to the challenges in-school HIV-positive young people may face. This chapter therefore responds to the need for relevant evidence by exploring the experiences of HIV-positive adolescent boys and girls in primary and secondary schools in Uganda from the perspectives of school officials and teachers, the general student body, as well as adolescents perinatally infected with HIV. It specifically focuses on: (1) school attendance and experiences with class repetition; (2) experiences of stigma and discrimination within the school environment; and (3) availability of school-based health and psychosocial support programs and services for HIV-positive students. It ends with a discussion of the implications of these experiences for addressing the needs of in-school HIV-positive young people by the education sector not only in Uganda but in SSA countries affected by the pandemic.

2. Context

Uganda had an estimated population of 33.8 million people as of mid 2010 with the majority (87%) living in rural areas and nearly half (49%) being below 15 years of age (Population Reference Bureau, 2010). The first AIDS case was diagnosed in the country in 1982 and by 1986, it had reached the level of a generalized epidemic with the predominant mode of transmission being heterosexual contact (Ministry of Health & ORC Macro, 2006; Serwadda et al., 1985). The sentinel surveillance system from which national HIV prevalence estimates were initially derived was established in 1989 starting with six clinics in urban areas but later expanded to include clinics from peri-urban and rural areas (Garbus & Marseille, 2003). HIV prevalence was estimated at 15% among all adults (15-49 years) in 1991-1992 which was considered to be the peak of the epidemic in the country (Kirungi et al. 2006; Stoneburner & Low-Beer, 2004). This, however, declined to 7% in 2001 and was still at this level in 2009 (Joint United Nations Programme on HIV/AIDS [UNAIDS], 2010; Kirungi et al. 2006; Stoneburner & Low-Beer, 2004). As in other sub-Saharan Africa countries affected by the epidemic, HIV prevalence is higher among women than among men and in the urban compared to rural areas. In 2004-2005, for example, 8% of women aged 15-49 years were HIV-positive compared to 5% of men of similar age groups while prevalence was nearly twice as high in the urban compared to rural areas (10% versus 6%; Ministry of Health & ORC Macro, 2006). Similarly in 2009, prevalence among young people aged 15-24 years was 5% for women and 2% for men (UNAIDS, 2010).

The first AIDS control program was set up in the country in 1987 with emphasis on abstinence, being faithful to one partner, and condom use (Ministry of Health & ORC Macro, 2006). This prevention strategy—referred to as ABC—has since been expanded to include voluntary counselling and testing (VCT), prevention of mother-to-child transmission (PMTCT) of the virus, antiretroviral treatment (ART), and HIV care and support services (Ministry of Health & ORC Macro, 2006). The Ministry of Health started a voluntary door-to-door HIV screening programme in 1999 and has also begun implementing provider-initiated testing and counselling (PITC) at health facilities (Menzies et al., 2009; Wanyeze et al., 2008). By 2009, HIV testing and counselling services were available in 1,215 health facilities representing an increase from 812 facilities in 2008 and 554 in 2007 (World Health Organization [WHO] et al., 2009, 2010). Free ART has been available since 2004 and by 2009, 39% of adults in need of treatment were receiving it (WHO et al., 2010). The Ministry of Health began offering free PMTCT services in 2000; the proportion of HIV-positive mothers receiving PMTCT services increased from 12% in 2005 to 53% in 2009

(WHO et al., 2009, 2010). However, challenges still remain with respect to reaching all those in need of treatment due to limited human resource capacity to provide the services, and lack of efficient management of funds and supplies (Onyango and Magoni, 2002).

With respect to education, Uganda implemented the Universal Primary Education (UPE) programme in 1997 which removed fees for enrolment in primary schools and resulted in substantial increases in enrolments (Deininger, 2003; Murphy, 2003; Nishimura et al., 2008; UBOS and Macro International, 2007). This was followed ten years later (in 2007) with the introduction of Universal Secondary Education (USE) whose impact is yet to be systematically evaluated (Chapman et al., 2010). Estimates of HIV prevalence among members of the school community (students and teachers) are unavailable. However, realizing the challenges posed by HIV to the education sector, the Ministry of Education and Sports issued the *Education and Sports Sector National Policy Guidelines on HIV/AIDS* in 2006 to provide a framework for responding to the epidemic within the sector. The objectives of the policy are to: (1) raise knowledge of students, education managers and other sector employees on HIV/AIDS; (2) ensure that students, education managers, and educators access prevention, treatment, care and support services; (3) eliminate all forms of stigma and discrimination; (4) mitigate the impact of HIV/AIDS that impede access to and provision of quality education; (5) strengthen the education sector's capacity to effectively respond to HIV/AIDS; and (6) contribute to the knowledge base on HIV/AIDS through research (Ministry of Education and Sports- Uganda, 2006).

3. Data

The data are from a study conducted in Uganda in 2009 whose objective was to understand the needs of in-school HIV-positive young people. The study involved two major components. The first component was a survey among 718 young people aged 12-19 years (of school-going age) who were perinatally infected with HIV (had been living with the virus since infancy) and who knew their sero-status. The sample members were identified and recruited through existing HIV/AIDS treatment, care and support programs/centres selected by The AIDS Support Organization (TASO)-Uganda in four districts (Kampala, Wakiso, Masaka and Jinja). Thirteen such centres participated in the study. All adolescents who received services from the centres and satisfied the eligibility criteria in terms age, perinatal infection, and awareness of sero-status were targeted for inclusion in the study. TASO counsellors assisted with the identification and mobilization of the eligible respondents. The process involved obtaining clearance from the management of the centres, identifying the target sample from the existing records, and making calls to their parents to request them to come to the centres or targeting days when they visit the centres for routine reviews or drug re-fills.

Information was collected using a structured questionnaire which was translated into *Luganda* and *Lusoga*, the two dominant local languages. Interviews were partially completed with 6 of the participants. Information was gathered on the respondents' background characteristics, educational attainment, school attendance (absenteeism, repetition, changing of schools, and drop-out), motivations for being in school or dropping out, disclosure of HIV status within the school environment and the reactions of others to the disclosure, availability of support programs for HIV-positive young people within schools, psychosocial feelings in school and whether these affected school attendance, and experiences of physical or verbal abuse, discrimination and stigma in school. For adolescents aged 12-17 years, written consent to participate in the study was sought from parents/guardians and assent was sought from the adolescents themselves. However, for adolescents aged 18-19 years, the study obtained individual written consent only. The TASO Internal Review Board, the Uganda National Council for Science and Technology (UNCST), and the Population Council's Institutional Review Board granted ethical clearance for the study.

Female respondents comprised more than half (59%) of the survey participants. There was, however, no significant difference in the distribution by sex according to most of the background characteristics such as age, district of residence, whether the respondent lived with a biological parent, and the living arrangements of the biological parents (Table 1). The majority (65%) of the respondents were aged below 18 years, hence considered minors while slightly more than one-third (37%) were from Kampala district. Besides, 80% of the respondents reported that one or both parents had died, which suggests that the majority of them might lack proper support not only in school but also at home.

Characteristics	Male (N=294) %	Female (N=424) %	Both sexes (N=718) %
Age group			
12-14	31.0	38.4	35.4
15-17	31.0	28.1	29.3
18-19	37.4	33.3	35.0
Don't know	0.7	0.2*	0.4
District			
Jinja	21.1	27.6*	24.9
Kampala	40.1	34.0	36.5
Wakiso	7.1	5.2	6.0
Masaka	31.6	33.3	32.6
Lives with a biological parent			
Yes	39.8	39.4	39.6
No	58.8	58.0	58.4
Missing/no answer	1.4	2.6	2.1
Parents' living arrangements			
Married/living together	11.2	10.9	11.0
Divorced/separated	3.7	6.6	5.4
Mother dead	16.3	10.9	13.1
Father dead	27.2	24.3	25.5
Both parents dead	39.1	44.1	42.1
Don't know/missing	2.4	3.3	2.9

Notes: Percentages may not add up to exactly 100 in some cases due to rounding; Differences between male and female proportions are statistically significant at: **$p<0.01$; *$p<0.05$.

Table 1. Percent distribution of survey participants by various background characteristics

The second component of the study involved in-depth interviews with school officials to assess the school environment and their preparedness to support in-school HIV-positive young people. A total of eight schools (four primary and four secondary) in five districts (Kampala, Jinja, Wakiso, Mukono and Iganga) were included in the assessment. Two of the primary and two of the secondary schools were mixed day while one school in each category was a boys' only and the other a girls' only boarding institution. The schools were purposively selected in consultation with the Ministry of Education and Sports. The Ministry granted the research team permission to visit the schools and talk to the officials. The research team obtained oral consent for participation in the study from the school officials. Information was collected through in-depth interviews to determine the operationalization of the HIV/AIDS policies in schools, perceptions and practices of teachers and school management towards in-school HIV-positive young people, the existence of support programs, and possible responses by the education sector to the needs of infected students. A total of 52 in-depth interviews were conducted with head teachers (7), deputy head teachers (4), director of studies (1), deans of students (2), senior teachers (12), Presidential Initiative on AIDS Strategy for Communication to Youth (PIASCY) teachers (3), school nurses/clinical officers (8), school matron (1), peer counsellor (1), health prefects (8), and club patrons and members (5) from the selected schools.
In addition, a total 1,012 students in Senior Three and Five from the four secondary schools wrote essays on specified themes. These included the perceived and actual attitudes and practices of students towards peers who are HIV-positive as well as possible responses by fellow students and the school administration to the needs of HIV-positive students. The essays were anonymous-- students were asked to indicate only their age, sex, and class but not their names-- and were administered to the students as a class exercise. It was explained to them that the exercise was voluntary and that they had the freedom not to participate in it if they did not wish to. Twenty nine (3%) of these essays were, however, discarded because it was apparent the students did not understand the nature of information required. Participants whose essays were analyzed were aged between 11 and 25 years, 71% of them were females (1% of the students did not indicate their sex), and about two-thirds (63%) were in Senior Three.

4. Analysis

The first part of analysis involves cross-tabulations with Chi-square tests and significance tests of proportions to examine differences in schooling, experiences of stigma and discrimination, and availability of school-based support programs and services by various background characteristics of the respondents including age, sex, district, and whether the respondent lived with a biological parent. In the second part of the analysis, random-effects logistic regession models are estimated to predict the likelihood of HIV-positive adolescents being in school at the time of the survey, experiencing stigma and discrimination in school, and receiving any form of support from school. The choice of the analysis technique is guided by the need to account for unobserved characteristics of individuals identified from the same HIV/AIDS treatment, care and support program/centre. The model is of the form:

$$\log it(\pi_{ij}) = X_{ij}\beta + \mu_j \quad (1)$$

where π_{ij} is the probability of a given outcome for individual i identified from facility j; X_{ij} is the vector of covariates; β is the associated vector of parameter estimates; and μ_j is the disturbance term due to unmeasured characteristics that may also affect the outcome for individuals identified from facility *j*.

The first dependent variable is measured by whether the respondent was still in school at the time of the survey conditional on having ever attended school. Stigma and discrimination, on the other hand, refer to whether those attending school had ever been teased, called nasty names, or suspected that rumours were spreading about them because of their HIV status. The third dependent variable is measured by whether the respondent received any support from groups, clubs or the school. The models control for age (single years), sex (male or female), district of residence (Kampala, Jinja, Masaka, Wakiso), and whether the respondent lived with a biological parent (yes or no).

5. Results

5.1 School attendance

Nearly all (99%) of adolescents perinatally infected with HIV had ever attended school with no significant difference between male and female respondents. In addition, 44% of those who had ever attended school reached secondary and above level of education (41% of male and 46% of female respondents; p=0.19). Most of those who had ever attended school (82%) were still in school at the time of the survey (81% of male and 83% of female respondents; p=0.49). As expected, current school attendance was significantly associated with age and whether the respondent lived with a biological parent (Table 2). In particular, older HIV-positive adolescents were significantly less likely to be in school compared to their younger counterparts (p<0.01) while those living with a biological parent were significantly more likely to be in school compared to those who did not live with a biological parent (p<0.05).

Covariates	Currently attending school[a]	Indicator of stigma/ discrimination[b]	Any support from groups/clubs/ school[b]
Age (single years)	-0.47** (0.06)	0.01 (0.05)	0.08 (0.06)
Sex (Female = 1)	0.04 (0.22)	-0.05 (0.18)	-0.27 (0.21)
District (ref = Kampala)			
Jinja	-0.51 (0.53)	0.08 (0.26)	-0.72 (0.41)
Wakiso	-0.71 (0.87)	-0.10 (0.42)	-0.03 (0.96)
Masaka	-0.84 (0.59)	0.84** (0.24)	0.21 (0.38)
Lives with any biological parent (Yes = 1)	0.62* (0.24)	0.04 (0.18)	0.28 (0.21)
Number of respondents	710	583	583

Notes: [a]Among those who ever attended school; [b]Among those currently attending school; Estimates are based on equation (1) in the text; Standard errors are in parentheses; ref: reference category; *p<0.05; **p<0.01.

Table 2. Coefficient estimates from random-effects logit models predicting current school attendance, experiences of stigma/discrimination, and receipt of any support from school

Slightly more than half (52%) of the respondents attending school at the time of the survey missed going to school the previous term (Table 3) with no significant variations by age, sex or whether the respondent lived with a biological parent. Nonetheless, the proportion that missed school the previous term was significantly lower in Jinja compared to other districts. Further analysis shows that illness was the major reason for missing school (cited by 57% of those who missed school) followed by lack of school fees or education materials (23%), and going for treatment/ medication (12%). There were also significant variations in the major reasons for missing school by sex and district of residence ($p<0.05$ in each case). For instance, 60% of female respondents cited illness as the major reason for missing school the previous term compared to 51% of male respondents. In contrast, slightly more than twice as many male as female respondents cited going for treatment/medication as the major reason for missing school (18% versus 8%). Similarly, the proportion mentioning illness was about 10 percentage points higher in Jinja and Masaka (61% in each case) compared to Kampala and Wakiso districts (52% and 50% respectively) while the proportion citing treatment/medication was nine times higher in Kampala compared to Jinja district (19% versus 2%).

Background characteristics	Missed school previous term (%)	Ever repeated a class (%)	Considers schooling very important (%)
Age group	p=0.24	p=0.42	p=0.46
12-14	55.3	56.1	96.2
15-17	48.5	59.1	93.6
18-19	50.3	50.3	95.4
Sex	p=0.32	p=0.66	p=0.39
Male	49.2	56.3	94.1
Female	53.3	54.5	95.7
District	p<0.01	p<0.01	p<0.01
Jinja	37.2	64.1	98.6
Kampala	58.7	45.8	95.6
Wakiso	52.9	52.9	79.4
Masaka	54.1	60.2	94.5
Lives with a biological parent	p=0.75	p=0.13	p=0.18
Yes	52.4	51.6	96.4
No	51.1	58.0	94.0
All respondents	51.6	55.2	95.2
Number of respondents	585	585	585

Notes: p-values are from Chi-square tests.

Table 3. Percentage of survey participants who missed school the previous term, percentage that ever repeated a class and percentage that considered schooling very important by background characteristics

More than half (55%) of the respondents who were still in school at the time of the survey reported ever repeating a class (Table 3). The proportion having repeated a class did not significantly vary by age, sex or whether the respondent lived with a biological parent. It, however, significantly differed by district of residence with the lowest proportion being in Kampala (46%) and the highest in Jinja (64%). Results of further analysis show that poor performance and illness were the major reasons for repeating a class the last time (cited by 35% of the respondents in each case) followed by lack of fees or education materials (20%). There were also significant variations in the major reasons for repeating a class by age ($p<0.01$) and district of residence ($p<0.05$). For example, the proportion of adolescents aged 12-14 years who repeated a class because of poor performance was more than twice as high as that of those aged 18-19 years (49% versus 22%). In contrast, the proportion of those aged 18-19 years who cited lack of fees or education materials was about four times higher than that of those aged 12-14 years (35% compared to 9%). Similarly, the proportion that repeated a class because of poor performance was highest in Jinja (42%) and lowest in Kampala district (22%) while the proportion that repeated a class because of illness was highest in Kampala (41%) and lowest in Jinja district (28%).

Background characteristics	Future career prospects (%)	Encouraged by others (%)	Gain new knowledge (%)
Age group	$p<0.05$	$p=0.49$	$p<0.01$
12-14	64.6	16.9	16.5
15-17	67.3	20.5	10.5
18-19	77.1	21.1	5.7
Sex	$p=0.72$	$p=0.13$	$p<0.01$
Male	68.1	22.3	6.7
Female	69.5	17.3	15.0
District	$p<0.01$	$p=0.14$	$p=0.08$
Jinja	86.2	14.5	9.7
Kampala	74.7	19.1	9.8
Wakiso	64.7	14.7	5.9
Masaka	48.6	24.3	16.6
Lives with a biological parent	$p=0.18$	$p=0.57$	$p=0.85$
Yes	66.7	20.1	11.9
No	71.8	18.3	11.4
All respondents	68.9	19.3	11.6
Number of respondents	585	585	585

Notes: p-values are from Chi-square tests.

Table 4. Percent distribution of survey participants by three most commonly cited motivations for schooling according to background characteristics

In spite of the challenges with absenteeism and class repetition, nearly all respondents who were still in school (95%) considered education very important to them with no significant variations by age, sex or whether the respondent lived with a biological parent (Table 3). Nonetheless, a significantly lower proportion of respondents from Wakiso compared to those from the other districts recognized that education is very important to them ($p<0.01$). Their major motivations for continuing with education included future career prospects (mentioned by 69% of the respondents), encouragement from others (19%) and the urge to gain new knowledge (12%; Table 4). A significantly higher proportion of older (18-19 years) compared to younger respondents mentioned future career prospects as a motivation for schooling ($p<0.05$). In contrast, the proportion of respondents from Masaka district mentioning future career prospects was nearly half of that of respondents from Jinja district ($p<0.01$). There were, however, no significant variations in the proportion of respondents mentioning encouragement by others as a motivation for schooling by the background characteristics considered. But a significantly higher proportion of younger (12-17 years) and female respondents cited the urge to gain new knowledge as a motivation compared to older and male respondents respectively (Table 4).

Further analyses show that among respondents who had ever attended school but were out of school at the time of the survey, 63% cited lack of fees or education materials as the major reason for non-attendance followed by illness (16%) while 8% mentioned death of parent/guardian. There were no significant variations in the major reasons for non-attendance by age, sex or district of residence. However, the reasons differed significantly by whether the respondent lived with a biological parent ($p<0.05$). In particular, the proportion of those not living with a biological parent that cited lack of fees or education materials as the major reason for non-attendance was 24 percentage points higher than that of those who lived with such a parent (69% versus 45%). In contrast, the proportion of those living with a biological parent who mentioned illness as the major reason was more than three times higher than that of those not living with such a parent (32% versus 10%).

5.2 Stigma and discrimination

Findings from in-depth interviews with school officials indicate that students with full-blown AIDS face greater challenges in school compared to those who are HIV-positive but asymptomatic. The challenges include being isolated and withdrawn as well as being shunned and stigmatized by other students. The existence of self-imposed stigma and discrimination as well as discrimination by others was also evident from the student essays. For instance, among students who knew a fellow student in their school who was HIV-positive, the reported actual reactions by students and teachers towards the HIV-positive students is at variance with reports of how they would react in the hypothetical case (Table 5). In most cases, the proportions reporting actual positive reactions towards HIV-positive students are significantly lower than those reporting similar possible reactions to a hypothetical case. In contrast, whereas only 2% reported that they would discriminate, isolate or stigmatize a fellow student who is HIV-positive, nearly half (47%) acknowledged that such students face considerable discrimination, isolation and stigmatization not only from fellow students and teachers but also self-imposed. This is further supported by the following excerpts from the essays representing the perspectives of both male and female students:

Reactions	Possible reaction[a] (%)	Actual reaction[b] (%)
Show love, compassion, friendship, kindness	60.7	56.4[ns]
Provide hope, encouragement, advice/counsel for positive living	46.9	12.9**
Show pity, sympathy, feel bad, sad or sorry	43.9	56.8**
Discourage sexual activity/relationships	32.3	5.0**
Encourage to pray and/or trust in God	22.8	5.6**
Encourage/remind to take ARVs and other medicines always	23.1	6.3**
Encourage balanced diet	17.2	0.3**
Encourage/support to seek medical treatment including lab tests	15.2	0.7**
Stop sharing sharp instruments and other things	13.2	2.6**
Assist with class or house work	11.9	4.3**
Keep information confidential/secret	11.6	4.0**
Discriminate, isolate, stop friendship, stigmatize	2.0	46.9**
Tell others/gossip about it	1.7	5.9**
Number of students	303	303

Notes: [a]Possible reaction refers to the hypothetical case whereby students were asked how they would react if they found out that a fellow student was HIV-positive; [b]Actual reaction refers to how the students themselves, other students, and teachers react to the presence of an HIV-positive student; ARVs: antiretroviral drugs; Differences between proportions for possible and actual reactions are statistically significant at: **$p<0.01$; *$p<0.05$; ns: not significant.

Table 5. Distribution of most commonly cited possible and actual reactions as expressed in the essays by students who knew of a fellow student living with HIV in their school

"Yes we have someone in our school who is HIV-positive. I don't like to even touch her I think I can even get tempted to loving her and get infected. Other students don't want to talk to her." (17-year old male student).

"At first I did not like her and any person around her because I thought they also had the virus." (14-year old female student).

"Yes I know someone in the school with AIDS ... some students isolate him some are friendly to him. But even some do not share with him, some beat him up, some do not want to be nearer to him." (20-year old male student).

"Students always feel disgusted with her sickness and tend to keep a distance from her." (17-year old female student).

"Students tend to nickname such student for example there's a boy who was nicknamed 'woliru woofira' [poison]." (18-year old male student).

"Her dormitory mates normally insult her when they see her going back home on a monthly basis for treatment, for example they say 'kigenze kuleta biweke' ['she has gone to get medication' but in a derogatory manner]." (19-year old female student).

"They don't associate with us and always make insulting comments... Even teachers should stop back-biting us." (17-year old HIV-positive male student).

"Teachers have also resorted to nick-naming him like for example 'musuja' [fever] and rebuke him in public." (18-year old male student).

"I know of a boy in our school who is HIV-positive...However much other students try to comfort him, he always wants to be alone." (18-year old female student).

"Yes, I know one boy with HIV and he is not always healthy. He does not associate with others. Every time he is in a bad mood." (16-year old male student).

Adolescents perinatally infected with HIV who participated in the survey and were still in school were asked whether they had been teased or called nasty names because of their HIV status and whether they suspected rumours spreading about their sero-status. Sixteen percent reported being teased because of their HIV status (similar proportions of male and female respondents), 19% reported being called nasty names (22% of male and 16% of female respondents; $p=0.07$), and close to a quarter (24%) suspected that rumours were spreading around in school about their sero-status (23% of male and 25% of female respondents; $p=0.56$). Results from the random-effects logit model predicting the likelihood of experiencing any of the three indicators of stigma and discrimination show no significant differences by age, sex, or whether the respondent lived with a biological parent (Table 2). District of residence is, however, significantly associated with experiencing stigma and discrimination ($p<0.01$) with those from Masaka being significantly more likely to report such experiences compared to their counterparts from Kampala ($p<0.01$), Jinja ($p<0.01$), and Wakiso districts ($p<0.05$).

5.3 School-based support

Only 16% of in-school HIV-positive adolescents reported having support groups or clubs for HIV-positive students in their learning institutions (18% of male and 14% of female respondents; $p=0.19$). Of those who had, 73% belonged to and received support from the groups/clubs (74% of male and 71% of female respondents; $p=0.75$). In addition, only 15% reported receiving any kind of support from school (19% of male and 13% of female respondents; $p<0.05$). Results from the random-effects logistic regression model predicting the likelihood of receiving any support from the groups, clubs or school show no significant differences by age, sex, district of residence, or whether the respondent lived with a biological parent (Table 2). However, nearly all those who received some kind of support from the groups/clubs (94%) or schools (92%)—where these exist—were satisfied with it. Additional analysis shows that the kind of support provided by the groups, clubs or schools mostly included taking medicine, counselling or moral support, basic needs, and life skills training.

School officials also reported during in-depth interviews that once they found out that a particular student had HIV or other chronic illness, they exempted them from engaging in heavy extra-curricular activities, provided them with special meals where possible, and reminded them to take medicine in cases where they were aware that the children were on antiretroviral drugs (ARVs). Nonetheless, the interviews revealed that the support was mainly non-formal and a lot seemed to depend on the goodwill of particular head teachers, other teachers, and school nurses who sometimes use their own resources. In one school, for example, a teacher reportedly helped HIV-positive students to pick their monthly refill of ARVs so that they did not miss lessons while in another, the head teacher invited the guardian of one of the students to the school, counselled them, and connected them to a treatment centre. As one senior female teacher in one of the primary schools explained:

"Sometimes their guardians do not genuinely have the money but others [guardians] are just negligent they feel that 'after all the child may not have long to live'. In cases where the child knows that they are HIV positive this adds to their psychological stress. At school we ask them 'where are the materials we sent you for'; at home they are being told 'we do not have money'. When we do not know their special circumstances we think they are just being stubborn and not informing their parents. But when we find out, we try as a school to see how best to help them. Some teachers even buy them the materials using their own money but this is after they have found out the circumstances."

Findings from the in-depth interviews further show that HIV-positive young people in boarding institutions face additional challenges such as poor diet, adherence to ARVs, and taking cold showers. Whereas these have implications for their academic performance, schools lack formally established mechanisms for meeting these needs. For instance, sick-bays—where they exist in schools—are ill-equipped; they do not commonly stock antibiotics, have no full-time nurses while the available staff members are equipped to provide First Aid treatment only. Moreover, school-based caregivers (school nurses, guidance and counselling teachers, and senior teachers) are inadequately trained to handle the healthcare needs of HIV-positive students.

6. Discussion and implications

This chapter examined the schooling experiences of HIV-positive adolescent boys and girls in Uganda from the viewpoints of not only perinatally infected in-school young people but also school officials, teachers, and the general student body. As expected, most of the adolescents living with HIV are vulnerable on account of both their young age and the fact that the majority had lost one or both parents. Thus, although nearly all of them had ever attended school and most of them were still in school at the time of the survey, issues of absenteeism, class repetition, stigma and discrimination (by others or self-imposed) remain a challenge. These challenges cut across adolescents of various groups, that is, age, sex and whether they live with a biological parent. Moreover, the most commonly cited reasons for missing school and repeating a class are lack of fees or education materials, illness, going for treatment, and poor performance. Those who are in boarding institutions face additional challenges including poor diet, cold showers, and adherence to treatment for fear of being stigmatised.

The above challenges have implications for the academic performance and educational attainment of HIV-positive young people. Schools, however, lack formally established mechanisms for addressing these needs. Formal access to treatment, counselling, care and support at school or through school is almost non-existent. Sick-bays—where they exist in schools—are not equipped with essential medicines while school-based caregivers (school nurses, guidance and counselling teachers, and senior teachers) are inadequately trained to handle the healthcare needs of HIV-positive students. Existing attempts at addressing the needs of in-school HIV-positive young people are ad hoc, at individual level, and crisis-driven. The absence of formally established mechanisms could also partly be due to non-disclosure of students' sero-status by parents/guardians during admission given that in certain cases, school authorities often discovered when the student became symptomatic while at school or because of continued absenteeism or seeking permission to go for treatment on specific days.[1]

These findings have important programmatic implications for the education sector not only in Uganda but other SSA countries affected by HIV/AIDS. Specifically, they suggest the need for: (1) school-based programs to assist orphans and other vulnerable children, including those living with HIV, so that they do not miss attending school for lack of essential materials; (2) strengthening the school-based healthcare program including treatment, care and support for HIV-positive students, encouraging in-school young people to undergo testing and counselling for HIV, and equipping sick-bays—where these exist—with essential medicines; (3) pre- or in-service training for school-based caregivers (school nurses, guidance and counselling teachers, and senior teachers) on HIV counselling, care and support; (4) putting in place psychosocial support mechanisms for HIV-positive young people, orphans and other vulnerable children in schools, which should be expanded to incorporate all students irrespective of their HIV status in order to reduce stigma and discrimination through innovative ways such as child-to-child communication; and (5) putting in place measures to discourage stigma and discrimination against HIV-positive students through sensitizing school officials and students on the consequences of the same on those who are exposed to them.

Although this chapter identifies possible responses by the education sector to the needs of in-school HIV-positive young people, its major limitation is that it does not consider acceptable, feasible and effective strategies for addressing these needs. This is largely because it relies on data from an exploratory study whose aim was to provide a better understanding of the schooling experiences of this subset of the population. Operations research is best suited for providing answers regarding acceptable, feasible and effective strategies for responding to these needs. Operations research can, for instance, provide answers to the following questions: What school-based support programs are appropriate and effective in meeting the education needs of orphaned and vulnerable children, including those living with HIV? How can school-based health care programs be strengthened to better meet the needs of in-school HIV-positive young people? Does training of school-based caregivers improve the provision and quality of care and support for HIV-positive learners? What strategies and psychosocial support mechanisms can

[1]In Uganda, parents/guardians complete medical forms upon student admission so that the information can be used to identify those with needs that might require special attention. However, most parents/guardians tend to conceal certain ailments including HIV, perhaps, for fear that their children might not be admitted if their conditions are known or to protect them from stigma and discrimination.

effectively reduce stigma and discrimination in schools? These are questions which are beyond the scope of the present chapter.

7. Conclusion

In-school HIV-positive young people in Uganda face a number of challenges including: (1) high rates of absenteeism and class repetition because of illness, having to go for drug re-fills regularly for those on ART, or socio-economic hardships at home; (2) stigma and discrimination from fellow students, teachers or self-imposed; and (3) poor diet, cold showers, and non-adherence to ART because of fear of stigma and discrimination from fellow students among those in boarding institutions. At the same time, schools are not adequately prepared to respond to their special needs. Key actors in the education sector (government, private sector, non-governmental organizations, and donors) should therefore consider appropriate interventions aimed at enhancing the capacity of schools to respond to the unique needs of HIV-positive learners.

8. Acknowledgement

The study that provided the data for this chapter was funded by the Ford Foundation and implemented by the Population Council in collaboration with the Child Health and Development Centre- Makerere University, The AIDS Support Organization (TASO)-Uganda, and the HIV/AIDS Unit in the Ministry of Education and Sports- Uganda. Florence Baingana of the Institute of Public Health- Makerere University conducted the in-depth interviews with school officials. The TASO Internal Review Board, the Uganda National Council for Science and Technology (UNCST), and the Population Council's Institutional Review Board granted ethical clearance for the study. The views expressed in this chapter are, however, those of the authors.

9. References

Bennell, P., Hyde, K., & Swainson, N. (2002). T*he impact of HIV/AIDS epidemic on the education sector in sub-Saharan Africa: A synthesis of the findings and recommendations of three country studies*, Centre for International Education, University of Sussex Institute of Education.

Birungi, H., Mugisha, J.F., Nyombi, J., Obare, F., Evelia, H., & Nyinkavu, H. (2008). *Sexual and reproductive health needs of adolescents perinatally infected with HIV in Uganda.* FRONTIERS Final Report, Population Council, Washington, DC.

Chapman, D.W., Burton, L., & Werner, J. (2010). Universal secondary education in Uganda: The head teachers' dilemma. *International Journal of Educational Development*, 30(1):77-82.

Cohen, D. (2004). HIV and education in sub-Saharan Africa: Responding to the impact. In: *The HIV challenge to education: a collection of essays*, Carole Coombe (ed.), pp. 60-80, International Institute for Educational Planning, Paris.

Deininger, K. (2003). Does cost of schooling affect enrollment by poor? Universal primary education in Uganda. *Economics of Education Review*, 22(3):291-305.

Garbus, L. & Marseille, E. (2003). *HIV/AIDS in Uganda.* AIDS Policy Research Center, University of California, San Francisco.

Joint United Nations Programme on HIV/AIDS [UNAIDS]. (2010). *2010 Report on the Global AIDS epidemic*, UNAIDS, Geneva.

Kelly, M.J. (2003). The Development of HIV/AIDS Policies in the Education Sector in Africa. *DPMN Bulletin, Volume X, Number 1.*

Kelly, M.J. (2000). Standing education on its head: Aspects of schooling in a world with HIV/AIDS. *Current Issues in Comparative Education*, 3(1):28-38.

Kirungi, W.L., Musinguzi, J., Madraa, E., Mulumba, N., Callejja, T., Ghys, P., & Bessinger, R. (2006). Trends in antenatal HIV prevalence in urban Uganda associated with uptake of preventive sexual behaviour. *Sexually Transmitted Infections*, 82(Suppl 1):i36-i41.

Menzies, N., Abang, B., Wanyenze, R., Nuwaha, F., Mugisha, B., Coutinho, A., Bunnell, R. Mermin, J., & Blandford, J.M. (2009). The costs and effectiveness of four HIV counseling and testing strategies in Uganda. *AIDS*, 23(3):395-401.

Ministry of Education [Kenya]. (2004). *Republic of Kenya: Education Sector Policy on HIV/AIDS*, Ministry of Education, Nairobi.

Ministry of Education and Sports [Uganda]. (2006). *Education and Sports Sector National Policy Guidelines on HIV/AIDS*, Ministry of Education and Sports, Kampala.

Ministry of Health (MOH) [Uganda] and ORC Macro. (2006). *Uganda HIV/AIDS Sero-behavioural Survey 2004-2005*, Ministry of Health & ORC Macro, Calverton, Maryland, USA.

Murphy, L. (2003). Does increasing access mean decreasing quality? Paper commissioned for the *EFA Global Monitoring Report 2003/4: The Leap to Equality*, UNESCO, Paris:.

Nishimura, M., Yamano, T., & Sasaoka, Y. (2008). Impacts of the universal primary education policy on educational attainment and private costs in rural Uganda. *International Journal of Educational Development*, 28(2):161-175.

Onyango, S. & Magoni, M. (2002). Implementing PMTCT program in Uganda: Challenges and lessons learned. *Proceeding of the XIV International AIDS Conference*, Barcelona, July 2002.

Population Reference Bureau. (2010). *2010 World Population Data Sheet.* Population Reference Bureau, Washington, DC.

Rugalema, G. & Khanye, V. (2004). Mainstreaming HIV/AIDS in the education systems in sub-Saharan Africa: Some preliminary insights. In: *The HIV challenge to education: a collection of essays*, Carole Coombe (ed.), pp. 81-103, International Institute for Educational Planning, Paris.

Serwadda, D., Sewankambo, N.K., Carswell, J.W., Bayley, A.C., Tedder, R.S., Weiss, R.A., Mugerwa, R.D., Lwegaba, A., Kirya, G.B., Downing, R.G., Clayden, S.A., & Dalgleish, A.G. (1985). Slim disease: A new disease in Uganda and its association with HTLV-III infection. *Lancet*, 2(8460):849-852.

Stoneburner, R.L. & Low-Beer, D. (2004). Population-level HIV declines and behavioral risk avoidance in Uganda. *Science*, 304(5671):714-718.

Uganda Bureau of Statistics (UBOS) & Macro International Inc. (2007). *Uganda Demographic and Health Survey 2006*, UBOS & Macro International Inc., Calverton, Maryland, USA.

Wanyenze, R.K., Nawavvu, C., Namale, A.S., Mayanja, B., Bunnell, R., Abang, B., Amanyire, G., Sewankambo, N.K., & Kamya, M.R. (2008). Acceptability of routine HIV counselling and testing, and HIV seroprevalence in Ugandan hospitals. *Bulletin of the World Health Organization*, 86(4):302-309.

Ward, V. & Mendelsohn, J. (2009). *Supporting the educational needs of HIV-positive learners in Namibia.* United Nations Educational, Scientific and Cultural Organization, Paris.

World Health Organization [WHO], Joint United Nations Programme on HIV/AIDS [UNAIDS], & United Nations Children's Fund [UNICEF]. (2010). *Towards universal access: Scaling up priority interventions in the health sector.* WHO, UNAIDS, & UNICEF, Geneva.

World Health Organization [WHO], Joint United Nations Programme on HIV/AIDS [UNAIDS], & United Nations Children's Fund [UNICEF]. (2009). *Towards universal access: Scaling up priority interventions in the health sector.* WHO, UNAIDS, & UNICEF, Geneva.

5

An Institutional Analysis of Access to GBV/HIV Services in Rural KwaZulu-Natal, South Africa

William Boyce, Sarita Verma, Nomusa Mngoma and Emily Boyce
Queen's University,
Canada

1. Introduction

The health systems context in rural South Africa presents significant challenges for addressing the intersecting problems of HIV/AIDS and Gender Based Violence (GBV). In KwaZulu-Natal Province, district level government responses to these issues are principally focused in urban, higher population areas. Rural health systems rely more heavily on non-governmental organizations (NGOs), which have serious time limitations and insecure external funding. Weak management skills, and insufficient capacity to design and monitor services, are key problems. There is also a shortage of health personnel in rural areas, and high attrition rates due to poor work conditions, substandard accommodation environments, inadequate pay and benefits, and illness and stress resulting from to the high demands posed by the HIV/AIDS epidemic and other primary health care issues. Overall, the rural health structure is very under-developed, under-staffed, under-resourced and under-trained around issues of GBV and HIV/AIDS.

There is a pressing need for rural health services to focus on health promotion and prevention - including violence prevention - and to develop new strategies for coordinating the activities of health professionals with voluntary associations and NGOs. This paper presents an institutional analysis of why access to GBV and HIV/AIDS services is low in rural KwaZulu-Natal, with a focus on understanding existing professional structures and community beliefs that act as barriers to health system development. Such an understanding can also reveal how existing strengths and resources may be harnessed to encourage changes in the cultural attitudes and structures that support the gender violence-HIV/AIDS nexus, and identify salient points of entry at which interventions can be designed.

1.1 An institutional perspective on "Access"

1.1.1 The health system as "Institution"

It is well recognized that the health sector faces certain institutional characteristics that distinguish it from other sectors of society [Jan et al., 2008; Mooney, 1994]. Specifically, these characteristics include the role of institutions in providing access to health benefits, or more exactly, preservation from ill health or health losses. In this view, institutions are not organizations per se, but are the 'rules' that govern the conduct of players, whether individuals or organizations, within society [North, 1993]. Thus, institutions include formal rules such as legislation concerning resource allocation to health and the regulation of professionals, and informal rules such as social customs and community norms that shape

health care practices. An institutionalist analysis views interventions as more than a simple balancing of inputs and outputs (or costs and benefits) and thus provides a more complete account of health decision-making. Such an analysis requires a coherent theory of how health services work in a specific context.
The development of health programs in areas of restricted resources often involves 'institution building' and this paper provides an analysis of how this occurs in the context of HIV/AIDS and gender violence in South Africa. Other recent institutional analyses that have focused on this problem expose implicit costs and values from the perspective of health economics [Jan et al., 2008]. Institutional development may also be concerned with issues of health service quality. However, the current analysis is focused on concepts of equity in access to these important health and social services.

1.1.2 Institutional access

Health systems research is increasingly focused on issues of inequity in access to underlying determinants of health, as well as to curative services. Access is understood to be amenable to policy decisions about the supply of health care. Access barriers deter, delay and minimize the search for health care solutions to HIV/AIDS and gender violence. However, it is important to note that access is also limited by demand-side factors that are less than optimal.
Gilson and Schneider [Gilson et al., 2007] have summarized three key dimensions in defining access, or the degree of fit between the health system and those it serves. These domains concern a dynamic process of interaction between health institutions and individuals or households. 'Availability', or physical access, refers to whether the appropriate health services are in the right place at the right time. 'Affordability', or financial access, refers to the relationship between the cost of health care and individuals' ability to pay. Finally, 'acceptability', or cultural access, refers to the social and cultural distance between health care systems and their users [Guilford et al., 2002; Delius et al., 2002]. Studies of how these dimensions interact with each other are particularly needed, as interventions to address single issues of access may be ineffective in reducing inequity. Within an access framework and from an institutional perspective, we examine the interactions of various material and operational, or procedural, barriers to accessing HIV/AIDS and gender based violence services in an under-resourced rural area in KwaZulu-Natal. This multi-dimensional analysis will hopefully provide the basis for multi-level interventions.

1.2 Literature review

The issue of gender violence and its links to HIV/AIDS in rural settings has not been addressed in a substantive way. There are several complex issues in rural health systems that interact to present significant institutional problems to health and safety. Material barriers to health for poor rural women have been noted to include lack of physical access to public health clinics, low levels of resources and staff in existing clinics, and the high costs of treatment [Delius et al., 2002]. Further, considerable operational or procedural problems exist in terms of staff awareness and training around GBV and HIV/AIDS issues, as well as negative attitudes and gendered discrimination against women seeking contraceptives, HIV/AIDS tests, or HIV/AIDS treatment [MacPhail et al., 2001]. These general structural and operational problems are exacerbated in rural locations, which also have problems of inattention by the government, lack of training and resources, and poor staff recruitment and retention. In rural areas, traditional socio-cultural norms, practices and beliefs at once inhibit women from seeking health care around GBV and HIV/AIDS, and can produce institutional resistance to the restructuring of health services in ways that might facilitate better patient access.

1.2.1 Location, mandate, resources and organization of public health clinics

Women in rural areas of South Africa may have considerable difficulty accessing public health clinics for several reasons. First, significant variability in access and availability of clinical services mean that some women must travel long distances to reach the nearest clinic. This is physically impossible for many women with disabilities, illness, or who are sick with HIV/AIDS, who may otherwise have reached the clinic by walking or other forms of transportation. Women without economic means cannot pay for the costs of transport, creating a key structural barrier to their ability to access free contraceptives, receive HIV/AIDS testing and counseling, or access treatment if they are HIV/AIDS infected. The nature of voluntary testing and counseling in public health clinics requires multiple visits: formerly in KwaZulu-Natal, HIV test results took an average of three weeks to be processed, for example, and many patients never returned to receive their results [Campbell et al. 2002]. Treatment and counseling may also require multiple visits, which means that women without physical and economic access to clinics may not attend initially or make return visits. Finally, some community-based service providers who would have provided home visits to isolated women have reported that they do not do so because of their own limited funding and access to transport [Russel et al., 2000].

Public health clinics are also very uneven in terms of resource and staff availability across the country, with rural areas suffering the most [Delius et al., 2002; Kelly et al., 2001]. In some rural areas of KwaZulu-Natal, voluntary counseling and testing is not available at all [Kelly et al., 2001]. Many primary health care clinics in rural KwaZulu-Natal are organized to render antenatal services to pregnant women on one specific day of the week, and 40-60 pregnant women often require services on that particular day [Ngidi et al., 2002]. These demands create major challenges in terms of offering adequate Voluntary Counseling and Testing (VCT) follow-up services to these same women.

The physical and organizational structure of clinics is also a component in the improvement of VCT services, as well as for increasing the likelihood that people will feel comfortable attending clinics for HIV/AIDS related reasons [Senderowitz, 1999]. Van Dyk's [Van Dyk, 2002] survey of over 1400 men and women found that 33% preferred to go to an unknown clinic (i.e., not in their community) for voluntary counseling and testing. Of these, 50% do "not trust health care workers to keep a secret", 30% prefer "total confidentiality" which they may not receive at their local clinic, and 13% "fear prejudice and rejection" from going to the local clinic. These fears are highly attributable to the public nature of many clinics, in which there is a lack of privacy and individuals' problems or reasons for coming to the clinic can easily be discerned by onlookers [Senderowitz, 1999; Van Dyk, 2002].

Finally, state provision of free and/or low cost accessible services and drugs to HIV/AIDS patients has long been identified as a crucial step in the prevention and treatment effort [Joint Monitoring Committee on the Improvement of the Quality of Life and Status of Women, 2001a]. However, the roll-out of antiretroviral therapy (ART) is still far from even or universal, despite the fact that the government began providing it through the public health system in 2003. Rural areas continue to experience the least access to publicly-provided ART [Human Rights Watch, 2008]. In areas where clinics do not offer ART, many people cannot afford the cost of accessing treatment privately. Poor rural women with HIV/AIDS are unlikely to access these drugs for a variety of reasons, including lack of transportation to clinics offering ART, fear of stigma, inability to maintain the level of health (nutrition, clean water, adequate rest) required to take the drugs as prescribed, and a lack of other services or support in the community to help them comply with their medication regimen. Although ART was not available in the public health system when this study was conducted, the same issues around uneven provision of ART by clinics, and lack of training, expertise, equipment and attention to guidelines among health professionals, are still very relevant today.

1.2.2 Community, legal and public health handling of violence against women

Vetten & Bhana [Vetten et al., 2001] outline several problematic and gender-blind aspects of traditional VCT models. VCT and mother-to-child-transmission (MTCT) programmes usually promote partner-notification when a woman tests positive for HIV/AIDS. Such disclosure is encouraged to promote safer sex practices and partner testing. The potential for violent partner reactions to women's disclosure is rarely taken into account; similarly, VCT counselors may suggest couple counseling which may also trigger male violence and abuse. VCT/MTCT counselors or nurses may have little knowledge of domestic violence or expertise in determining if certain patients come from abusive relationships which will place them at even greater risk for abuse upon disclosure. Finally, HIV/AIDS testing is often done in public antenatal clinics without the patients' consent. Patients are often informed of their HIV/AIDS status in non-private settings, where the likelihood of others hearing is high.

Vetten & Bhana also argue that rape crisis centres in public hospitals and/or nurses and counselors on staff who deal with rape victims - are similarly lacking in training on the links between rape and HIV/AIDS. Rape victims are not always referred to HIV/AIDS counseling and testing centres, and nurses are often ill-equipped to counsel the women themselves, as they do not have the proper information or knowledge about the risk of HIV/AIDS following rape (i.e., when can the victim be tested, how long does HIV/AIDS take to incubate) [Vetten et al., 2001; Gernholtz, 2002]. At the time of this study, most clinics in rural KwaZulu Natal were not providing post-exposure prophylaxis (PEP) to rape survivors, and most women faced barriers of lack of transportation, stigma, discrimination and negative attitudes by health professionals, among others, when it came to accessing this life-saving drug. In 2002, the South African government committed to providing post-exposure prophylaxis (PEP) to rape survivors through the public health system. Like ART, however, this roll-out has been slower than desired and uneven, with rural areas being slower to offer PEP to rape survivors (Human Rights Watch, 2008]. A corresponding protocol was released by the Department of Health [Department of Health, South Africa, 2003], which requires that all rape survivors be provided with counseling around HIV and PEP, and that referral systems be in place so that survivors of rape can access longer-term counseling. However, preliminary findings have shown that there is a lack of coordination among service providers and poor knowledge among health professionals of PEP guidelines [Birdsall et al., 2004]. A recent Bill [Republic of South Africa, 2007] legislated the provision of PEP to sexual assault providers, but added the requirement that a woman press criminal charges in order to access the life-saving drugs. No references to other treatment or counseling for rape survivors were made in the Bill. It has yet to be seen how these gaps and the requirement that women report to police will influence women's access. The Bill at once requires coordination between police and health services while eliminating the need for collaboration between health services and voluntary organizations or NGOs that provide other supports. Women who fear further violence from perpetrators or who do not want to go "public" about the rape for fear of stigma, will choose not to file charges and so will be denied access to PEP. It will also be less likely that health professionals will be compelled to refer them to support services or counseling. Pre-existing inefficiencies with service coordination, and gender-blind aspects of post-sexual assault care in rural areas, may be perpetuated as a result of the new Bill.

Many researchers argue that a gap clearly exists in public health clinics and VCT programs in terms of staff training, awareness, attitudes, and overall handling of violence against women in the context of HIV/AIDS; conversely, HIV services have not been adequately integrated into public services provided to survivors of sexual violence [Vetten et al., 2001; Joint Monitoring Committee on the Improvement of the Quality of Life and Status of Women, 2001b; France et al., 2000]. This lack of integration works as a barrier to HIV/AIDS prevention and treatment for survivors of rape, and may put HIV/AIDS infected women at increased risk for violence. For example, non-governmental rape crisis centres and women's shelters require more resources and training around the issues of HIV/AIDS. Shelters for abused women are not always accessible to HIV/AIDS infected women: many of these shelters will not allow HIV/AIDS infected women to reside there, which puts women at risk of more violence at the hands of their partners. Women's shelters and clinics that do address issues of HIV/AIDS are often poorly resourced to do so. Non-governmental rape crisis centres often do not have the resources, knowledge or capacity to give HIV tests, administer PEP, or provide counseling around HIV and PEP.

1.3 Research question

Overall, there are significant barriers documented regarding access to the health system response to GBV and HIV/AIDS. How do these material and procedural barriers to availability, affordability and acceptability interact together in rural areas to aggravate the gender violence and HIV/AIDS nexus?

2. Methods

The Health District Sisonke (DC43) in KwaZulu-Natal was the site for this study. Located in the foothills of the southern Drakensberg mountains, about 90 kms from Pietermaritzburg, this area has a demographic profile with a variety of rural communities broadly representative of the country as a whole. It also has a history of public health involvement and innovation dating back to the 1940s [Jeeves, 1998]. The legacy of apartheid has created a highly uneven landscape, with marked inequalities in access to land, resources, employment, income and services. Migration remains a commonly practiced response to extreme poverty and unemployment in large parts of the district under study, continuing a long-established tradition of migrant labour.

The study setting is a traditional tribal area with poor secondary roads and almost complete lack of public/private transport. There are health clinics at Pholela, Bulwer, Underberg and Ixopo, a district mission hospital at Centacow, as well as a larger referral hospital in the town of Edendale. From these locations, a sample of 46 key informants was drawn that included doctors, nurses, and VCT counselors. Semi-structured interviews were taped and administered by trained medical students, in Zulu, English or Xhosa, as appropriate. Interviews were done with fully informed consent and the right to refuse consistent with Research Ethics Board approval of universities in Canada (Queen's University) and South Africa (University of KwaZulu-Natal). The overall purpose of the interviews was to understand health workers' attitudes towards HIV/AIDS and GBV and how it affected their own work. However, a subset of questions focused on their experiences and roles, responsibilities and capacities in HIV/AIDS-GBV service delivery, which are reported here. In addition, relevant material was utilized from other interviews done for a larger study with local women, men, faith leaders and traditional healers.

Transcripts were analyzed and categorized according to concepts and issues derived from the literature review.

- distance, transport and public health
- service availability, volunteers
- physical space and confidentiality
- costs and poverty
- compatibility in public health practices versus safety practices
- compatibility in social versus clinical responses to violence
- ignorance and bias
- lack of integrated care

3. Results

3.1 Issues of availability

3.1.1 Variety in optimal settings for public health care

Respondents identify two principal and linked dynamics in the impact of rurality on HIV/AIDS care. Interestingly, public health care is perceived to be both a 'place' and a 'service'. Public knowledge in rural areas about HIV/AIDS is low, as it is for many health problems in a traditional rural environment. Negative community attitudes and stigma around HIV/AIDS have a profound impact in small, cohesive rural communities such that a more distant 'place' for testing is preferable to many community members. However, such attitudes also result in late recognition of HIV and delayed decisions to be tested. As the disease progresses, the capacity for ill people to travel declines further. At this point, and as HIV status becomes known to neighbours, a 'service' approach to public health is more preferred by community members. However, lack of transport for health care workers in remote areas affects HIV/AIDS awareness building, case identification, and follow-up services. Further, a service approach might alleviate the problem of limited space at hospitals, as noted below.

3.1.2 Limitations in quantity and scope of practice of professional personnel

The extreme conditions of HIV/AIDS clearly affect the adequacy of rural health care.

Nurses and VCT counselors are very overloaded and underpaid. Adding nursing staff is often considered to be a solution, but there are also practical barriers such as the need to share accommodation. As well, the limitation in types of South African health human resources is a severe problem. Marriage counselors and social workers are particularly lacking. Doctors are not only in short supply, but many are temporary. South African medical practitioner licensing requires a one year community residency [Republic of South Africa 1997] which has increased the number of young doctors in rural areas, but often leaves gaps in service:

Doctors here are very nice but very junior. I think for them it's "let's stick some chest drains in, put a CVP line in and do a 'caesar'. It's because we are only here for a year ...let's turn it into an educational experience. I'm going to do all these courses and come up with these skills."

Distinctions between various medical professions and their scope of practice also creates service lacunae:

These patients need to have their bloods taken for CD4 counts, as a nurse I have to do that but it's not within my scope.

Additionally, strict clinical guidelines for administering ART and considerable job stress creates problems in quality of care:

When I'm giving everybody else their medication usually at 1800h, the HIV patient won't take it because they have to take it at 2000h. Who is going to sit down and wait for 2000h to give them their treatment? So they must remember for themselves because if they don't then they won't be taking their medication properly.

3.1.3 Lack of physical space, resources and confidentiality

Having sufficient working space is a concern for all hospital and clinic staff:

Our ward accommodates 26, especially female medical, so we have floor beds and there we nurse some conditions, and now you as a nurse will have to be on your knees, and how can you put up a drip on the floor?

However, respondents hold differing views regarding the treatment of patients within the physical space of clinics. Some value the use of physical space for purposes of 'integration' of HIV/AIDS patients, while others value it for the purpose of 'separation'. Both views are linked to issues of ethics. Integration of HIV/AIDS patients with the general outpatient population is recommended by some respondents for the purpose of maintaining privacy of HIV status. Integration is also preferred to maintain equity of service for non-AIDS patients. For others, separation of HIV/AIDS outpatients is desirable for confidentiality of information. Most respondents recommend the separation of inpatients to ensure such privacy:

The sad thing with HIV positive patients is that they are not protected. We don't have an isolation ward for them, the medical patients are mixed with them ... There is no confidentiality for the HIV patients.

Numerous respondents identify problems related to the lack of essential medical equipment and supplies for HIV/AIDS care. First, there is a basic lack of equipment (e.g., suction machines, blood pressure instruments) for various clinic locations and needs. Further, existing equipment is not well maintained, or may be lost or stolen. Second, protective supplies (e.g., masks, gloves) that are necessary for working in a HIV/AIDS environment are lacking, especially in the communities. Basic supplies such as HIV test kits, oxygen and medications are not always available. Third, preventive immunizations (e.g., for hepatitis) are not routinely provided to health workers without cost. Although PEP is provided adequately to health workers, it is not necessarily provided to members of the public who might be exposed to the virus through caring for an HIV positive person. Finally, there is lack of coordination in using the available resources. A significant example is the lack of transport for delivery of blood samples to regional laboratories.

3.2 Issues of affordability

3.2.1 Poverty is an over-riding risk factor in HIV/AIDS and GBV

Rural incomes are low and provide only marginal resources for health care or for maintaining health. However, the bureaucracy required to supplement rural incomes reflects an interaction between affordability and availability issues:

I think more funds need to be allocated for them so they'll be able to buy enough formula for the babies and immune boosters for the HIV patients. There needs to be enough funds for them, food like porridge, beans…foods that have protein….We have just one social worker, and it's hard for our HIV patients to access disability grants, and the orphans too, you know getting these grants take a long time.

Volunteers in the community who participate in essential home care activities find that the costs are too high:

When this thing started home based carers used to love their job but now they do not get paid and they no longer like it, these people used to help the pensioners a lot but now do not because there is no pay.

3.3 Issues of acceptability

3.3.1 Complex health care concepts and rural people

In environments of socially mediated disease, there is often a tension between public health protocols and community knowledge and priorities. In this study area, clinical criteria for HIV/AIDS treatment occasionally conflict with community understandings of the disease and with their readiness to act:

Why it is necessary for a person to have an ID for a CD4 count, meaning without an ID you cannot check CD4? Since people need to start treatment when their CD4 count is less than 200, you get people that come in very sick but they can't attend the sessions.

Similarly, ART compliance is more complicated for rural patients living at home:

Maybe if they were like other pills and were being taken in the morning, midday, and night without specific times, it would make life easier especially those who are not educated. It would be so much better if the government could change the policy on taking ARVs, and not have a specific time.

Rural persons are among the last to learn about treatment complexities, or contradictions between earlier medical advice and current practice. For example, breastfeeding had been strongly promoted in rural areas in the past. Then it was not recommended for HIV positive mothers. Similarly, modern methods of birth control can lead to increased risks of HIV infection:

The rate of HIV would go down if the prevention methods used (Depo-provera), were to be reduced, because you find that people don't want to use condoms.

Communication of complex health care concepts to rural people can be hindered by the mandate for training new professionals, illustrating the link between acceptability and availability of professional care:

That's partially medicine. It's got a history of using funny abbreviations that nobody understands but it doesn't improve communication with people… But within the hospital, if you can't have clear communication between all the different health professions and patients, how can we expect the patients to disclose to their partners or families?

At the same time, language differences between Zulu, Xhosa and English-speaking staff and patients limit effectiveness:

We are all from different cultures, backgrounds and communication is via translators and it can be difficult. You notice a huge shift in thought and a shift in the doctor/patient relationship as a result of that.

3.3.2 Appropriate social care

Counseling is considered to be a lynch pin in HIV/AIDS and GBV social care. It is an evolving practice that originated in the West and is a common response to post-traumatic stress disorder. In rural South Africa, confidential counseling is increasingly intended to minimize the risks of HIV transmission, to prepare people for medical and social consequences of the disease and to increase treatment compliance. However, counseling may not be viewed in the same way by rural people themselves:

Our people do not understand the idea behind the concept of counseling. Even when you explain it to them they don't see the benefit of going there. People do not see how their problems can be solved by just talking.

Community based volunteers for public education, support or home care are often an essential adjunct in integrated HIV/AIDS care. It is rare for adult men or younger women to volunteer, however, as they are usually pre-occupied with wage labor and subsistence activities. In the rural area, the HIV/AIDS volunteers are often older women or unemployed youth, that is, groups having lower community status. Such secondary status and varying concepts of privacy can affect the effectiveness of these volunteers and their acceptance by the community, as noted by one volunteer:

The problem is that we wouldn't be able to tell the community members what to do...they will say we think we are better. People who do counseling are those that you are close to, you come from the same neighbourhood, so it becomes hard to open up to them; especially if the families are not on good speaking terms. You go and share your story and the counselor will share it with everyone she knows, those are the reasons we fear going for counseling. People who do counseling are not well trained.

3.3.3 Acceptability of health care in the context of violence

Rural communities, in turn, may not be supportive of women who experience violence. Fear of stigma and rejection by partners, family and community members inhibit women from disclosing rape to others and seeking out health care. Lack of knowledge of the risk of contracting HIV and other sexually transmitted infections (STIs) through rape means women do not necessarily consider health care an urgent priority following sexual assault:

She will not go to the police station because she might be afraid that her neighbours will laugh at her.... I think that she wouldn't go. Before a woman can go for medical help she has to tell certain people. If she does not want her rape ordeal to be known in the area, she can just let it slip. It is difficult for women to go to hospital without telling their mothers first. Moreover, if the raped woman lives with her partner and has not told him about the rape, it would be impossible to seek help. Also, not all women know the dangers inherent in rape. Some forget that the long term effects of rape can be catastrophic (i.e., contracting HIV/AIDS).

Even violence towards young children elicits contradictory responses. On the one hand, there is a feeling that child rape should be hidden to maintain a girl's reputation for future marriage. At the same time, children are considered to be especially vulnerable to the psychological consequences of rape, particularly stranger rape, and are in need of counseling. Women's susceptibility to GBV and HIV/AIDS due to poverty is clear:

Look, you know, I'm unemployed. I'm the one without a job and my boyfriend is paying for me too, for my drugs and I must' absorb' a lot.

Even with a broad understanding of GBV-HIV links and their effects on communities, rural community women often have more immediate priorities than HIV testing and care:

So hunger is first, violence and a fear of violence is second, generalized poverty is third, ("How am I even going to get to the clinic to get care? I don't have bus fare.") and then fourthly HIV. So sometimes people behave in a risky way because they have to deal with the first and second need and the third need. ("HIV will kill me six years from now, but hunger will kill me in a short while from now.")

Ironically, in the context of a conservative rural health care environment, gender violence may be viewed as a legitimating pre-condition for a woman to get prompt sexual health care. Exposure to HIV as a result of violence is more accepted in a clinical setting than is exposure due to consensual unsafe sex, which is often considered by health care staff to be preventable.

3.3.4 Poorly integrated care for HIV/AIDS and GBV

In this locale, there is a marked inability to integrate social-psychological, medical and legal processes for HIV/AIDS and GBV care. The rural communities are used to their traditional laws and have poor knowledge of the formal systems for addressing GBV:

The people from the 'bundus' (olden days) ... most of them don't even know that they must report. The ones that are not informed don't know what to do, especially those from rural areas.

Police have little experience or sensitivity-training when it comes to dealing with inter-personal issues that are considered to be private matters:

Police officers will show up at a school and say "I have come here to see the rape child" in a big loud voice so that everyone will know, so that is very poor sensitivity. It's just another crime which I think needs to be investigated.

The medico-legal system in rural South Africa faces enormous capacity and coordination challenges, both in terms of fulfilling women's rights to adequate post-sexual assault care, and bringing perpetrators of rape to justice:

There is definitely a problem with logistics though and follow up of these rape cases.... With the junior doctor, the counseling is good, but who will take the specimens? It's the junior doctor, who by the way doesn't know how to do it properly. And then two years later the magistrate throws it out because the examining doctor is now in Canada, and that's it.

Overall, the rural context of HIV/AIDS and GBV amplifies the impact of availability, affordability and acceptability barriers to health system access:

Post-prophylactics in this society is a tragedy because women are raped routinely in this country and they rape very violently and they rape the people who are at the highest possible risk for HIV and there isn't a way that a woman can rush somewhere to get access to PEP. It doesn't exist. If you had money, and you had understanding, you could rush to a pharmacist. You could get a script there, pay for it and pay for prophylactics and start your treatment. But if you didn't have knowledge and you didn't have money, there absolutely isn't a way for you to get PEP.

Many respondents suggest that a local rape crisis centre is the solution.

4. Discussion

Adequate access to health services can be conceptualized as the fit between population health needs and health system resources. Health needs are multi-dimensional and multi-causal, and encompass environmental, physical, psychological, economic and political agents. Consequently, to meet these needs, the development of health system resources must go beyond improving financial and human capacities, and also address suitable socio-cultural-political conditions, operational plans and understandings of professional health care from community perspectives. These elements are particularly important for preventive health care in situations of GBV and HIV/AIDS.

While the access framework used in this paper is useful for categorization of different dimensions of access, there is also a need for exposure of underlying mechanisms that contribute to these barriers. Three major mechanisms affecting access to HIV/AIDS and GBV services in the KwaZulu-Natal rural health care system may be posed from this study.

First, due to many years of isolation during the apartheid era, the health professions maintained many traditional features. They were less influenced by broader paradigmatic and practice shifts occurring in health systems in other parts of the world. There continues to be considerable role differentiation and a clear medical hierarchy in South Africa. At best, the health professions are just emerging from a model of health that minimizes a social or community perspective on causes or solutions for health problems. Such medical elitism leads to hierarchies of treatment modalities, for example, an overdependence on post-infection testing and pharmaceutical treatments over the prevention and promotion of healthy social environments. Second and third tier health workers (nurses and VCT counselors) expect full health services (e.g., PEP) for themselves, yet there is not an effective system in place to similarly protect or treat community members. Individual social work professionals are viewed as primarily responsible for managing the consequences of gender based violence, but are restricted to working in clinical settings and are rarely exposed to community conditions that underlie such violence. Overall, traditional power differentials continue to separate health professionals from each other and from the communities they serve. Those who work in areas that carry elements of cultural stigma or shame (GBV or HIV), and more generally, in counseling, prevention or palliative roles (as opposed to curative), experience lower status and professional devaluation. These power dynamics, combined with overwork and lack of resources, is leading to ever-increasing burn-out among those providing GBV and HIV/AIDS related care. This situation is not unique to South Africa and has been recognized by the World Health Organization in its Integrated Management of Adult and Adolescent Illness model that promotes task shifting from doctors to nurses and from nurses to community health workers [World Health Organization, 2004].

Second, there is considerable stereotyping of rural and poorly educated populations. Gender based violence victims may be viewed by health staff as being in primitive social relationships that condone male violence as normative. The female victim is often seen as sharing responsibility since she has stayed in an abusive relationship. Alternately, women are viewed as being victims of an accepted rural tradition of rape. There is little understanding of a middle dynamic that is neither collusive nor coercive, but relational. Generally misunderstood is the victim's deeply ingrained role in 'absorbing' her male partner's anger, frustrations, and violent reactions to persistent social and economic deprivation.

Third, rural South African society presents differing perspectives on appropriate hierarchies for action related to HIV/AIDS and gender based violence. The health care worker considers the proper order of priority to be actions within their scope of practice and experience, that is, HIV/AIDS testing, treatment and prevention education. Poverty alleviation and addressing the social causes of violence are given much lower priority by health workers as these are more distal in the causal chain. Community members, however, consider hunger relief and safety from violence as their most immediate priorities, without which, longer term poverty relief and HIV/AIDS treatment implementation become meaningless. From both perspectives, within a limited resource environment, only the higher priorities are addressed. Consequently, there is a lack of capacity to address population level solutions to causal indicators and determinants of HIV/AIDS and GBV. For example, there is a lack of understanding of concepts such as community viral load and infectiousness, community safety mechanisms and practices, adaptation of community social standards, and the importance of support groups and counseling in a socially-mediated epidemic.

In this study, the relationship between the formal health structures and traditional ones, and between the government legal structures and the customary ones, were porous. This situation compromises access to the full spectrum of care that can be informed by a social understanding of rural communities and their realities, leaving the great possibility that many patients will fall between the cracks. There is a significant absence of collaboration between traditional and modern structures, which creates problems for access into the health care system and access to the police and magistrates. More positively, health care workers themselves identify the need for help in addressing the alleviation of basic risk factors for AIDS such as poverty, unemployment and poor education in rural settings. For them, training about safe water supply and nutrition were sometimes viewed as more important than specific training in HIV/AIDS management.

These findings suggest that an institution building approach to interventions would be useful in addressing HIV/AIDS and GBV issues in rural areas. Jan et al. [2008] suggest that such an institutional perspective would address individual (agency), household (power relations, communication, well-being), community (networks, norms, relationships and responses) and organizational (resources, coordination) levels. These interventions might include formal legislation, specifically for rural and under-serviced areas, concerning resource allocation to health services and the regulation of professionals. These interventions might also include more training regarding social customs and cultural norms that shape rural sexual practices and traditional health care.

Petersen [1999] suggests that a 'reorientation programme' in the new South Africa is necessary to address neglected issues, such as mental health.. Such reorientation initiatives could also be applied to the context of HIV/AIDS and GBV to address the following:

- the role and functions of the primary health care nurse within a district HIV/AIDS system;
- problems with a narrow biomedical approach to identify and manage HIV/AIDS problems at the primary level of care;
- nursing ideology and its sub-ordination to the medical system;
- culturally congruent care;
- a framework for assessing problems from the perspective of comprehensive care; and
- skills for comprehensive care, including the socio-medical relationship with community members.

Perhaps of highest priority is the need to conceptualize the institutional role of the community in HIV/AIDS and GBV services. According to the originator of the institutionalist approach [Tool, 1977], as well as others who have used it in the health sector [Jan, 1998], the social value of any intervention should be judged in terms of how well an action contributes to the 're-creation of community', as opposed to simple incremental health gains for individuals. Thus, interventions should also have ongoing value to the community, in this case by affecting the capacity of the rural community to transform itself to a new context.

Concrete examples of such transformation are already being achieved in urban South Africa with regard to HIV/AIDS services. These include the establishment of anonymous, rapid VCT sites that are crucial for HIV/AIDS prevention and treatment programs [Joint Monitoring Committee on the Improvement of the Quality of Life and Status of Women, 2001a]. Also, Senderowitz [1999] identified several physical and operational characteristics that transform health facilities to being "youth-friendly". These include the creation of a separate space and special times for adolescent clients; hours that are convenient for school-going youth; the establishment of clinics in locations convenient for youth; adequate space and sufficient privacy in clinics; and comfortable, youth-oriented surroundings (posters, audio-visual material on youth issues, avoid overly "sanitized" décor). Finally, the Community Agency for Social Enquiry [Community Agency for Social Enquiry, 2001] determined through its survey of urban HIV/AIDS service organizations that government could establish or fund HIV/AIDS information/resource drop-in centres to take the burden off clinics, develop programs focusing on AIDS discrimination and stigma, and develop clear policy guidelines that standardize training for health care workers. Similar recommendations could be adapted for the South African rural environment.

Urban South Africa is now making advancements in terms of providing comprehensive GBV services, again drawing on an integrated and collaborative approach to care. Many urban areas of South Africa have medico-legal clinics which have evolved into "one-stop clinics". Also called Thutheleza Centres (TTCs), these clinics provide medical treatment, police services, HIV and PEP counseling, PEP and STI prophylaxes and emergency contraceptives, and referrals to NGOs and voluntary organizations for longer-term counseling, all under one roof. TTCs are considered to be "best practices" in post-rape care. However, there is a major service gap in rural areas, where TTCs have yet to be rolled out fully. As respondents for this study indicated, such centres would be invaluable in their communities given existing service gaps.

Other major programmatic shifts in the sexual assault arena in recent years include the emergence of Community Forums (some are called "community policing forums" or "medico-legal forums"). In the absence of TTCs, communities have organized regular meetings between governmental and non-governmental service providers (including police stations, health clinics, gender violence and women's NGOs, children's services, Department of Welfare units, and other community organizations). These meetings provide a forum for information-sharing, the development of a comprehensive referral system, identification of problems that still need to be addressed to meet the needs of the community, and the development of strategies (task delegation as well as collaborative activities) to deal with the problems identified. Intersectoral collaboration has become a goal in the area of GBV in informal settlement and township communities, pointing to the beginnings of transformation of traditional hierarchies and structures of service delivery in urban areas.

Both TTCs and Community Forums are good examples of actions contributing to the "re-creation of community". With proper adaptation to the rural context, the replication of similar structures and/or forums in rural areas could improve community capacity to facilitate improved access (in terms of availability, affordability, and acceptability) to GBV and HIV/AIDS services. They would contribute to the breaking down of traditional power hierarchies and the division of labour. They might also encourage health and community professionals at all levels to see their work as complementary and mutually beneficial, and to view service integration and collaboration as a key strategy for delivering quality and accessible GBV and HIV/AIDS services in a resource-scarce environment.

5. Conclusions

The main problems related to availability, affordability and acceptability of HIV/AIDS and GBV services in this rural south African setting included many *material* limitations: variations in optimal settings for public health care; limitations in quantity and scope of practice of professional personnel; lack of physical space, resources and confidentiality; and poverty as an over-riding risk factor in HIV/AIDS and GBV. Similarly, *operational* limitations included the complexity of modern health care concepts for rural people; lack of appropriate models for rural social care; acceptability of health care in the context of violence; and poorly integrated care for HIV/AIDS and GBV. These problems may arise from health professions' maintenance of traditional features, stereotypes of rural and poorly educated populations, and differing perspectives on appropriate action related to HIV/AIDS and gender based violence. Interventions for complex social health issues such as HIV/AIDS and GBV should be judged in terms of how well they contribute to the 're-creation of community' through addressing both material and operational limitations of public health systems, as opposed to simple incremental health gains for individuals.

6. Acknowledgement

This chapter reports some of the findings from a larger programme of research entitled "Transforming Violent Gender Relations to Reduce Risk of HIV/AIDS Infection among young Women and Girls." The following gave valuable support to the project as research assistants: Diane Davies, Owen Gallupe, Ncedile Mankahle, Vuyelwa Mkhize, Tobias Mngadi, S'thembile Ngidi, Cyril Nkabinde, Hana Saab, Sid Sahay and Siduduziwe Zulu. The research could not have been carried out without the co-operation of community members in the Centocow, Underberg, and Pholela areas of Sisonke District, Kwa-Zulu/Natal. In particular, we would like to thank: Gcina Radebe, District Health Manager, Sisonke; Fritse Muller and the team at RapeCrisis/Lifeline, Pietermaritzburg; the Turn Table Trust, Bulwer; the community at the Centocow Mission, especially the home-based HIV/AIDS care volunteers of Izandla Zothando, and youth of the Centocow Leadership Training Group; and the staff of the Pholela Clinic, St Apollinaris Hospital (Centocow) and Christ the King Hospital (Ixopo), and associated clinics.

7. References

Birdsall, K., Hajiyiannis, H., Parker, W. & Nkosi, Z. (2004). *Post-exposure prophylaxis (PEP) in South Africa: Analysis of calls to the National AIDS Helpline.* Communicating AIDS Needs Project (CAN). Durban: Centre for AIDS Development, Research and Evaluation (CADRE).

Campbell, L.M., Colvin, M. & Hausler, H.P. (2002). *Lessons learned from a voluntary HIV counselling and testing programme in rural South Africa [abstract].* Barcelona: 14th International Conference on AIDS.

Community Agency for Social Enquiry (2001). *CASE report on HIV/AIDS - 2001.* Johannesburg: Centre for the Study of Violence and Reconciliation.

Delius, P. & Walker, L. (2002) *AIDS in context. African Studies,* 61: 5-11.

Department of Health, South Africa (2003). *Policy guideline for management of transmission of human immunodeficiency virus (HIV) and sexually transmitted infections in sexual assault.* Johannesburg: Department of Health.

France, N., Djeddah, C & Suwanjandee, J. (2000). *Violence: A gender-based barrier to HIV prevention and care [abstract].* Durban: 13th International Conference on AIDS.

Gerntholtz, L. (2002). *The provision of post-exposure prophylaxis for survivors of sexual violence in South Africa [abstract].* Barcelona: 14th International Conference on AIDS.

Gilson, L. & Schneider, H. (2007). 'Understanding health service access: concepts and experience.' in *Global Forum Update on Research for Health. Volume 4.* London: Pro-Book Publishing, pp. 28-32.

Guilford, M., Figueroa-Munoz, J., Morgan, M., Hughes, D., Gibson, B., Beech, R. & Hudson, M. (2002). What does 'access to health care' mean? *Journal Health Services Research Policy,* 7(3): 186-188.

Human Rights Watch (2008): *Universal periodic review of South Africa: Human Rights Watch's submission to the Human Rights Council [press release].* London: Human Rights Watch.

Jan, S. (1998). A holistic approach to the economic evaluation of health programs using institutionalist methodology. *Social Science & Medicine,* 47: 1565-1572.

Jan, S., Pronyk, P. & Kim, J. (2008). Accounting for institutional change in health economic evaluation: A program to tackle HIV/AIDS and gender violence in Southern Africa. *Social Science & Medicine,* 66: 922-932.

Jeeves, A. (1998). *Public health and rural poverty in South Africa: "Social medicine" in the 1940s and 1950s.* Johannesburg: Institute for Advanced Social Research, University of the Witwatersrand.

Joint Monitoring Committee on the Improvement of the Quality of Life and Status of Women. (2001a) *How best can South Africa address the horrific impact of HIV/AIDS on women and girls?* Johannesburg: Centre for the Study of Violence and Reconciliation.

Joint Monitoring Committee on the Improvement of the Quality of Life & Status of Women. (2001b). *Taking steps to address the links between violence against women and HIV and AIDS in South Africa.* Johannesburg: Centre for the Study of Violence and Reconciliation.

Kelly, K. & Parker, W. (2001) *From people to places: Prioritising contextual research for social mobilisation against HIV/AIDS (abstract).* Johannesburg: AIDS in Context Conference.

MacPhail, C. & Campbell, C. (2001). 'I think condoms are good but, aai, I hate those things': Condom use among adolescents and young people in a Southern African township. *Social Science & Medicine,* 52: 1613-1627.

Mooney, G. (1994). *Key issues in health economics.* London: Harvester Wheatsheaf.

Ngidi, A.C., Myeni, Z.E., Bland, R.M. & Rollins, N.C. (2002) *Acceptability and limitations of HIV group pre-test counselling for pregnant women in rural KwaZulu Natal, South Africa [abstract].* Barcelona: 14th International Conference on AIDS.

North, D.C. (1993) Institutions and credible commitment. *Journal of Institutional Theory & Economics,* 149(1): 11-23.

Penchansky, R. & Thomas, J.W. (1981). The concept of access: Definition and relationship to consumer satisfaction. *Medical Care*, 19: 127-140.

Petersen, I. (1999). Training for transformation: Reorientating primary health care nurses for the provision of mental health care in South Africa. *Journal of Advanced Nursing*, 30(4): 907-915.

Republic of South Africa (1997). *No. 89 of 1997: Medical, dental and supplementary health service professions amendment act, 1997*. Cape Town: Government Gazette.

Republic of South Africa (2007). *No. 32 of 2007: Criminal law (sexual offences and related matters) amendment act, 2007*. Cape Town: Government Gazette.

Russel, M. & Schneider, H. (2000). *A rapid appraisal of community-based HIV/AIDS care and support programs in South Africa*. Johannesburg: Centre for Health Policy, University of the Witwatersrand.

Senderowitz, J. (1999). *Making reproductive health services youth friendly*. Washington: FOCUS on Young Adults.

Tool, M.R. (1977). A social value theory in neoinstitutional economics. *Journal of Economic Issues*, 11: 823-847.

Van Dyk, A.C. (2002). *Voluntary counselling and testing in South Africa: Challenges and opportunities [abstract]*. Barcelona: 14th International Conference on AIDS.

Vetten, L. & Bhana, K. (2001). *Violence, vengeance and gender: A preliminary investigation into the links between violence against women and HIV/AIDS in South Africa*. Johannesburg: Centre for the Study of Violence and Reconciliation.

World Health Organization (2004). *Acute care: Integrated management of adolescent and adult illness*. Geneva: WHO.

6

Education Against HIV/AIDS

Abdulbaset Elfituri, Fadela Kriem, Hala Sliman and Fathi Sherif
Faculty of Pharmacy, University of Zawia, Zawia
Libya

1. Introduction

The sexually transmitted diseases (STDs) represent one of the major health problems worldwide today. The characteristics of human immunodeficiency virus (HIV) and acquired immunodeficiency syndrome (AIDS) demarcate the pandemic from the other communicable diseases, including the STDs. These include the rate of the virus spread, reaching epidemic proportions in some parts of the world, the magnitude of its infection and the inordinately long incubation period before symptoms development. These are in addition to the lack of curative therapy and lack of a preventive vaccine. Apart from its health and social implications, it has a huge burden on the affected patient, family and society. Thus, a global increasing attention is being paid to the prevention and control of HIV/AIDS. Furthermore, it is alarming for a global more coordinated education strategies against HIV/AIDS.

2. Adolescence risk for HIV/AIDS

Adolescents are at high risk of STDs, including HIV/AIDS. Evidence shows that age between 15 and 24 years is the highly vulnerable one for the infection. About one third of HIV infection cases occur in this age group and most of them are women (CDC, 2008). The adolescents and youth are among the high risk groups, because of their propensity in indulging in risky sexual activities and drug abuse. Negative attitudes regarding prevention misconceptions of HIV/AIDS reflect a false perception of the disease among these vulnerable groups. Strong well organized actions to increase awareness and improve behaviors are imperative. This calls for a wide comprehensive information, education and communication strategies targeting the youngsters as early as possible.

3. Education against HIV/AIDS

Since STDs, particularly HIV/AIDS, represent such a major health problem, more resources need to be devoted. There are several complementary ways in which STDs, including HIV/AIDS, can be controlled. Education of the public is an important control measure. The epidemic will not subside until most people around the world know how HIV is transmitted, understand how to prevent the spread of the infection and practice healthy safe behaviors (United Nations, 2002). The level of knowledge on STDs, including HIV/AIDS, and the attitudes of people are vital in preventing and eradicating the virus and disease (Binswanger, 2000). Hence, accurate and timely information, education and communication represent the best opportunity for changing life-styles and acting towards combating

HIV/AIDS. These should cover a wide range of sexual and social attitudes and behaviors. Therefore, the best way to avoid HIV/AIDS is to change those attitudes and behaviors, including avoidance of unsafe sexual practices.

3.1 Health education

Health education can be regarded as the communication of knowledge and the provision of experiences to help individuals to develop attitudes and skills which will assist their adopting behaviors to improve and maintain health for themselves and their fellows. The preventive model of health education adopts behaviors which will prevent infections and/or diseases, such as HIV/AIDS, at all levels. However, the self-empowerment model seeks to facilitate choice, not merely by providing understanding, value clarification and practice in decision making, but by attempting to empower the individual. Empowerment is about increasing people's power to change or improve their health. It includes motivation which is the inner force that drives the individual to a certain action. The process of self-empowering people involves modifying the way people feel about themselves, through improving their self-awareness and self-esteem. It involves supporting and encouraging them to think critically about their own concerns and gain the skills and confidence to build up their own values and beliefs system and to make a responsible action upon them (Tannahill, 1990; Downie et al., 1996).

3.2 Levels, approaches and categories of health education

Primary level health education is the type of education that is utilized for the prevention and control of HIV/AIDS. Different from the secondary and tertiary levels, it is directed at healthy people and aims to help individuals or groups learn how to keep healthy and how to prevent the onset of infection, disease and disability. Health education for primary prevention encourages people to develop behavior conductive to good health, such as that prevents contracting HIV infection. Primary prevention should aim at educating individuals, groups and communities about the advantages of prevention, including behaviors of discriminate and safe sex. It has to be accepted, however, that there is no agreement on the principles of normal sexual behavior.

Primary prevention is the level at which health education is able to encompass its role and function, not only to influence individual behavior change but also to influence group and community action. These include environmental, economic and organizational alterations to protect and promote health. HIV/AIDS prevention and control represent an appropriate example. Several approaches may be utilized separately or in combination. The persuasion or directive approach is the deliberate attempt to influence the individual to do a certain action or to follow a certain practice. The informed decision-making approach is about giving people information, problem-solving and decision-making skills to make decisions, but leaving the actual choice to the individual.

Furthermore, health education can be conducted on the basis of three categories. ***Disease-oriented health education*** is still utilized by several health education programs despite the improvements in the field. It has a negative focus, merely aiming at the prevention of specific diseases, with an emphasis on progress towards target rates of morbidity and mortality. Major preventable diseases, such as AIDS, are dealt with by specific preventive programs aimed at reducing relevant 'risk factors'. This orientation of health education works on single topics in isolation from one another, with an incomplete view of health.

However, it should be mentioned that most of the current health education programs are ***Risk factor-oriented***. It aims at eliminating particular risk factors in order to prevent associated diseases. Its main advantage is the recognition that a single risk factor can be linked to more than one disease category. The connection between unsafe sex and the STDs represents an example. But the model's view of health is inadequate; educational interaction is limited; and experts dominate. On the other hand, the relatively new ***Health-oriented health education*** has a dual focus. Its aim is to enhance positive health as well as to prevent ill-health. The physical, mental, and social components of health are recognized. Thus, the positive focus enhances the educational validity by developing comprehensive programs of health education in key people and key settings. Multidisciplinary and intersectorial collaboration is facilitated. Obviously, the health-oriented approach should be the preferred model for planning health education programs, including those to prevent and control HIV/AIDS.

3.3 Health promotion

Health education used to be seen as concerned mainly with personal health actions. It was perceived as a series of messages about healthy practices and the avoidance of risk behaviour. Though these kinds of health messages remain important today and should not be neglected, it is equally important to direct education towards collective action. Empowering people to take responsibility for collective health is a challenge that has to be met. Health promotion, on the other hand, is a broader term which covers all aspects of those activities that seek to improve the health status of individuals and communities. It starts out by considering the whole population in the context of their everyday lives, not selected individuals or groups. Its goal is to enhance collective health.

Health promotion had probably developed from health education. The latter is seen as a very important element in health promotion. It is one route to the improvement of people's health, encompassing all those activities which aim to provide health via learning of one kind or another. Therefore, health promotion can be regarded as health education 'plus'. Health promotion includes health education and other proactive aspects of health. Health promotion can be the umbrella term for three elements; health education, disease prevention and health protection. The three of them are essential elements in combating HIV/AIDS. The term health promotion is not synonymous with the term public health. Health promotion, however, constitutes a dynamic and interactive process based on person-empowerment, whereas public health focuses on the crucial issue of health-engendering social structures. Health promotion can be considered as the new public health. It is defined by the World Health Organization (WHO, 1984) as the process of enabling people to increase control over and to improve their health. The concept of HIV/AIDS control and prevention represents a component of this enhanced collective health and health promotion. To demonstrate the shift from individual to collective and societal action to improve health, Ewles and Simnett (1996) described five approaches to health promotion. These are:

1. Medical; to prevent or ameliorate ill-health, in order to achieve freedom from medically defined disease.
2. Behaviour change; to adopt healthy life-styles and change attitudes and behaviour.
3. Educational; to impart knowledge and act on well-informed decisions.
4. Client centred; to enable people to make their own decisions and choices according to their own value systems.

5. Societal change; to help people take control over their own lives and make choice easier to change the environment.

3.4 Communication

Provision of information is the principle of health education. Thus, it is vital for the prevention and control of HIV/AIDS within the communities and worldwide. In this respect, its aim is to protect and promote the health of the healthy individuals. In addition, communication aims at assisting HIV infected patients to recognise symptoms of the diseases and, by identifying the early onset of illness, to enable them to seek measures to control the problem. Furthermore, communication is to provide AIDS patients with self-care education, in order to learn about their illnesses, treatments and available health services.

Communication is conducted using a number of components. These are the receiver or the audience, the source or the provider, the message and the media or channels. A message or a medium that is effective with one audience may not succeed with another. The same applies to the source or the provider of the message. Empathy is used to describe the process by which the message provider learns to understand how others feel and think. The message will only be effective if the provided advice is valid, relevant, appropriate and understandable. Furthermore, efficiency relies on the appeal, which is the way providers organize the content of the message to persuade or convince individuals. Communication uses a variety of communication media. They can be classified according to two main groups; interpersonal (face-to-face) and impersonal (mass media). Interpersonal media include, but not limited to, school classes, university lectures, public small group discussions and doctor-patient counseling. Mass media include broadcast media, such as radio, television or social communication electronic networks; as well as print materials, such as books, booklets, magazines, newspapers, press releases, posters, leaflets or reports. McGuire's analysis of effective communication and persuasion methods (McGuire, 1969) suggests that messages that are more closely suited to the values and attitudes of those to whom they are directed will be more effective than other types of messages.

4. Means of individuals and community action

Although the many factors affecting health are beyond the reach of the individual, some individual choices or life-styles, such as the unsafe sexual practice, can influence health and well-being. Such choices can be influenced by action to empower the most vulnerable. The distinction between individual and collective empowerment is more theoretical than real. In particular, understanding a problem and acquiring the personal ability to deal with it are the basis of collective action for social change. In a social support network, each individual keeps his or her identify while receiving material support, services, information and new social contacts. These may also exist within a scope called social marketing. That is to describe the application of principles and methods of marketing to the achievement of socially desirable goals, such as health promotion or disease prevention, including HIV/AIDS control. Social marketing can be defined as the design and implementation of programs aimed at increasing the voluntary acceptance of social ideas or practices.

The framework for countrywide plans of action for health promotion (WHO & IUHPE, 2000) pointed out that community action is a concept that is both exciting and complex. In fact, the term community can mean different things in different contexts. The traditional notion of community is a well-defined geographical area with formal institutions such as school, church, mosque and town hall, where families live whose values are rooted in a shared history. This has begun to change in places where geographical barriers have been overcome by communications and transport. People no longer live where they work and their support networks do not coincide with any geographical boundaries. These considerations must be taken into account when the activities of groups, communities or social support networks in a given area are analysed and evaluated.

Empowerment gives a sense of personal control and the ability to bring about change in the social and health conditions through collective mobilisation. Participation in the decision-making process is desirable, not only from the ethical point of view but also in order to guarantee effectiveness.

Furthermore, various mechanisms or strategies for individuals and community action exist. Each of them is different, but all of them are complementary. The five complementary mechanisms for action proposed by the Ottawa Charter (1986), in addition to the above, include creating supportive environments, building healthy public policy and reorientation of health services.

5. Education towards behavior change

Education about STDs, including HIV/AIDS, should cover a wide range of attitudes and behaviors. Some believe that usually the mere presence of knowledge is sufficient to motivate healthy behaviors. Hence, motivation can lead to health-influencing behavior. This is known as ***the knowledge-action model*** of behavior change. However, in some cases, knowledge may be sufficient to elicit changes in behavior, but in other cases, it may not. Therefore, behavior may not change as a result of providing facts. The transfer of knowledge into action is dependent on a wide range of internal and external factors, including values, attitudes and beliefs. The communication of information can create, affect or change people's attitudes. Attitude is defined by Ribeaux and Poppleton (1978) as a learned predisposition to think, feel and act in a particular way, towards a given object or class of objects. Often, values and attitudes change precedes behavioral change. Attitudes can be transferred or reflected to behaviors or feelings. In many cases, people's attitudes are taken to determine their behaviors. Therefore, proper understanding of knowledge-attitude-behavior change models and theories provides guidelines for information, communication and education planning towards community health promotion and HIV/AIDS prevention and control.

Social scientists have evolved a number of models to explain the process of change influenced by personal and interpersonal communications within an individual. Stage models view behavior change as a series of actions or events. ***The health-belief model*** can be the best to explain the modification towards an AIDS-related protective behaviour. Rosenstock (1974) suggested that preventive health behavior can be understood as a function of perceived self-susceptibility of acquiring the disease, perceived severity of the disease, perceived benefits to be realized by engaging in particular preventive behaviors. Health-related action, then, is hypothesized to depend upon the simultaneous occurrence of three classes of action:

- the extent of sufficient motivation (or health concern) to make health issues relevant;
- the belief that one is susceptible (vulnerable) to a serious health problem (i.e., the perceived threat); and
- the belief that doing something would reduce the perceived threat at a subjective acceptable cost.

The transtheoretical model or ***the stages of change theory*** is among the simple models that can be applied in the field of HIV/AIDS prevention and control (Prochaska & Di Clemente, 1983). According to this model, people appear to pass through a series of distinguishable stages before they adopt a new practice. These stages are: *Pre-contemplation,* not recognizing the problem or the need to change; *Contemplation,* seriously thinking about the problem and the possibility of change; *Preparation,* making a commitment to change and taking steps to prepare for that change; *Action,* successful modification of behavior for a period of one day to six months; and *Maintenance,* continuation of change from six months to an indefinite period. Research has shown that relapse and recycling through the stages of behavior change happens often as individuals try to stop or change particular behaviors.

The knowledge-attitude-behavior change (or AIETA) model (Park & Park, 1997) is a simple and similar model to the one described above to explain the process of change. The stages of change in this model are: *Awareness:* At this stage the individual comes to recognize the new idea or practice. He/she has only some very general information about it and knows little about its usefulness, limitations and applicability to him/her. *Interest:* This is the stage when the individual seeks more detailed information. He/she is willing to listen or read or learn more about it. *Evaluation:* During this stage, the individual weighs the pros and cons of the practice and evaluates its usefulness to him/her or his/her family. Such an evaluation is mental exercise and results in a decision to try the practice or reject it. *Trial:* This is the stage when the decision is put into practice. He/she would need additional information and help at this stage so as to overcome the problems in implementing the idea. *Adoption:* At this stage, the individual decides that the new practice is good and adopts it.

6. Response to adolescence needs

Adolescence is a period of dynamic change during which the differences between males and females become more apparent, especially with regard to sexual characteristics and reproductive capacity. In all societies, some form of courtship takes place during which adolescents may began to form lasting relationships, which commonly lead to marriage and family formation. During the different phases of adolescence, adolescents have different needs. For instance, early on, they need to understand the nature of changes that are taking place in themselves, as well as the new demands and expectations that are placed upon them. In addition, they may be aware of anything which may be a cause of concern. As they move through later adolescence, as well having new kinds of relationships with adolescents and adults of both gender, they need to have responsible and satisfying relationships with others. Ultimately, in adulthood, they benefit from their capacity to form lasting relationship and have good parenting skills.

In order to meet the natural needs of adolescents, a response is required which is promotive or preventive in nature. In early adolescence, this will include appropriate education and health screening. In middle adolescence, it may include guidance, support and empowerment. In late adolescence or adulthood, it includes preparation for marriage and parenthood. Those people in a position to help the young are likely to be those who are close to them and whom they trust. Such people must be adequately prepared, whether formally or informally. The important figures include the parents, other family members, teachers, social workers, youth leaders, health professionals, role players and other popular figures. Those who determine policy in the key sectors such as health, education, culture, religious or ethnic affairs, youth and social welfare will be needed to facilitate appropriate training for adolescent health and development, including protection from HIV/AIDS (WHO, 1993).

7. Effectiveness of school education against HIV/AIDS

Health literacy is explained by competence in critical thinking and problem solving, responsible and productive, self-directed learning, and effective communication. School health education is to teach students the information and skills they need to be literate and maintain and improve their health, prevent disease and reduce their health-related risk behaviors, including those related to HIV/AIDS. School planned comprehensive curricula, covering health education and promotion, including HIV infection prevention, now represent a prerequisite. Students should comprehend concepts related to HIV/AIDS prevention and health protection and promotion. Schools and universities are settings that most children and many young people, respectively, attend. This provides an opportunity for knowledge and skills provision and accordingly for changing behaviors and modeling healthy practices. Therefore, schools and universities are a crucial setting for health promotion and HIV/AIDS control.

Schools and universities represent an effective and efficient means to reach a large proportion of young people and, in turn, their families and communities (Kore et al., 2004; Naidu & Aparna, 2008). Several researchers proved that students' HIV/AIDS education interventions improve knowledge (Svenson et al., 1997; UNAIDS, 2008; Ahmed et al., 2009). This in turn increases personal concern about the risk and possible disease contraction, and thus leads to disease prevention behavior. Educated students succeeded in developing skills for negotiating prevention and risk reduction, and resisting peer pressure to engage in risk-related behaviors (Becker & Maiman, 1975; Hingson et al., 1990; Svenson & Varnhagen, 1990; Svenson et al., 1997). Nevertheless, other researchers reported that school or university education courses do not necessarily affect students' behaviors (Baldwin et al., 1990; DiClemente, 1992).

The International Union for Health Promotion and Education (IUHPE, 1999) demonstrated that schools are cost-effective sites for health promotion interventions. The effectiveness and sustainability of school health is governed by how closely health promotion interventions are linked to the primary business of schools in developing the educational skills and knowledge base of young people. Schools can create an educated population who are the better able to make use of any health education they receive in later life from sources such as newspapers, magazines, books and booklets or leaflets. Provision of education concerning sexual health and of HIV/AIDS education is best started at school. The United Nations Program on HIV/AIDS (UNAIDS, 1999) showed that responsible and safe behavior can be learned. Reaching the adolescents as early as possible is arguably the highest HIV/AIDS prevention priority. This includes protection from other sexually transmitted diseases.

8. Appropriate students HIV/AIDS education

Students empowerment, including teaching of appropriate skills, combined with proper provision of HIV preventive knowledge and acquiring healthy attitudes, can motivate practicing healthy behaviors even when students are outside of the school or university setting (Svenson et al., 1997). Several health issues, such as HIV/AIDS control, can be integrated within and into the different subjects, including biology, sociology, environment, physical education, economics, mathematics and languages or linguistics. In addition to classroom lessons and activities, practical in-school and in-community activities and programs have to be organized. Examples include the school club, the school theatre, the school fraternity, the scouts activities and the local community cultural and entertainment programs. In addition to these, schools and universities influence students, through the values they teach, including respect, gender equality and human rights. Education settings can also create an environment that is safe from abuse and fosters understanding, caring and no-discrimination. These are well applied within the concept of 'health-promoting schools'. Furthermore, the student-to-student, child-to-child and peer-led projects or programs encourage the adolescents to undertake community projects. Older and trained peers can be selected as health guides and are then involved in teaching other pupils. The involvement of adolescents themselves in developing messages and approaches is a critical element. The UNAIDS (1999) has demonstrated that these projects and programs have greater credibility and acceptance.

Internations and intercommunities differences, including cultural and religious perspectives, need to be taken in consideration when deciding on the timing for the introduction of components of reproductive health and HIV/AIDS education in schools and universities. A number of other factors will also need to be considered when defining the minimum set of interventions that can be implemented, including the reality and diversity of educational settings, capacity of education system, levels of enrollment and retention and the continuum of the system. The strategies to increase the knowledge of children and youth to prevent and control HIV/AIDS will be highlighted at the "Discussion" section of this chapter.

An important base for designing proper prevention programs is to assess people's knowledge and attitudes towards HIV/AIDS. University students, especially in medical faculties, represent a primary resource. A number of studies have been conducted in several countries to assess medical students' knowledge and attitudes about HIV/AIDS. However, to the authors' knowledge, this is the first study to include Libyan university students at the final year of the faculties of medical sciences.

9. Study to assess HIV/AIDS awareness among medical sciences university students

Research should play an important part in the prevention and control of HIV/AIDS. Information on the size of the problem, infectivity, aetiology and behavioral determinants have to be gathered first. Evidence based planning, as well as, appropriate assessment and monitoring of the conducted programs and activities are crucial for fruitful actions.

9.1 Aim

The aim of this study was to assess the knowledge and attitudes of final year medical sciences university students on HIV and AIDS at the University of Zawia, Zawia, Libya.

9.2 Objectives

The study was designed to assess the current knowledge of final year undergraduate university students regarding various aspects of HIV and AIDS. These include general knowledge about the virus and the disease, and routes of transmission of the virus. It was also to assess attitudes towards prevention and treatment. It was to identify differences in knowledge and attitudes by gender and by different medical sciences faculties; medicine, pharmacy, dentistry and medical technology. The study was also designed to identify areas of misconceptions, gaps in knowledge and discussion, as well as, conclusions and recommendations on the basis of outcomes.

9.3 Methods

Study ethical approval was obtained from the local Scientific Committee, at the Faculty of Pharmacy, University of Zawia, Zawia, Libya, on March 2010. A WHO approved, pre-tested and previously utilized standard closed-end questionnaire was used. The questionnaire included 39 statements, divided to three parts. These are general knowledge about HIV/AIDS, knowledge on the routes of transmission and attitudes towards prevention and treatment. The questionnaire was piloted for feedback and validation. Simple random sampling method was applied to recruit 400 final year (BSc) university students, 100 from each faculty. These are faculties of medicine, pharmacy, dentistry and medical technology. The targeted participants were requested to tick their gender and to tick one of the given choices in front of each statement; 'Yes', 'No' or 'I don't know'. Then, only the response of the correct answer was considered. The answer 'I don't know' was considered as a wrong answer. The questionnaire was self administered by the participants colleagues, within their regular university classes, during May 2010. Study objectives and method were explained to each. Verbal consent was obtained accordingly. Validity and reliability of attitude measuring questions were found satisfactory. Questionnaires were answered anonymously and confidentiality was assured. Fifteen minutes were given to each participant to complete the questionnaires.

9.4 Statistical analysis

All data were statistically described and analyzed with the statistical package for social sciences (SPSS) for windows, version 13.0. Data obtained were evaluated by frequency and percentage of responses of correct answers, and t-test was used to find the difference at p value < 0.05.

9.5 Results

The 100 handed over questionnaires in each faculty were completed and returned. Total returned questionnaires were 400. Males represented 16.75% of all study participants; 23% at the faculty of medicine, 12% at the faculty of pharmacy, 16% at the faculty of dentistry and 16% at the faculty of medical technology. Percentage of responses of correct answers in all faculties participants was 74.21%. Percentages of responses of correct answers were 72.1%, 69.2%, 75.8% and 74.6% in the faculties of medicine, pharmacy, dentistry and medical technology respectively. Comparison of responses to groups of statements according to faculties is given in Table 1. Percentages of responses of correct answers of students of the four faculties to all given statements are shown in Table 2. Responses comparison (in terms of Mean $\pm$SD & range in parenthesis), among the four studied faculties, is presented in Table 3.

10. Discussion

Several studies and surveys, in different parts around the globe, have attempted to assess knowledge and attitudes related to HIV/AIDS among university students. To the authors' knowledge, this study was the first one in Libya to assess those of final year medical sciences students. Self administration of the questionnaire led to 100% response rate. Gender participation was representative of the faculties composition. The study revealed several interesting findings. All study participants (100%), in the four studied faculties, had heard of AIDS. Most (94%) believed that they are aware about the causative agent of AIDS and almost all (98%) indicated that they are aware how HIV is transmitted. However, they demonstrated lower level of deeper knowledge on routes of virus transmission. Moreover, only 58.8% of the participants indicated that they have enough knowledge about AIDS. Percentages of responses of correct answers of students of the different faculties have varied greatly, from 8% to 99%. Mean percentage of responses of correct answers in all faculties participants is 74%. For instance, within responses to statements related to general knowledge, only 13% of the study participants indicated that HIV infected person becomes a source of infection after some period of time from getting the infection. Moreover, only about a third believed that primary symptoms of AIDS do not necessarily occur immediately after infection with HIV. On the other hand, 96% knew that it is possible that any ordinary person can get HIV infection from someone who is infected, while more than 17% did not think that someone who looks healthy but is HIV infected may infect others.

Similar university students assessment studies that were conducted in several countries around the world showed similar results. These studies demonstrated lack of good knowledge on various aspects of HIV/AIDS and revealed the presence of apparent unease or lack of positive attitudes (Al-Owaish et al., 1999; Ahmed et al., 2009; Albrektsson et al., 2009). Kore and others (2004) found that knowledge and awareness about HIV/AIDS among university students is grossly inadequate. On the other hand, some studies found that most students have a relatively good knowledge, with positive attitudes, but with some misconceptions and risky behaviors (Svenson et al., 1997; Tan et al., 2007). Another study showed satisfactory findings, despite some disappointing facts on basic knowledge (Al-Jabri & Al-Jabri, 2003). Only 6% of the students, of Al-Jabri study, either thought that AIDS is not caused by HIV or they did not know. Most of the respondents to that study showed a moderate knowledge regarding the routes of HIV transmission. The earlier United Nations General Assembly Special Session (UNGASS) Libya Progress Report 2010 (UNAIDS, 2010) showed that 87% of Libyan students, aged 15-25 years, stated that they knew what HIV and AIDS are. Furthermore, Greenlee and Ridley (1993) found that only 61% of university students knew that HIV infected individuals do not necessarily lock sick.

In this current study, there was an uneven knowledge in the subcategories of routes of transmission of the virus. As high as 69% of the targeted students believed that mosquitoes are vectors of HIV and more than half of the students thought that it is risky to share swimming pools or toilets with infected people respectively. This might be due to the controversy of some of these modes of transmission and the lack of solid scientific evidence around some of them. Furthermore, almost all study participants pointed out that HIV is sexually transmitted, while only 92% agreed that homosexuality can lead to virus transmission. Almost all (98%) assumed that sharing drugs needles with an infected person represents a source of infection. On the other hand, 96% and about 90% knew that the virus can be transmitted by sharing razor blades or toothbrushes with an infected person respectively. Receiving blood from an infected person was seen by 97% as a possible source of infection. However, some of the studied students lacked knowledge regarding the relationship between sharing clothes, plates or cups with infected people and increased HIV transmission, at which about a quarter of them thought that the virus can be transmitted through these ways of sharing.

Group of statements	Faculty of Medicine	Faculty of Pharmacy	Faculty of Dentistry	Faculty of Medical Technology
1. General knowledge	68.8 +31.5 (11-100)	66.1 +32.1 (12-100)	69.2 +29.5 (15-100)	70.7 +28.4 (8-100)
2. Routes of transmission	83.2 +16.9 (40-100)	77.9 +23.0 (25-100)	81.5 +21.5 (32-100)	83.1 +20.2 (29-100)
3. Prevention and treatment	63.6 +22.4 (40-88)	52.3 +23.1 (31-92)	53.1 +20.4 (37-89)	57.0 +20.3 (35-86)

Data presented as Mean +SD, range in parenthesis.
No statistical difference was found between groups.

Table 1. Comparison of responses to groups of statements according to faculties.

Statements	All	Faculty of Medicine	Faculty of Pharmacy	Faculty of Dentistry	Faculty of Medical Technology
1. General knowledge					
I am aware about AIDS	100.0	100.0	100.0	100.0	100.0
I have enough knowledge about AIDS	58.8	52.0	55.0	60.0	68.0
I know the name of the causative agent for AIDS	94.3	97.0	93.0	91.0	96.0
Primary symptoms of AIDS occur immediately after infection with HIV	30.0	11.0	12.0	22.0	75.0
An HIV infected person can have no symptoms	86.0	86.0	81.0	92.0	85.0
HIV infected persons are expected to die because of the virus infection itself	37.8	38.0	29.0	39.0	31.0
AIDS patients are expected to die because of the disease itself	41.3	37.0	23.0	37.0	36.0
AIDS patients are expected to die because of the disease complications	85.8	88.0	87.0	89.0	79.0
The HIV infected woman is able to become pregnant	89.8	94.0	88.0	86.0	91.0
Someone who looks healthy but is HIV infected may infect others	82.3	84.0	77.0	84.0	84.0
I am aware how HIV is transmitted	98.0	99.0	98.0	99.0	96.0
I know the vulnerable groups of people to HIV	88.0	92.0	90.0	85.0	85.0
It is possible that any ordinary person can get HIV infection	74.8	68.0	76.0	80.0	75.0
It is possible that any ordinary person can get HIV infection from someone who is infected	95.5	99.0	96.0	94.0	93.0
HIV infected person becomes a source of infection immediately after getting the infection	36.3	41.0	39.0	35.0	30.0

Statements	All	Faculty of Medicine	Faculty of Pharmacy	Faculty of Dentistry	Faculty of Medical Technology
HIV infected person becomes a source of infection after some period of time from getting the infection	13.0	15.0	14.0	15.0	8.0
2. Routes of transmission The HIV virus can be transmitted by:					
Touching an HIV infected person	82.0	88.0	69.0	82.0	89.0
Sharing plates or cups with an infected person	73.5	74.0	64.0	86.0	70.0
Sharing clothes with an infected person	74.3	76.0	71.0	69.0	81.0
Sharing swimming pools with an infected person	53.8	68.0	49.0	45.0	53.0
Sharing toilets with an infected person	51.3	59.0	41.0	40.0	65.0
Receiving blood from an infected person	96.5	98.0	92.0	98.0	98.0
Sharing medications needles with an infected person	98.5	100.0	95.0	100.0	99.0
Sharing drugs needles with an infected person	98.0	99.0	96.0	100.0	97.0
Sharing razor blades with an infected person	95.8	95.0	97.0	93.0	98.0
Sharing toothbrushes with an infected person	90.3	87.0	90.0	93.0	91.0
Sharing cupping tools with an infected person	95.8	93.0	95.0	97.0	98.0
Sharing circumcision tools with an infected person	94.3	90.0	99.0	96.0	92.0
Being bitten by a mosquito	31.5	40.0	25.0	32.0	29.0
Mother to fetus	93.8	91.0	94.0	95.0	95.0
Mother to breastfed infant	64.8	65.0	61.0	69.0	64.0
Making sex with an infected person	99.5	98.0	100.0	100.0	100.0
Male making sex with an infected male (homosexuality)	91.5	94.0	87.0	91.0	94.0
3. Prevention and treatment					
HIV infected persons should be isolated to avoid virus transmission to others	34.3	46.0	33.0	37.0	35.0
AIDS patients should be isolated to avoid virus transmission to others	33.3	45.0	42.0	38.0	40.0
Ordinary people can avoid the risk of HIV infection by behavior change	88.8	88.0	92.0	89.0	86.0
Ordinary people can avoid the risk of HIV infection by using condoms during sexual intercourse	39.0	40.0	31.0	40.0	45.0
Ordinary people can avoid the risk of HIV infection by using the HIV vaccine	62.5	87.0	51.0	50.0	62.0
It is possible that HIV infected persons can be cured using relevant treatment	70.0	76.0	65.0	65.0	74.0

Table 2. Percentages of responses of correct answers of students of the four faculties to the given statements.

Faculties	Males	Females
1. General knowledge		
Medicine	70.6 +31.3 (13-100) n= 23	68.2 +31.9 (10-100) n= 77
Pharmacy	67.1 +31.5 (8-100) n= 12	66.2 +32.7 (13-100) n= 88
Dentistry	66.4 +36.4 (0-100) n= 16	67.6 +28.6 (13-100) n= 77
Medical Technology	64.9 +36.4 (0-100) n= 16	71.9 +27.1 (10-100) n= 84
2. Routes of transmission		
Medicine	85.2 +15.4 (48-100) n= 23	82.7 +18.1 (34-100) n= 77
Pharmacy	82.8 +18.7 (50-100) n= 12	77.4 +23.9 (22-100) n= 88
Dentistry	82.8 +17.9 (43-100) n= 23	81.5 +27.4 (16-100) n= 77
Medical Technology	73.6 +28.3 (19-100) n= 16	84.3 +19.1* (31-100) n= 84
3. Prevention and treatment		
Medicine	71.2 +9.6 (61-83) n= 23	61.7 +27.7 (31-94) n= 77
Pharmacy	55.5 +15.6 (33-75) n= 12	51.8 +24.6 (27-94) n= 88
Dentistry	55.1 +17.2 (35-83) n= 23	52.6 +21.7 (135-91) n= 77
Medical Technology	52.1 +19.7 (31-88) n= 16	57.8 +20.9 (36-86) n= 84

Data presented as Mean +SD, range in parenthesis.
*$P < 0.05$, $t = 2.5$.

Table 3. Gender distribution and comparison of responses to groups of statements.

The present data are consistent with those of other studies (Al-Jabri & Al-Jabri, 2003; Tan et al., 2007; UNAIDS, 2010). UNGASS Libya Progress Report (UNAIDS, 2010) showed that there is a high degree of misconception amongst secondary school Libyan students with regards to modes of transmission and prevention. Only 42% of those previously surveyed students, aged 15-25 years, agreed that HIV can be transmitted through use of public toilets, while 31% stated that HIV infection can be transmitted by getting near to an HIV-infected individual while sneezing or coughing and 30% stated that HIV can be transmitted by looking after an HIV-infected individual (UNAIDS, 2010). Tan and colleagues (2007) demonstrated that most university students were also aware that HIV can be transmitted by unsafe sex (99%), by sharing needles with infected drug users (98%), or by receiving blood from an infected person (97%). However, only 90% agreed that swimming pools do not transmit the virus, and only 40% understood that mosquito does not carry risk. University students that were studied by Al-Jabri and Al-Jabri (2003) showed that they very strongly agreed that sex (98%) and drug needles (99%) are modes of virus transmission. However, 19% thought a person may get HIV by a mosquito bite and 46% believed that blood donation leads to a risk of infection.

In this present study, although about 90% thought that ordinary people can avoid the risk of HIV infection by behavior modification, a large proportion of the students had poor attitudes. Only 39% of them believed that condom use during sexual intercourse is essential for the prevention of HIV transmission. Furthermore, results revealed that there is a high level of stigma among the students towards HIV infected individuals. About two thirds agreed that isolation of HIV positive or AIDS patients is necessary to achieve protection. Negative attitudes regarding prevention misconceptions of HIV/AIDS reflect a false perception of the disease among these university students. On the other hand, the authors of this study see it is disappointing that about a third of the studied medical sciences university students thought that there is a vaccine to protect from the risk of HIV infection (37.5%) or that it is possible to cure an HIV infected person (30%).

These findings on university students attitudes towards HIV/AIDS are in line with those found by other researchers (Al-Jabri & Al-Jabri, 2003; Kore et al., 2004; Tan et., 2007; Ahmed et al., 2009; Albrektsson et al., 2009; UNAIDS, 2010). For instance, an earlier study revealed that 61% of the Libyan students strongly agreed or agreed that HIV infected individuals are dangerous and believed that they should be banned from entering into the country (UNAIDS, 2010). Moreover, about one third of Omani students believed that HIV infected individuals should be separated from others, and nearly a quarter of them thought that AIDS patients should always kept at hospitals, not at home (Al-Jabri & Al-Jabri, 2003).

This is probably because the conservative school education was not able to cover certain sensitive issues around HIV/AIDS. Moreover, mass media education could not be thorough enough and was not able to cover such issues. In addition, the coverage of such content in public remains low. The UNAIDS Report (2010) demonstrated that there is a lot of cultural sensitivity associated with the issue. There is a probable difficulty, even in permissive Western societies, to discuss sensitive issues related to HIV prevention, such as the importance of use of condoms, with the adolescents in schools. Hence, some specialists in the field call for a more liberal ideology can be promoted. Teachers and social workers require greater skills in tackling such sensitive issue areas, and as such students are may not be receiving the information that they need.

In this study, in general, there were no statistically significant differences, neither by faculty nor by gender, regarding the groups of statements of HIV/AIDS general knowledge, routes of transmission, or prevention and treatment. A small significant difference was found between males and females of the faculty of medical technology in respect to the group of statements related to the routes of transmission. Ahmed and colleagues' similar university students study (2009) revealed similar findings. However, other studies demonstrated some significant gender differences; some favored males and others favored females. For example, one study showed that only 36% of males have comprehensive knowledge about HIV/AIDS, whereas only 20% of females do so (IIPS & ORC Macro, 2008). On the other hand, Kore and others' study (2004) pointed out that 53% males and 62.0% females knew that AIDS is an infective communicable disease. The aetiology of AIDS, being the HIV virus was known by 55% male and 69% female students. Moreover, 18% and 13% male and female university students respectively thought that HIV is a bacteria (Kore et al., 2004). Albrektsson and colleagues (2009) have also found that female students had better knowledge than male students.

Being medical sciences university final year students, responses of this study participants are assessed by the study authors as unsatisfactory. Many of them do not have a good level of understanding and attitudes towards HIV/AIDS. Similarly, much research from around the world has demonstrated gaps in health care students knowledge about HIV transmission and patients' treatment. Moreover, some medical sciences university students hold negative attitudes and risk perceptions that could become barriers in their eventual professional care of HIV/AIDS patients (Ahmed et al., 2009). It can be argued that medical schools disease orient their students, and at the best, they risk-factor orient their students. They concentrate on clinical sciences and conduct their training programs on the various branches of curative medical services, at university hospitals. Many of the medical schools around the globe prepare doctors not to care for the health of the people or to promote the individual's or the community's health. They engage them in a medical practice that is blind to any thing but disease and the technology for dealing with it. Therefore, students get less orientation towards health promotion, health protection and disease protection.

On the other hand, other researchers (Al-Jabri & Al-Jabri, 2003; Tan et al., 2007; Gopal et al., 2010) revealed that medical faculties' students acquired more accurate and complete information regarding HIV/AIDS, compared with students from other faculties including science. In fact, health professionals, in general, are at high occupational risk for contracting HIV, since they have a high exposure to HIV and AIDS patients. Therefore, health care students need to stay knowledgeable and aware of all relevant issues around HIV and AIDS and must receive an improved HIV/AIDS training. However, education against HIV/AIDS is not only required for medical and paramedical students, but also to a large extent, for all university level students, in addition to the basic education to those in the primary and secondary levels.

Findings of this study highlight the need for immediate general public education actions, within a wide comprehensive strategy. At which, if HIV/AIDS awareness is left unaddressed can permit the virus to spread considerably in the coming years. The most effective and efficient way to combat HIV/AIDS is through interventions for information, education and communication that target most at-risk populations and groups. Emphasis is to be made on children and youth. Schools and universities represent the most critical setting.

Several studies stressed that there is an immense need to conduct awareness programs about HIV/AIDS at schools and universities (Svenson et al., 1997; IUHPE, 1999; Al-Jabri & Al-Jabri, 2003; Kore et al., 2004; Elfituri et al., 2006). These have to be extended beyond formal education to reach teachers and parents. A previous Libyan study demonstrated that the general public ranked education against HIV/AIDS as one of top three priority issues of the national health education programs (Elfituri et al., 2006). The general public and the health officials agreed that children and youth represent the vital groups to be targeted and that schools and universities are the appropriate settings. Moreover, many HIV/AIDS educational interventions in different parts of the world have shown promising outcomes (Becker & Maiman, 1975; Hingson et al., 1990; Svenson & Varnhagen, 1990; Svenson et al., 1997; UNAIDS, 2008; Ahmed et al., 2009).

Prevention efforts, around most nations, including Libya, have been geared to providing accurate knowledge on HIV/AIDS through the school based health education system. However, similar to several other populations, only about half of the Libyans considered school health education as an effective medium of health education to raise the public health knowledge and to influence healthy behaviors (Elfituri et al., 1999). Furthermore, only one third of Chinese university students have received their first information on HIV/AIDS from schools (Tan et al., 2007), while more than 75% of them received information at university (Albrektsson et al., 2009). Moreover, the school and university settings were not the main sources of information for the Indian students (Kore et al., 2004).

11. Summary, conclusions and recommendations

Several studies to assess knowledge and attitudes of university students towards HIV/AIDS were conducted in different countries around the world. This current study was the first one to assess knowledge and awareness of final year medical sciences students. Participants were final year students from the faculties of medicine, pharmacy, dentistry and medical technology.

The study revealed several interesting findings. Although every student participated in the study believed that he/she is aware about what HIV/AIDS mean, only 94% of the students thought that they know what agent that causes AIDS. Study results indicated that the majority of the students had a moderate level of HIV/AIDS knowledge and of its routes of transmission. 98% believed that they know how HIV is transmitted. Only 59% of the participants indicated that they have enough knowledge about AIDS. Percentages of responses of correct answers of students of the different faculties have varied greatly. Only 13% of the study participants indicated that HIV infected person becomes a source of infection after some period of time from getting the infection. Moreover, only about a third believed that primary symptoms of AIDS do not necessarily occur immediately after infection with HIV. On the other hand, 96% knew that it is possible that any ordinary person can get HIV infection from someone who is infected, while more than 17% did not think that someone who looks healthy but is HIV infected may infect others.

This study demonstrated that there was an uneven knowledge in the subcategories of routes of transmission of the virus. As high as 69% of the targeted students believed that mosquitoes are vectors of HIV and more than half of the students thought that it is risky to share swimming pools or toilets with infected people. Furthermore, some of the studied students lacked knowledge about the relationship between sharing clothes, plates or cups with infected people and increased HIV transmission, at which about a quarter of them thought that the virus can be transmitted through these ways of sharing.

Although 89% thought that ordinary people can avoid the risk of HIV infection by behavior modification, a large proportion of the students had negative attitudes. Only 39% of them believed that condom use during sexual intercourse is essential for the prevention of HIV transmission. Furthermore, about two thirds agreed that isolation of HIV positive or AIDS patients is necessary to achieve protection. Negative attitudes regarding prevention misconceptions of HIV/AIDS reflect misconceptions about the virus and disease among these university students.

This study showed that participants' awareness and attitudes on HIV/AIDS are not satisfactory, especially for final year medical sciences university students. General public education, with a focus on the adolescents, should represent a fundamental role of the national, regional and international HIV/AIDS control programs. Schools and universities are strongly recommended to be the priority setting. Peer education programs are suggested to be utilized, as they demonstrated success worldwide. Moreover, it is important to build learning experiences into students' active participation programs at all levels. In this way, students will be able to understand more about the different factors that influence their health and how to be safe from all sexually transmitted diseases, including HIV/AIDS. Furthermore, university students have a vital role in the community prevention and control of HIV/AIDS, at which, social changes are commanded and transmitted from schools.

Educational interventions, in addition to providing HIV/AIDS prevention knowledge, have to emphasize on students' empowerment and motivation. It is important to use students-centerd approaches that develop a critical awareness of the situation and empower the students to work together for their personal, family and community improved awareness and behavior change. Development of appropriate skills for behavior modification should be included. Ensuring the greatest success involves a multifaceted and coordinated effort.

At the education settings, group techniques offer an intermediate approach between the one-to-one interaction and the wider community or mass media communications. As the required HIV prevention behavioral modification is complex, experiential group learning can be performed. The didactic approach can then be utilized. It includes content knowledge, lecturing skills and the ability to answer questions clearly. The didactic approach generally is individualistic and can be directed at groups to bring about such individual and community behavior change.

Finally, individuals' knowledge, attitudes and behaviors change over time. Therefore, repeated surveys and evaluation studies of the effectiveness of educational interventions by monitoring changes in health knowledge, attitudes and behaviors are necessary. Then, health education, disease prevention and health promotion should be planned, implemented and continuously evaluated and updated to meet the changes and developments.

12. References

Agrawal, G., Ahmad A. & Zubair M. (2010) Knowledge, attitude and beliefs towards HIV/AIDS among youth students in India. World Family Medicine Journal. Vol. 8(3): 10-15.

Ahmed, S., Hassali, M. & Abdul Aziz, N. (2009) An assessment of the knowledge, attitudes and risk perceptions of pharmacy students regarding HIV/AIDS, *American Journal of Pharmaceutical Education*. Vol. 73(1) (15): 1-7.

Albrektsson, M., Alm, L., Tan, X. & Andersson, R. (2009) HIV/AIDS awareness, attitudes and risk behavior among university students in Wuhan, China, *The Open AIDS Journal*. Vol.3: 55-62.

Al-Jabri, A. & Al-Jabri, J. (2003) Knowledge and attitudes of undergraduate medical and non-medical students in Sultan Qaboos University toward Acquired Immune Deficiency Syndrome. *Saudi Medical Journal*. Vol. 24(3): 273-277.

Al-Owaish, R., Moussa, M., Anwar, S., Al-Shoumer, H. & Sharma, P. (1999) Knowledge, attitudes, beliefs and practices about HIV/AIDS in Kuwait. *AIDS Education & Prevention*. Vol.11: 163-173.

Baldwin, J., Whiteley, S. & Baldwin J. (1990) Changing AIDS and fertility related behavior; the effectiveness of sexual education. *Journal of Sex Research*. Vol.27: 245-262.

Becker, H. & Maiman, A. (1975) Sociobehavioral determinants of compliance with health and medical care recommendations. *Medical Care*. Vol.13: 10-24.

Binswanger H. (2000) Scaling up HIV/AIDS programs to national coverage. *Science*. Vol.23: 2173-2176.

CDC (2008) HIV/AIDS Among Youth; Revised. Centres for Disease Control and Prevention, USA.

Downie, R., Tannahill, C. & Tannahill, A. (1996). *Health Promotion: Models and Values*. Oxford University Press. ISBN 0-19-262591-8, Oxford, UK.

DiClemente, R. (1992) Pscychosocial determinants of condom use among adolescents, *in* DiClemente R. (ed.) *Adolescents and AIDS: A Generation in Jeopardy*. Sage, Newbury Park, CA, USA.

Elfituri, A., Elmahaishi, M. & MacDonald, T. (1999) Role of health education programs within the Libyan community. *Eastern Mediterranean Health Journal*. Vol.5(2): 268-76.

Elfituri, A., Elmahaishi, M., MacDonald, T., & Sherif, F. (2006) Health education in the Libyan Arab Jamahiriya: assessment of future needs. *Eastern Mediterranean Health Journal* Vol.12 (2): S147-56.

Ewles, L. & Simnett, I. (1996). *Promoting Health: A Practical Guide*. Bailliere Tindall, ISBN 1-873853-17-3, London, UK.

Hingson, R., Strunin, L. & Berlin, B. (1990). Acquired immunodeficiency syndrome transmission; changes in knowledge and behaviors among teenagers, Massachusetts Statewide Surveys, 1986-1988. *Pediatrics*. Vol.85, 24-29.

IIPS & ORC Macro. (2008) *National Family Health Survey-3, 2005-06*. International Centre for Population Sciences, Mumbai, India.

International Union for Health Promotion and Education (1999) *The Evidence of Health Promotion Effectiveness: A Report for the European Commission*. Brussels, Belgium.

Kore, S, Pandole, A., Nemade, Y., Putharaya S. & Ambiye, V. (2004) Attitude, knowledge, beliefs about HIV/AIDS in college going adolescents: BHJ. Vol.(46)2: 11.1-4.

McGuire, W. (1969) The nature of attitude and attitude change *in* Lindzey, G. & Aronsen, E. (eds.) *Handbook of Social Psychology*. Addison Wesley, Reading, UK.

Ottawa Charter for Health Promotion, The First International Conference on Health Promotion. (1986) Ottawa, Canada.

Park, J. & Park, K. (1997) *Park's Textbook of Preventive and Social Medicine*. Jabalpur, Banarsidas Bhanot.

Prochaska, J.& DiClemente, C. (1983), Stages and process of self change of smoking: Towards an integrative model of change. *Journal of Consulting and Clinical Psychology*. Vol.51: 390-395.

Ribeaux, S. & Poppleton, S. (1978) *Psychology and Work- An Introduction*. Macmillan, London, UK.

Svenson, L., Carmel, S. & Varnhagen, C. (1997) A review of the knowledge, attitudes and behaviors of university students concerning HIV/AIDS. *Health Promotion International*. Vol. 12(1), 61-68.

Svenson L. & Varnhagen C. (1990) Knowledge, attitudes and behaviors related to AIDS among first year university students. *Canadian Journal of Public Health*. Vol.81, 139-140.

Tannahill, A. (1990) Health education and health promotion: planning for the 1990s. *Health Education Journal*. Vol.49(4): 194-8.

Tan, X., Pan, J., Zhou, D., Wang, C. & Xie, C. (2007) HIV/AIDS knowledge, attitudes and behaviors assessment of Chinese students; a questionnaire study. *International Journal of Environmental Research and Public Health*. Vol.4(3): 248-253.

United Nations (2002) *HIV/AIDS awareness and behavior*. Department of Economic and Social Affairs. Population Division. UN, 2002. ST/ESA/SER.A/209: 29. New York, USA.

UNAIDS (United Nations Program on HIV/AIDS) (1999) *Children and HIV/AIDS; UNAIDS Briefing Paper*. Geneva, Switzerland.

UNAIDS (United Nations Program on HIV/AIDS) (2008) *Monitoring the declaration of commitment on HIV/AIDS: Country Report of Malaysia*. http://data.unaids.org/pub/Report/2006/2006_country_progress_report_malaysia-en.pdf. Accessed February 5, 2011. Geneva, Switzerland.

UNAIDS (United Nations Program on HIV/AIDS) (2010) *United Nations General Assembly Special Session (UNGASS) Country Progress Report of Libya 2008-9*. Geneva, Switzerland.

WHO (World Health Organization) (1984) *Health Promotion: a W.H.O Discussion Document on Concepts and Principles*. Geneva, Switzerland.

WHO (World Health Organization) (1993) *Counselling Skills Training in Adolescent Sexuality and Reproductive Health*. Geneva, Switzerland.

WHO & IUHPE (World Health Organization & International Union for Health Promotion and Education) (2000) *Framework for Countrywide Plans of Action for Health Promotion.* A conference document, Fifth Global Conference on Health Promotion, Mexico City, Mexico.

Part 2

Psychological Aspects of HIV/AIDS

Psychosocial Needs and Support Services Accessed by HIV/AIDS Patients of the University of Ilorin Teaching Hospital, Nigeria

Yahaya, Lasiele Alabi and Jimoh, A.A.G.
[1]*Department of Counsellor Education, University of Ilorin, Ilorin*
[2]*Department of Obstetrics and Gynaecology*
University of Ilorin Teaching Hospital, Ilorin
Nigeria

1. Introduction

HIV/AIDS has become a threat to public health in Nigeria as a result of its devastating consequences, which are manifested in forms of prolonged sickness, deaths and increase in number of orphans and widows/widowers. Nigeria has an estimated population of about 150 million of which about 3.5 million are infected by HIV/AIDS (FMINO, 2007). HIV/AIDS was first identified in Nigeria in 1985 and reported at an International Conference in 1986 (Adeyi et al, 2006). The HIV/AIDS pandemic led to the death of 170,000 Nigerians in 2007 (UNAIDS, 2008). According to Edewor (2010), Nigeria has already surpassed the 5 percent explosive prevalence phase and the disease has killed more than 1.3 million people and orphaned more than 1 million children (FMINO, 2007). The infection rates of HIV/AIDS vary across the six geopolitical zones of Nigeria. According to Edewor (2010), the mode of HIV transmission in Nigeria is mainly through unprotected sex, and other factors which contribute to the spread of the virus include poverty, Sexually Transmitted Infection (STI), social and religious norms and political and social changes (National AIDS/STD Control Programme, 1999).

Parke and Aggleton (2007) noted that negative social attitudes toward marginalised populations, policies mandating the testing of high risk groups and limited legal protections based on HIV status may exacerbate stigma. They stressed further that increase vulnerability to discrimination complicates the social and psychological adjustment of Persons Living With HIV/AIDS (PLWHA). The victims require necessary assistance to be able to live happily and contribute meaningfully to the development of the society. Thus, they need psychosocial supports to be able to cope with their challenges.

Psychosocial needs can be described as social, mental and spiritual requirements of PLWHA in order to live quality life and contribute to development of the society. The needs can be viewed from a psychological theory propounded by Abraham Maslow in 1943. According to Maslow (1954), the hierarchy of needs is often portrayed in the shape of a pyramid, with the largest and most fundamental levels of needs at the bottom, and the need for self-actualization at the top. The most fundamental and basic four layers of the pyramid contain what Maslow called "deficiency needs" or "d-needs", esteem, friendship and love, security, and physical needs. With the exception of the most fundamental (physiological) needs, if these "deficiency needs" are not met, an individual's body gives no physical indication but the individual feels anxious and tense. Maslow's theory suggests that the most basic level of needs must be met before an individual strongly desires (or focuses motivation upon) the secondary or higher level needs. Maslow also coined the term "Metamotivation" to describe the motivation of people who go beyond the scope of the basic needs and strive for constant betterment. "Metamotivated" people are driven by B-needs (Being Needs), instead of deficiency needs (D-Needs)(Wikipedia, 2011). For the purpose of this study, the psychosocial needs adopted comprise physiological needs, safety needs, belongingness needs, esteem needs, aesthetic needs and self-actualization as propounded by Maslow. Physiological needs include food, air and water; safety needs involve housing and security; belongingness implies social interaction and group affiliation; esteem needs involve high regard for self and others; aesthetic needs deal with love of beauty while self-actualization involves becoming what one desires to be in life.

Psychosocial support can be described as a process of providing for the emotional, social, mental and spiritual needs of clients or patients. It is an essential element of promoting human development. Support services are the social facilities which are available and provided by an organization or a community to those in need of such supports in order to assist them to live a good life. The supports can be grouped into spiritual, moral, social, psychological/counselling and financial supports. Spiritual support involves prayer and meditation, moral support implies identification with someone's concerns and encouragement, financial support connotes provision of monetary assistance while psychological support comprises guidance and counselling. In order to meet the needs of PLWHA, an emergency action plan was prepared by the National Action Committee on AIDS in 2001 with a view of institutionalizing best practices in care and support for Persons Living With HIV/AIDS (PLWHA). The plan was designed to mitigate the effects of the disease on the victims, orphans and other affected groups and stimulate research on HIV/AIDS (USAID, 2002). According to the World Health Organization (WHO, 2011), psychosocial supports address the on-going concerns and social problems of HIV infected individuals, their partners and caregivers. WHO stressed that HIV infection affects all dimensions of the victims' life such as physical, psychological and social. The infection could result in stigma and fear for those living with the virus, as well as for those caring for them and the entire family. Infections often result in loss of socio-economic status, employment, income, housing, health care and mobility.

WHO (2011) observed that counselling and social support can help people and their carers to cope more effectively with each stage of the infection and enhances quality of life. The organisation noted that with adequate support, PLWHA are more likely to respond adequately to the stress of being infected and are unlikely to develop serious mental health problem.The psychological supports provided by the patients' partners and their family members can assist them in making appropriate decisions, coping better with illness and dealing more efficiently with discrimination.

The community also has important role to play in assisting PLWHA. It could assist in adding quality to the life of HIV/AIDS patients through provision of economic, social and psychological supports. Thus, psychosocial supports for HIV/AIDS patients need to be scaled up and encouraged in any community.

Amirkhanian, Kelly and McAuliff (2003) conducted a study on the psychosocial needs, mental health and HIV transmission risk behaviour among people living with HIV/AIDS in

St. Petersburg, Russia. Sample of the study consisted of 470 persons with HIV/AIDS at St. Petersburg HIV care and service agencies. The participants completed anonymous self-administered questionnaires on social and psychological characteristics of HIV, serostatus disclosure, discrimination experience and risk practices. The study found that HIV infected persons in Russia experienced a wide range of social, psychological and care access problems.

Jordans, Kein and Pradhan (2007) investigated the counsellors' and beneficiaries' perception of psychosocial counselling in Nepal. Semi-structured interviews were conducted with clients, para-professional counsellors and managers of organisations in which psychosocial counselling was taking place. The study revealed that stakeholders generally presented a positive view of the significance and supportive function of psychosocial counselling, and the issues of training, supervision, confidentiality and integration of counselling within the mainstream care provision were emphasised.

Although, a lot of studies (Ostrow et al. 1992; Kelly, Murphy, 1992; Slugget, 2003; Amirkhanian, Kelly & McAuliff, 2003) have been conducted on the psychosocial needs and support services of PLWHA across the world, but little or no attention had been paid to the patients of the University of Ilorin Teaching Hospital, Nigeria in this direction. The need to make up for part of this gap provided the major impetus for this study. To this end, the study investigated the psychosocial needs and support services accessed by HIV/AIDS patients of the University of Ilorin Teaching Hospital, Nigeria. Kuh (1982) noted that assessment of clients' needs is crucial for effective determination of developing effective services to address the clients' needs. The objective of this study therefore, was to investigate the psychosocial support needs and support services being accessed by the HIV/AIDS patients at the University of Ilorin Teaching Hospital, Nigeria.

2. Research questions

1. What are the psychosocial needs of HIV/AIDS patients of the University of Ilorin Teaching Hospital, Nigeria?
2. What are the support services accessed by HIV/AIDS patients of the University of Ilorin Teaching Hospital, Nigeria?

3. Methodology

The study is a descriptive survey which employed quantitative and qualitative measures to obtain data from the respondents. An estimated 2,365 patients living with HIV/AIDS at the University of Ilorin Teaching Hospital, Nigeria constituted the study population while all the literate HIV/AIDS patients (i.e. those who can read and write in English) at the hospital constituted the target population. The sample for the study comprised 125 HIV/AIDS patients who indicated interest in participating in the study. Thus, a purposive sampling technique was adopted for the study. The researchers explained the purpose of the study to the respondents and emphasised that it aimed at identifying the needs of HIV/AIDS patients in order to provide better services and supports. The researchers obtained the list of HIV/AIDS patients at the Teaching Hospital, identified the educated ones through personal data and interactions. The consents of the respondents were sought before the questionnaires designed for the purpose of the study were distributed to them. This was followed by a scheduled interview with 15 randomly selected respondents. The interview was designed to obtain information from respondents on ways by which their needs could be met. In all, 125 patients voluntarily agreed to participate in the study after been assured of confidentiality. The instruments employed in carrying out the study are researchers' designed questionnaire and structured interview. The questionnaire has three sections. Section A elicits information on demographic data; Section B seeks information on psychosocial needs (i.e. esteem needs, physiological needs, belongingness needs, safety needs, aesthetic needs and self-actualization) while Section C contains items on support services (i.e. social, spiritual, psychological, financial and moral). In Sections B and C of the questionnaire, a list of 6 categories of psychosocial needs and a list of 5 support services were presented to the respondents respectively. The instruments were validated by three lecturers in the Departments of Sociology, Counsellor Education and Obstetrics and Gynaecology, University of Ilorin, Nigeria. The respondents were required to read through the questionnaire forms and indicate their responses by putting a tick (√) on any item that is applicable to them to indicate their psychosocial needs and the support services that are being accessed by them. Responses obtained were grouped on the basis of the number of respondents that ticked each of the items in sections B and C of the questionnaire and later converted to percentages. The percentages were also converted into bar chart as shown in Figs 1 and 2. The limitation of this study was manifested in the use of literate respondents as the study sample. This was designed to facilitate easy and proper understanding of the questionnaire.

4. Results

Table 1 indicates that the majority of respondents are between the ages of 21-40 years old (44%). Majority are also females (53.6 %), holders of secondary education certificates (44.8 %) and married (41.6%).

Variables	Frequency	Percent
Age		
1-20	32	25.6
21-40	55	44.0
41-60	31	24.8
61 and above	07	5.6
Gender		
Male	58	46.4
Female	67	53.6
Level of Education		
Tertiary Education	47	37.6
Secondary Education	56	44.8
Primary Education	22	17.6
Marital Status		
Single	45	36.0
Married	52	41.6
Divorced	10	8.0
Widow	18	14.4

Table 1. Demographic Characteristics of Respondents

Psychosocial Needs

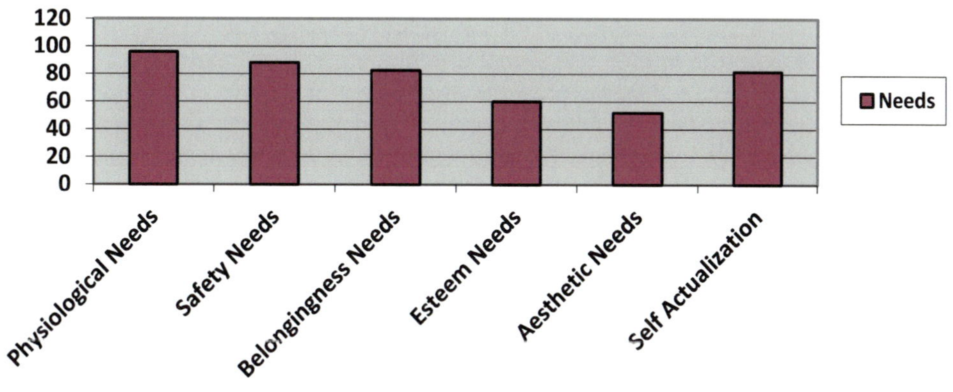

Fig. 1. Psychosocial Needs of Respondents

Source: Field survey, 2011

Fig 1 represents the respondents' psychosocial needs which are esteem needs, physiological needs, belongingness needs, safety needs, aesthetic needs and self-actualization. The figure shows that 120 (96%) respondents indicated physiological needs, 110 (88%) indicated safety needs, 103 (82.4%) indicated belongingness needs, 75 (60%) indicated esteem needs, 65 (52%) indicated aesthetic needs while 102 (81.6%) indicated self-actualization.

Psychosocial Supports

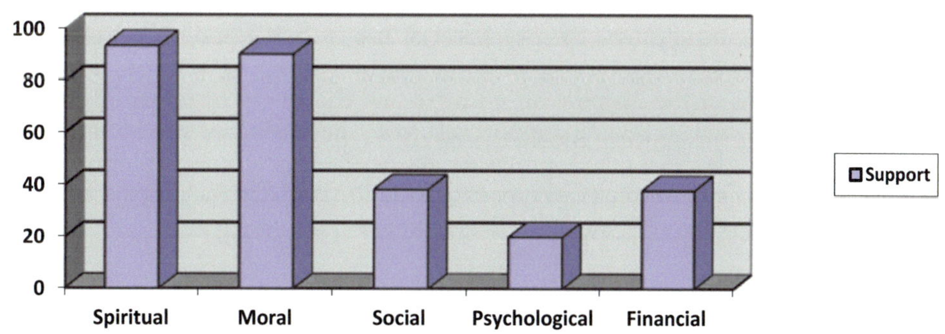

Fig. 2. Psychosocial Supports Accessed by Respondents

Source: Field survey, 2011

Fig. 2 represents the support services accessed by the respondents which are social, spiritual, psychological, financial and moral. The figure shows that 117 (93.6%) respondents indicated spiritual support, 113 (90.4%) indicated moral support, 48 (38.4%) indicated social support, 25 (20%) respondents indicated psychological/counselling support while 35 (28%) indicated financial support.

5. Discussion

The study indicated that majority of the respondents are between the ages of 21-40 years. This may be due to the fact that the age group is more actively engaged in risk behaviours. The finding also showed that the majority of respondents are females. Presumably, this could be as a result of their exposure to high risk sexual activities such as polygamy, circumcision, early marriages of young girls, and lack of power to insist on use of condoms during sex.

The findings also indicated the highest needs of the respondents as physiological needs which include food, water and air. The finding could be as a result of level of poverty in Nigeria. The least needs as identified by the respondents are aesthetic needs. This is in line with theoretical proposition of Maslow which proposed physiological needs as the most important.

The study also showed spiritual support as the most accessed by the respondents. This finding may be due to the fact that many Nigerians are religious as more than 90% of Nigerians are either Muslims or Christians. Psychological/counselling and financial supports are the least accessed. The economic recession in Nigeria may be responsible for the low level of financial support available to the respondents while the non-provision of professional counselling services in many Nigerian health centres may be a reason for the low level of psychological/counselling support. The implications of these findings are that there is the need to encourage aesthetic and esteem values among PLWHA. In addition, it is also essential to improve provision of social, psychological/counselling and financial supports to the PLWHA. The supportive role of religious organizations as well as peer groups in the use of antiretroviral (HAART) has been highlighted by previous studies in this environment (Jimoh et al, 2008). Similarly, Yahaya (2010) expressed the need for provision of counselling service to HIV/AIDS patients and stressed that with counselling support, PLWHA would be able to face the challenges of HIV/AIDS.

6. Conclusion

The study gave an insight into the psychosocial needs and support services accessed by HIV/AIDS patients of the University at Ilorin Teaching Hospital, Nigeria. It revealed that HIV/AIDS patients at the hospital are facing some challenges in terms of meeting their psychosocial needs and accessing support services. The areas that need attention include esteem and aesthetic needs and provision of psychological/counselling and financial supports. There is no doubt that if the needs of the PLWHA are met, they would be better equipped to adjust and contribute to the development of the society.

7. Recommendations

Based on the findings of the study the following recommendations are considered relevant:

a. Health counsellors should provide counselling services to the PLWHA and develop instruments to identify their psychosocial needs.
b. Health counsellors should encourage PLWHA to accept their conditions, identify their needs and acquire relevant skills in order to develop at t equal level with the other members of the community.
c. Counsellors and other health providers should collaborate and bring support services to the door steps of the PLWHA. This is necessary in areas of social and financial supports.

d. Non-Governmental Organizations, family members and other members of the community should empower PLWHA through job provision and financial support in order to assist them to meet their basic needs.
e. Medical and other health workers should display positive attitude towards PLWHA. This can be achieved, among others, by ensuring that PLWHA are not segregated in terms of services offered to them as currently practised at the University of Ilorin Teaching Hospital.

8. References

Adeyi, S., et al. (2006). AIDS in Nigeria: A nation on the threshold. In Adeyi S., & Ademo J. (Eds.). *The epidemiology of HIV/AIDS in Nigeria.* USA: Centre for Population and Development Studies.

Amirkhanian, Y. A; Kelly, J. A & Mcauliff, L. T. (2003). Psychosocial needs, mental health, and HIV transmission risk behaviour among people living with HIV/AIDS in St. Peterburg, Rusia. *AIDS*, 17, 2367-2374.

Edewor, N. (2010). Access to health information by People Living with HIV/AIDS in Nigeria. *Library Philosophy and Practice*. Retrieved from http://www.webpages.uidaho.edu/~mbolin/edewor.htm

Federal Ministry of Information and National Orientation (2007). *The Obasanjo reforms: HIV/AIDS response.* Federal Ministry of Information and National Orientation: Abuja.

Jimoh, A.A.G; Agbede, O.O; Abdurraheem, I. S; Saidu, R. et al. (2008). Antiretroviral treatment among students of tertiary institutions in Ilorin: Assessment of knowledge, attitude and practice. *Nigerian Medical Practitioner, 53* (6): 94-98.

Jordans, M. J., Keen, A. S., Pradhan, H., & Toi, W. A. (2007). Psychosocial counselling in Neptal: Perspectives of counsellors and beneficiaries. *International Journal of Advanced Counselling,* 29, 57 68.

Kelly, J. A, Murphy, D. A. (1992). Psychological interventions with AIDS and HIV: Prevention and treatment. *J Consult Clin Psychol,60*:576–585.

Kuh, G.D. (1982). Purposes and Principles for Needs Assessment in Student Affairs. *The Journal of College Student Personnel, 23*, 202-209.

Maslow, A. (1954). *Motivation and Personality.*: Harper.ISBN 0060419873. New York.

National AIDS/STD Control Programme/Federal Ministry of Health (1999). *HIV syphilis sentinels sero prevalence survey in Nigeria* .Technical Report.

Ostrow, D. G, Monjan, A; Joseph, J.; VanRaden, M; Fox, R; Kingsley, L. et al.(1992). HIV-related symptoms and psychological functioning in a cohort of homosexual men. *American Journal of Psychiatry,* 146:737–742.

Parke, R & Aggleton, P. (2002). *HIV/AIDS related stigma and discrimination: A conceptual framework and an agenda for action.* The Population Council: New York.

Slugget, C. (2003). Mapping of psychosocial support for girls and boys affected by child sexual abuse. Four countries in South and Central Asia. Save the Children: Kathmandu.

USAID (2002). *HIV/AIDS in Nigeria*. Retrieved from www.usaid.gov/pop-health/aids

UNAIDS (2008). *Report on the global AIDS epidemic.* Retrieved January13, 2009, from http://www.avert.org

Wikipedia (2011). *Maslow's hierarchy of needs.* Retrieved from

http://en.wikipedia.org/wiki/Maslow%27s_hierarchy_of_needs
World Health Organization (WHO; 2011). *Psychosocial support.* Retrieved http://www.who.int/hiv/topics/psychosocial/support/en
Yahaya, L. A.; Jimoh, A. A. G & Balogun, O. R. (2010). Factors hindering acceptance of HIV/AIDS Voluntary Counselling and Testing (VCT) among youth in Kwara state, Nigeria. *African Journal of Reproductive Health, 14* (3) 159-164.

8

Triple Challenges of Psychosocial Factors, Substance Abuse, and HIV/AIDS Risky Behaviors in People Living with HIV/AIDS

Gemechu B. Gerbi, Tsegaye Habtemariam, Berhanu Tameru, David Nganwa, Vinaida Robnett, and Sibyl K. Bowie
Center for Computational Epidemiology, Bioinformatics and Risk Analysis (CCEBRA), College of Veterinary Medicine, Nursing and Allied Health (CVMNAH), Tuskegee University, Tuskegee, Alabama, U.S.A

1. Introduction

Thirty years ago, the first cases of Human Immunodeficiency Virus (HIV) and Acquired Immunodeficiency Syndrome (AIDS) garnered the world's attention. Since then, the lives of people living with HIV/AIDS (PLWHA), their families, communities, and the society as a whole are all affected by the HIV/AIDS pandemic. Not only does HIV/AIDS elicit detrimental physical manifestations but psychosocial health is affected negatively as well in PLWHA. Since the discovery of the Highly Active Antiretroviral Therapy (HAART) in the mid-nineties, PLWHA have overcome the fear of what previously was a certain death sentence. Their life expectancy, as a result of HAART, is now approaching that of the general population (The Antiretroviral Therapy Cohort Collaboration, 2008). However, many PLWHA confront a broad range of challenges that are multiple and chronic in nature. These challenges may yield adverse psychosocial consequences that can lead, eventually, to substance abuse and other HIV/AIDS-risky behaviors.

The discovery that one is infected with the HIV is associated with reduced psychosocial health in China, the United States (U.S), and South Africa (Freeman et al., 2007; Sun, 2007; Vanable, 2006). Studies show that PLWHA have complicated histories including substance abuse, mental illness, mood disorders, and social stigma (Stoskopf, 2004; Pence, 2007a; Whetten, 2006). These negative experiences have been seen across a wide range of populations including adult men and women (Kelly, 1993), men who have sex with men (MSM) (Martin, 1998, Strathdee, 1998), HIV-positive adults (Kelly, 1993), minority women (Champion, 2002), substance users (Camacho, 1996), gay and bisexual men (Rogers, 2003), adolescents, and young adults (Ramrakha, 2000). Furthermore, these negative experiences have been associated with psychosocial disorders which in turn can contribute to increased substance abuse and HIV/AIDS-risky behaviors among PLWHA (Pence, 2007b; Leserman, 2003; Tucker, 2003). Similarly, substance abuse can contribute to numerous problems for PLWHA. For example, alcohol abuse can modify liver drug metabolism, thus complicating treatment for patients with HIV/AIDS hepatitis C virus co-infection as alcohol may compromise pegylated interferon therapy and exacerbate the progression of liver disease (Kresina, 2002).

Since the first cases of HIV/AIDS emerged in the early 1980s HIV/AIDS-related stigma and its resulting discrimination continue to traverse across countries, religious groups, communities, and individuals. According to United Nations Secretary-General Ban Ki Moon, "Stigma remains the single most important barrier to public action. It is the main reason why too many people are afraid to see a doctor to determine whether they have the disease, or to seek treatment if so. It helps make AIDS the silent killer, because people fear the social disgrace of speaking about it, or taking easily available precautions. The stigma associated with it is a chief reason why the AIDS pandemic continues to devastate societies around the world" (Ban Ki-Moon, 2008). For example, if they feel a need to conceal their HIV-positive status within their social network, PLWHA may refuse to use protection during sex for fear that their partners may interpret condom use as a sign of being they are HIV positive (Klitzman, 2004). Stigmatization has been linked to higher risk behaviors in France, South Africa, and China (Mahajan, 2007).

The impact of HIV/AIDS is not only biological but psychosocial in nature. Increasingly it has become evident that psychosocial factors, substance abuse, and HIV/AIDS- risky behaviors co-exit together and therefore contribute to ongoing HIV/AIDS transmission pathways in many regions of the world. Importantly, as newer and more effective treatment therapies continue to evolve psychosocial factors, substance abuse problems, and other co-occurring risky behaviors in PLWHA must be addressed to develop more effective treatment protocols and to formulate highly-effective public health policies and prevention and control strategies to address the HIV/AIDS pandemic. Further, the high prevalence of comorbid medical and psychosocial conditions highlights the urgent need to co-locate varied health services and specialists who understand HIV/AIDS-related psychosocial factors in relation to HIV-risky behaviors so they can provide comprehensive care for the special needs of and overlapping medical and psychological conditions for PLWHA. Sweat and colleagues (2004) suggest a multidisciplinary, integrated approach to HIV/AIDS prevention be adopted to cater to the needs of PLWHA.

With this in mind, a study to address the triple challenges of psychosocial, substance abuse, and HIV/AIDS-risky behaviors among PLWHA has been conducted at the Center for Computational Epidemiology, Bioinformatics and Risk Analysis (CCEBRA), a research center located in the College of Veterinary Medicine, Nursing and Allied Health at Tuskegee University, Tuskegee, Alabama, USA. The specific objective of this study was to determine if significant differences exist in the prevalence of psychosocial factors and HIV/AIDS-risky behaviors before and after establishing HIV infection status among PLWHA.

The study hypothesis tested was: Multi-factorial and quantitative epidemiologic studies which interrelate multiple health determinants can be developed to extrapolate the quantitative contributions of each of these variables that affect the transmission of HIV/AIDS. Based on the epidemiological assessment of factors believed to influence HIV/AIDS-risky behaviors, three underlying assumptions were formulated: 1) With the exception of HIV/AIDS transmission via infected blood/blood products, tissues, or organs, all other HIV/AIDS transmissions occur only as a result of human behaviors; 2) The effects of psychosocial factors and substance abuse on HIV/AIDS-related risky behaviors are particularly pronounced among PLWHA; and 3) Psychosocial factors and substance abuse help to predict an increase or decrease in HIV/AIDS-related risky behaviors. It was hypothesized that psychosocial variables would be associated with substance abuse which in turn would be associated with HIV/AIDS-risky behaviors.

This chapter presents the findings of our original research with respect to triple factors that influence HIV/AIDS transmission among PLWHA. The research methodology and findings are presented under their respective sections. In addition, recommendations for a multidisciplinary approach to research and interventions are provided to address the triple challenges and interrelationships of psychological factors, substance abuse, and HIV/AIDS risky behaviors that are commonly seen in PLWHA.

2. The relationship between psychosocial factors and HIV/AIDS-risky behaviors

A substantial amount of literature indicates depression is one of the most commonly occurring mental disorders identified among PLWHA. HIV/AIDS, its related infections, and the anti-viral drugs used to treat these illnesses can cause depression along with number of other psychiatric disorders (Desquilbet et al., 2002). Psychosocial problems have been associated also with HIV/AIDS-risky behaviors, non-adherence to medications, and shortened survival (Farinpour et al., 2003; Cook et al., 2004). Despite the prevalence of psychosocial distress experienced by PLWHA, the available body of evidence indicates that depression is frequently undiagnosed and goes untreated on a large scale. For example, in a large cohort of patients undergoing care for HIV/AIDS in the U.S., nearly half of those who met the criteria for major depression had no mention of such a diagnosis in their medical records (Asch et al., 2003); and one-third of PLWHA who needed psychosocial health services were not receiving them (Taylor et al., 2004).

However, health care service providers and associated facilities may be unaware of the depressive experiences of their HIV/AIDS patients and the effects these experiences can have on both behaviors and health outcomes. As a result, prevention and treatment of depression and provision of psychosocial support are often neglected in PLWHA, despite the fact that they are critical components of their health care. So, to support and promote mental health throughout the lifespan of the illness a number of interventions, including psychosocial support and basic counseling for depression, are required. As the medical community adapts to managing HIV/AIDS as a chronic disease, understanding the conjoint influence of depression and substance abuse on HIV/AIDS risky behaviors is very important. Failure to recognize these variables may endanger both HIV/AIDS patients and others in the community.

Studies of patients who seek HIV/AIDS treatment or preventive health services have reported a fairly high prevalence of psychosocial problems including depression, anxiety, and hostility (Kalichman, 2000; Cohen et al., 2002). Other research shows that psychosocial variables, such as depression and other mental health problems, drug or alcohol addictions, or any combination of these are most commonly prevalent among PLWHA (Moore et al., 2008; Wyatt et al., 2002; Whetten et al., 2006). It is estimated that up to 50% of PLWHA suffer from a mental illness, such as depression, and 13% have both mental illness and substance abuse issues (Bing et al., 2001). The same study indicates also that one-half of adults living with HIV/AIDS had symptoms of a psychiatric disorder; 19% had signs of substance abuse; 13% had co-occurring substance abuse and mental illness (Bing et al., 2001); and one-half of PLWHA had depression (Lesser, 2008).

These psychosocial problems, in turn, have been shown to influence high-risk sexual behaviors and HIV/AIDS transmission (Benotsch et al., 1999). However, study findings have been inconsistent about the relationship between psychosocial problems and unsafe sexual practices. Some studies have failed to find any relationship (Kalichman, 1999) while other research has demonstrated a negative relationship between psychosocial problems and high-risk sexual behaviors (Robins et al., 1994). The inconsistency in these research findings may be related to the fact that the specific link between HIV/AIDS and psychosocial problems is still not clearly defined. For example, depressive symptoms may lead patients to engage in high-risk behaviors [(e.g., injection drug use (IDU)] and subsequently lead to HIV infection (Angelino, 2002)]. On the other hand, rather than being direct the relationship between negative mood states and high-risk behaviors might be mediated by cognitive factors: being infected may affect mood states which in turn might affect an individual's ability to consistently make rational decisions about safe sex which may then at times lead to high-risk sexual behaviors and eventually lead to HIV/AIDS transmission (Binson et al., 1993). Thus, further research is need to gain a clear understanding of how psychosocial problems are likely to influence PLWHA and impact their ability to consistently make rational decisions is required to fully understand high-risk sexual behaviors among PLWHA.

In addition, depression is noted to be oftentimes associated with substance abuse (Saylors & Daliparthy, 2005) and other HIV/AIDS risky behaviors (Kelly et al., 1993). Substance abuse can cause cognitive impairment (Rippeth et al., 2004) which could also lead to depression (NIDA, 2006). Bing and colleagues (2001) assessed a national probability sample of nearly 3,000 PLWHA and found that more than one-third screened positive for clinical depression, the most common disorder identified. These researchers also indicated that half of the 3,000 PLWHA who participated in the study reported use of illicit drugs. Drug use was associated with screening positive for depression. The study showed also that 36% of HIV-infected individuals screened positive for depressive symptoms in the previous year (Bing et al., 2001). Another study found similar levels, as 35% of participants screened positive for depression (Pence, et al., 2007a). Additionally, studies have indicated higher rates of depression symptoms, ranging between 26% and 49%, in HIV-positive people compared with HIV-negative control groups (Boarts et al., 2006; Spiegel et al., 2003; Ickovic et al., 2001; Pence et al., 2006). The association between depression and substance abuse in predicting HIV/AIDS-risky behaviors has been examined and presented in this chapter.

3. The relationship between substance abuse and risky sexual behaviors

Substance abuse or other drug-taking activities, such as IDU, have long been recognized for their role in HIV/AIDS transmission (National Institute of Drug Abuse, 2006). Sexual intercourse while under the influence of drugs and/or alcohol can generally lower the use of condoms which can increase the risk of HIV/AIDS transmission (Saylors & Daliparthy, 2005) and quite possibly disease progression is more rapid (Zablotska et al., 2006).

PLWHA are more likely to abuse alcohol at some time during their lives (Abderhalden, 2007). A study by the National Institute on Alcohol Abuse and Alcoholism (NIAAA), National Institutes of Health, U.S. Department of Health and Human Services (2008) shows that 80% of people infected with the HIV in the U.S. drink alcohol; between 30% and 60% have been diagnosed with an alcohol-related abuse disorder. In the U.S., a one-month national representative sample of current alcohol use among PLWHA showed a prevalence of 53%, with 8% classified as heavy alcohol consumers (Galvan et al., 2002).

Needles and syringes are the second most common route of HIV transmission in the U.S. [World Health Organization (WHO)/UNAIDS, 2004; WHO, 2005]. Each year more than 8,000 people are newly infected with HIV through the sharing of HIV-contaminated syringes and needles (CDC, 2005). Since the beginning of the HIV pandemic, the CDC (2005) estimates that IDU has directly and indirectly accounted for approximately one-third (36%) of AIDS cases in the U.S. Globally, approximately 10% of HIV infections are a direct result of transmission through IDU (Aceijas et al., 2004).

HIV/AIDS intervention studies that target risky behaviors in various groups have been conducted in an assortment of settings. A study in France, for example, found that the proportion of HIV-positive patients reporting sexual behavior at risk for HIV transmission increased from 5.1% in 1998 to 21.1% in 2001-2002 (Desquilbet, 2002). In addition it has been shown that risky sexual behaviors, including unprotected sex and multiple sexual partners, occur among PLWHA (Schiltz and Sandfort, 2000). For example, a study by Binson (1993) indicates that a considerable percentage of PLWHA (range of 10% to 60% depending on the specific sex acts) continue to engage in unprotected sexual behaviors that place others at risk for infection and place themselves at risk for contracting secondary STDs (e.g., syphilis) which may accelerate HIV infection (Lowry, 1994). In another study conducted between 1999 and 2001 in San Francisco, California, found that the proportion of MSM reporting to have had unprotected anal sex with two or more partners of unknown serostatus increased from 19% to 25% for HIV positive MSM, compared to an increase from 10% to 15% for HIV-negative MSM participants (Chen et al., 2002).

The reasons that underlie the correlation between substance abuse and high-risk behaviors among PLWHA have been described to include: decreased inhibitions and risk perception; belief that alcohol and other drugs enhance sexual arousal and performance; deliberate substance abuse as an excuse for high-risk behaviors; and the indirect association that bars (taverns) are common places to meet potential sexual partners. The mechanisms by which substance abuse influences risky behaviors are associated with situational factors, such as cognitive impairment, social modelling, or the fact that substance abuse and risk-taking behaviors often occur in the same social venues (Abderhalden, 2007).

4. Epidemiologic modelling to study HIV/AIDS dynamics at the macro-population level

Computational models and simulations are emerging as vital research tools in the fields of epidemiology, biology, and other sciences. Increasingly, scientific researchers are recognizing the enormous potential of these research tools to solve some of today's biggest and most complex health problems. Computational epidemiology permits the examination and investigation of diseases and risk agents in plants, animals, and humans without jeopardizing lives or creating hazards. This relatively recent branch of science is being used by researchers to understand the overwhelming complexity of the 21st century's health problems. In light of this, computational models that study HIV/AIDS viral dynamics at the macro-population levels by examining the dynamics of HIV/AIDS among different racial groups have been developed by the CCEBRA at Tuskegee University.

4.1 Systems dynamics modelling at the macro-population level

Systems dynamics (SD) is a concept based on systems thinking where dynamic interaction between the elements of the system is considered in order to study the behavior of the system as a whole. This methodology, introduced in the mid-1950s by Forrester and first described at length in his book *Industrial Dynamics* (1961) with some additional principles presented in his later works (Forrester, 1969; 1971; and 1980), involves development of causal diagrams and computer simulation models that are unique to each problem setting. A central principle of SD is that the complex behaviors of organizational and social systems are the result of ongoing accumulations of people, material or financial assets, information, or even biological or psychological states. Both balancing and reinforcing feedback mechanisms and the concepts of accumulation and feedback have been discussed in various forms for centuries (Richardson, 1991). However, SD uniquely enables the practical application of these concepts in the form of computerized models so that alternative policies and scenarios can be tested in a systematic way that answers the questions of "what if" and "why" (Sterman, 2001).

SD modelling is an iterative process of scope selection, hypothesis generation, causal diagramming, and quantification (Sterman, 2000); it consists of an interlocking set of differential and algebraic equations developed from a broad spectrum of relevant data. A completed SD model may contain scores or even hundreds of equations along with the appropriate numerical inputs. Importantly, epidemiologic SD models are designed to reproduce historical patterns and capable of generating useful insights. The data extrapolated from these epidemiological models are useful not only to study the past, but are reliable also to explore predictive and intervention possibilities (Forrester, 1980; Homer, 1996). With this in mind, a SD model incorporating various HIV/AIDS-risky behaviors has been developed by CCEBRA to model HIV/AIDS.

SD modelling, a tool widely used in epidemiological and mathematical modelling, allows researchers to study and develop a holistic way to assess not only the behavior of the system, but the relationships and interactions between different entities within the system so that scientists can predict what will happen if these systems behaviors persist into the future. If developed carefully, mathematical and statistical models can serve as tools to better understand the epidemiology of HIV/AIDS (Todd et al., 1999). Mathematical models of HIV/AIDS transmission dynamics also play an important role in understanding the epidemiological patterns and methods for disease control as they provide short- and long-term predictions of HIV and AIDS incidence, prevalence, and its dependence on various factors (Todd et al., 1999).

The principles of SD are well suited for modelling and are applicable to HIV/AIDS problems (Dangerfield et al., 2001). The dynamic systems analysis model developed by CCEBRA was performed using the Structural Thinking Experimental Learning Laboratory with Animations (STELLA) software (High Performance Systems, 2000). Applications of systems dynamics methodologies, which employ STELLA software to develop HIV/AIDS models (Dangerfield et al., 2001), addresses the utility of the software in a variety of modelling environments that are suitable for HIV/AIDS modelling purposes.

4.2 The equations that describe the changes in susceptible populations

The HIV infection rate in a given susceptible population directly depends on the proportion of people engaged in HIV/AIDS-risky behaviors. Equations defining all transition states, rates, and parametric variables are very critical in the development of an epidemiologic model. The proportion of people who are not using condoms is the primary focus addressed by this study. Manipulation of the condom use-related variable changes the behavior of the system and results in an increase or decrease of the incidence and prevalence of HIV infections; thus allowing the critical evaluation of alternative HIV/AIDS prevention and control strategies.

A number of basic assumptions are made in the development of the model. These include the assumptions that: 1) the number of susceptibles at a given time are the total population at that point in time; 2) a susceptible can become infected only if he/she engaged in HIV/AIDS-risky behaviors; 3) an individual can move from high HIV/AIDS-risky behaviors to low HIV/AIDS-risky behaviors or vice versa within the infective sub-populations; and 4) the changes in behavior from high-risk to low-risk may be as a result of educational programs that enhance awareness and counseling.

Mathematically, the model parameters are defined as follows. Three major ethnic populations were considered: white, black, and Hispanic, which are designated as ethnic, groups 1, 2, and 3 respectively. Within each group, an individual is considered to be in one of three sex-related statuses: female, heterosexual male, and bisexual/homosexual male, which are designated as sex-related statuses 1, 2, and 3 respectively. Each individual is also considered to be either a non-injecting drug user or injecting drug user. The HIV/AIDS infection rate in a given susceptible population directly depends on the proportion of injecting-drug users, proportion of homosexuals, proportion of people engaged in multiple sexual partnerships, and proportion of people not using condoms. Manipulation of one or several of these variables changes the trend of the system and results in an increase or decrease in the incidence of the HIV/AIDS, thereby supporting the critical evaluation of alternative disease prevention and control strategies.

Mathematically, let:

$S_{ijk}(a,t)$ denote the number of susceptible individuals of ethnic group i, sex-related status j, drug use status k, age a at time t,

$I_{ijk}(a,t,u)$ represent the number of incubating individuals of drug use status k (non-injecting drug user or injecting drug user), sex-related status j, ethnic group i, age a, at time t, who are infected by HIV at time t-u.

Similarly:

$A_{ijk}(a, t, v)$ denote the number of AIDS patients of ethnic group i, sex-related status j, drug use status k, age a, at time t, who become AIDS patients at time t-v.

The equations that describe the changes in susceptible populations, HIV-infected populations, and AIDS populations of ethnic group i, age a at time t were then defined as follows:

$$\frac{\partial S_{ijk}(a,t)}{\partial t} + \frac{\partial S_{ijk}(a,t)}{\partial a} = \{\sigma_{ijk}(a)[1-\gamma_{ijk}(a,t)]-1\}S_{ijk}(a,t) \quad (1)$$

$$\frac{\partial I_{ijk}(a,t)}{\partial t} + \frac{\partial I_{ijk}(a,t)}{\partial a} + \frac{\partial I_{ijk}(a,t)}{\partial \overline{u}} = \{\sigma_{ijk}(a,t)[1-tr(u)]-1\}I_{ijk}(a,t,u) \quad (2)$$

$$\frac{\partial A_{ijk}(a,t,v)}{\partial t}+\frac{\partial A_{ijk}(a,t,v)}{\partial a}+\frac{\partial A_{ijk}(a,t,v)}{\partial v}=\{\mu(v)-1\}A_{ijk}(a,t,v) \tag{3}$$

Where the indices i = ethnic group status, j= sex-related status, and k = individuals of drug use status:
$\sigma_{ijk}(a)$ is the age-specific survival rate of individuals of i, j, and k status;
$\gamma_{ijk}(a,t)$ is the HIV infection rate of individuals of age a at time t with i, j, and k status;
tr(u) is the probability that an individual infected by HIV at time $t-u$ becomes an AIDS patient at time t; and
$\mu(v)$ is the survival rate of individuals who become AIDS patients at time $t-v$.
The number of individuals of age a at time t who acquire HIV by sexual contacts and/or injecting drug use during $[t, t+dt]$ is defined as follows:

$$I_{ijk}(a + da, t + dt, 0) = \sigma_{ijk}(a)\, \gamma_{ijk}(a,t)\, S_{ijk}(a, t). \tag{4}$$

Note that I_{ijk} is the critical HIV infection rate and it relies either on injecting drug use and/or sexual contact. Since interest is to examine condom use as an intervention (HIV preventive approach), how the HIV infection rate via sexual contact is derived is shown.
Let $F_{ijk}(a,t)$ denote the events that an individual of age a, drug use status k, sex related status j, in ethnic group i is infected by HIV during $[t, t+dt)$ due to sexual contact. An individual may have sexual contacts with partners from different ethnic groups. The probability of HIV transmission due to sexual contacts is formulated in terms of the number of partners, number of sexual contacts with each partner, the probability that a partner is infected, and the probability that one contact with an infected partner will result in infection. Since three ethnic groups were considered in this study, each consisting of three sex-related sub groups, the HIV prevalence differs from group to group. The probability that an individual of age a, drug use status k, sex-related status j, in ethnic group i, is infected by HIV at time t, due to sexual contacts is given by:

$$P\left[F_{ijk}(a,t)\right]=1-\prod_{e=1}^{3}\left\{1-q_e(a,t)\right\} \tag{5}$$

Where:

$$q_e(a,t)=1-\left\{1-p_{je}(a,t)\left[1-(1-r)^{m_{ijk,e}}\right]\right\}^{n_{ijk,e}}$$

- is the probability that an individual of age a, drug use status k, sex-related status j, in ethnic group I, is infected by HIV during $[t, t+dt)$ due to sexual contacts with partners from ethnic group e,
- r is the probability of HIV transmission associated with a single sexual contact,
- $n_{ijk,e}$ is the number of sexual partners from ethnic group e,
- $m_{ijk,e}$ is the number of sexual contacts with a partner from ethnic group e, and
- $p_{je}(a,t)$ is the probability that a partner from group e is infected at time t.

If a condom is used during sexual contact, it is assumed to be 100% protective. Although low levels of condom breaks have been reported condom use is considered to be highly effective in preventing transmission of HIV and other sexually transmitted diseases. Three proportions of condom use at 25%, 50%, and 75% were considered, respectively, in each population to simulate and evaluate the impact on reducing the incidence of HIV by preventing disease transmission from infected to healthy individuals.

Once an individual is infected with HIV, after what is most often a long and varied incubation period, the disease advances to the stage of AIDS. The number of individuals of age a at time t, who progress to AIDS status during $[t,t+dt)$ is represented by:

$$A_{ijk}(a+da,t+dt,0)=\sum_{u=1}^{u_{\max}}\sigma_{ijk}(a)p(u)I_{ijk}(a,t,u) \tag{6}$$

Where u_{max} is the maximum incubating time, and $p(u)$ is the probability that an individual infected at time $t-u$ progresses to AIDS status at time t. The systems of equations for different ethnic groups are connected through the HIV infection rate, $\gamma_{ijk}(a,t)$. The results of the model simulations are shown in Figure 1.

4.3 Simulation results

Model parameters were estimated using CDC surveillance data. Computer simulations were carried out on a PowerPC with C as the programming language. In this study, focus was on the use of condoms and its impact on reducing the incidence of the transmission of HIV in sexually active adults in the U.S. The model (Figure 1) shows that if active HIV/AIDS prevention and control interventions are not pursued the HIV/AIDS incidence in the black population would increase from 60 per 100,000 in 1990 to 110 per 100,000 in 2020. In the Hispanic population, incidence would increase from 40 per 100,000 to 68 per 100,000 and in the white population it would increase from around 16 per 100,000 to 23 per 100,000, respectively. This represents an increase in AIDS incidence of 49%, 28%, and 21% for blacks, Hispanics and whites, respectively. As can be seen, these are significant increases for all populations but they are much more devastating for the black subpopulation. Condom use was evaluated in 25% (the status quo used until approximately 1995), 50%, and 75% of sexually active adult populations. The baseline of 25% was used in the model although the rates of condom use varied from low levels of 5% to 10% to 50% or more in previous surveys (CDC, 1996). Figure 1 shows that increased condom use in 50% - 75% of the sexually active population can decrease the rates to the pre-1991 levels, which were 47.9% for blacks, 27.5% for Hispanics, and 11.6% for whites respectively. By the year 2020, the percentage reduction of AIDS would be expected to be 53% in blacks, 49% in Hispanics, and 43% in whites. Previous meta-analysis indicated that condom use could reduce HIV/AIDS by about 69% to 87% (Weller, 1993). A meta-analysis showed that condom use could be effective when used consistently and could potentially reduce HIV by 90% – 95% (Pinkerton and Abramson, 1997). The model simulation examined the proportion of condom use of up to 75%, but if higher levels are evaluated the rate of reduction would be higher and more consistent with the reported findings in the meta-analysis.

Clearly, the significance of HIV/AIDS and its devastation of minority communities pose a great concern. Among racial/ethnic groups, the impact of HIV is greatest among Blacks. According to the CDC (2008), Blacks, who represent approximately 13% of the U.S. population (U.S. Bureau of Census, 2000), have an estimated rate of HIV diagnoses that is 9 times higher than that of whites and nearly 3 times higher than that of Hispanics. The lifetime risk for HIV infection is 1 in 16 for African American men and 1 in 30 for African-American women (Hall, 2008). Hispanics are also disproportionately impacted by HIV/AIDS, representing approximately 15% of the U.S. population but accounting for an estimated 17% of new HIV infections (Hall, 2008). The lifetime risk of an HIV diagnosis is 1 in 36 for Hispanic males and 1 in 106 for Hispanic females (CDC, 2010).

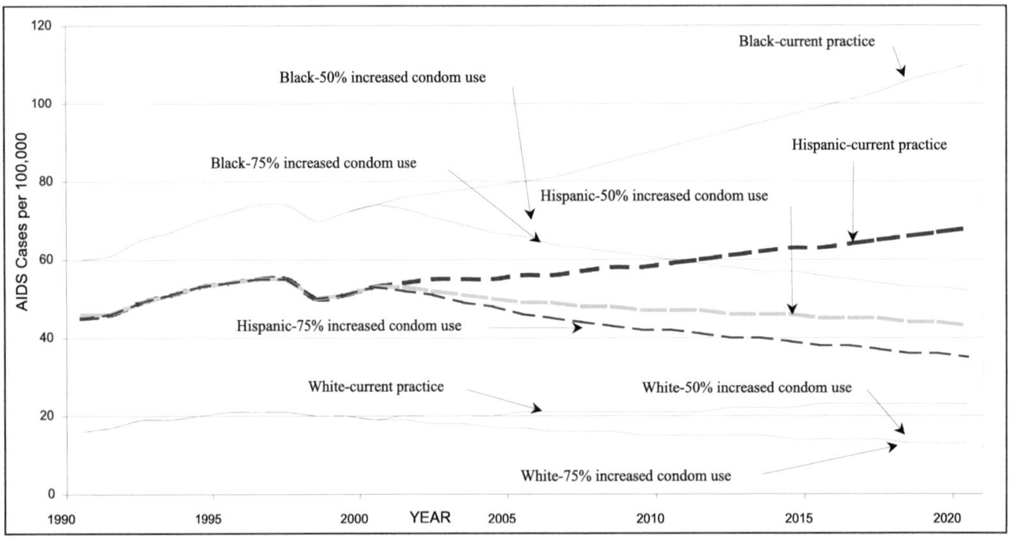

Fig. 1. Projections of AIDS Cases in blacks, Hispanics and whites (under various levels of condom use)

4.3.1 HIV/AIDS as a health disparity in the United States

Among diseases that disproportionately affect African Americans, the HIV/AIDS epidemic has been particularly devastating for this community at every stage of the disease. Despite extraordinary improvements in HIV treatment, African Americans accounted for 48% of new HIV or AIDS diagnoses in 2005 (CDC, 2007). AIDS remains the leading cause of death among black women between 25-34 years and the second leading cause of death in black men between 35-44 years of age (CDC, 2007). HIV infection levels are especially high (3.6%) among blacks aged 40-49, with males in this age group having an HIV prevalence (4.5%) (McQuillan et al., 2006) that approaches the region-wide prevalence in sub-Saharan Africa (5.0%) (UNAIDS, 2008). The rate of AIDS diagnoses for black adults and adolescents was 10 times the rate for whites and nearly 3 times the rate for Hispanics (CDC, 2007), and for black men it was 8 times more than the rate for white men (CDC, 2007). African-American women had a 23 times greater diagnosis rate than white women (Hader et al., 2001). More than 90 % of babies born with HIV belong to minority groups. African Americans are ten times more likely to die of AIDS than whites (U.S. Department of Health and Human Services, 2008).

Studies have also shown higher rates of HIV/AIDS in low-income populations, suggesting that this pandemic is spreading most rapidly among the poor (Hu et al., 1994). This is significant, especially for the South where half of all African Americans live below 200% of the poverty line. Notably, they have significantly less access to health care than people of other races and ethnicities (Preston et al., 2004; Whetten et al., 2005). In Georgia, Jackson,

Mississippi, and North Carolina, African Americans accounted for 70%, 84%, and 62%, respectively, of all PLWHA (Henry J. Kaiser Family Foundation, 2007).

Research suggests SES may affect the likelihood of contracting HIV/AIDS (Simon et al., 1995). In a cross-sectional study, Hargreaves (2002) found that men and women of low SES are at greater risk of newly acquired HIV infection. A study of HIV transmission among African-American women in North Carolina found that women with HIV infection were more likely than non-infected women to be unemployed, receive public assistance, have had 20 or more lifetime sexual partners, have used crack or cocaine, or have traded sex for drugs, money, or shelter (CDC, 1982). A lack of SES resources is linked also to HIV/AIDS-risky behaviors and leads to HIV infection (Simon et al., 1995). For each of the HIV/AIDS risk factors examined, low educational level was more common among minority populations and in women (Diaz et al., 1994).

SES is a key factor that determines the quality of life for PLWHA. Those individuals with fewer resources are often left with limited treatment options (Simon et al., 1995). A study by Diaz and colleagues (1994) indicated that HIV-positive people with lower SES also died sooner than HIV-positive people with higher SES because of their lack of access to medical care, the high cost of antiretroviral drugs, and a lowered immunity from other illnesses. SES is a correlate of behaviors that affect health, access to and use of health care, risk of disease, and mortality (Diaz at al., 1994). When HIV/AIDS rates are examined in light of SES both HIV/AIDS prevalence and incidence are found to be higher among minority populations experiencing high rates of unemployment (Aday, 2001; Fenton, 2001), and lower SES is among the most important determinants of HIV infection among African Americans (Diaz et al., 1994).

These findings have significant implications for the development of effective strategies to prevent and treat HIV/AIDS and other health disparities, particularly for the poor and racial and ethnic minority communities.

5. Community-based epidemiologic research to address the impact of psychosocial factors and substance abuse on HIV/AIDS-risky behaviors

This study is critical to the development of effective strategies to prevent and control a complex disease challenge such as HIV/AIDS, which is faced by millions of people globally. We conducted a community-based epidemiologic study that integrates multiple determinants - including psychosocial and SES factors - that facilitate HIV/AIDS transmission in all populations. The purpose of this study was to assess the quantitative contributions of each of these factors upon HIV/AIDS transmission. The objectives were: 1) to assess the relationships between psychosocial variables and HIV/AIDS-risky behaviors among PLWHA, and 2) to determine if significant differences exist in substance abuse among PLWHA both before and after their HIV infection status has been established.

Materials and methods

Study design

The data was collected by a questionnaire instrument survey of the HIV-positive clients of a community-based HIV/AIDS outreach facility (CBHAOF) located in Montgomery, Alabama, USA. The CBHAOF provides treatment and prevention services through education, quality services, and compassionate care for HIV/AIDS clients and their families in 27 counties in Alabama. In addition, the CBHAOF has a medical component/clinic that provides complete primary health care which includes physician visits and laboratory tests to diagnose HIV infection. The study questionnaire was designed to collect data on behaviors that could be associated with HIV/AIDS transmission in the Black Belt Counties (BBC) of Alabama, which stretch centrally across the state west to southeast. The BBC have a higher percentage (more than 50%) of African-American residents as compared to white residents. The questionnaire was pretested in collaboration with the CBHAOF to assess whether the materials were understood by and could be answered by the target participants. Tuskegee University's Institutional Review Board approved the final questionnaire, informed consent forms, and study protocol. The major modules of the questionnaire included: SES and demographic information; knowledge about HIV/AIDS and HIV testing; and substance abuse and other HIV/AIDS-risk behaviors before and after the knowledge of their HIV infection status. Participants filled out a questionnaire anonymously without any individual identifying information.

Data collection procedures

The data was collected in collaboration with the CBHAOF. The questionnaires and the informed consent forms were given to the facility staff to administer to and retrieve from study participants. The defined criteria to enroll study participants included: age equal to or greater than 18 years; being diagnosed as HIV positive by a laboratory test at the CBHAOF; or having AIDS diagnosed by a physician. A convenience sampling method was used to select the study group. During their regular medical visits eligible participants were informed about the study by the facility's staff. Each participant was approached individually at the end of his/her office visit by a trained interviewer who explained the goals of the study and requested consent for participation in the study. Although a convenience sampling method was used, almost all the clients approached were eligible and agreed to participate in the survey in one of two ways: 1) by signing or returning the consent form prior to their response to the questionnaire, or 2) by simply filling out the questionnaire at clinical sites. Participant's names were not included in the questionnaire, thus maintaining their anonymity.

A total of 341 questionnaires were distributed at the convenience of the participants and returned to CBHAOF staff in a sealed envelope. A total of 326 questionnaires were completed fully and returned; this represents a response rate of 96%. The remaining 15 questionnaires were returned to the facility but were not fully completed and as a consequence they were discarded and not used in the analysis. This represents a 4% refusal/dropout rate. Upon receiving the completed questionnaire CBHAOF staff gave each participant a Wal-Mart gift card valued at $15.00. Tuskegee University provided the gift card as an incentive and a token of appreciation for completing the questionnaire. Researchers at the CCEBRA collected the completed questionnaires from the CBHAOF staff, kept the surveys in a secured location, and entered data into a FileMaker Pro 6.0v4 database.

Statistical analyses

The data was analyzed using SAS System for Windows (SAS Institute Inc. Version 9.0.1 Software). Demographic variables were summarized using descriptive statistics. A path analysis model used the Analysis of Moment Structures (AMOS) version 17.0 Software (Arbuckle et al., 1999) to examine the relationships between all variables of the hypothesized model. A chi-square test was used to examine the association between depression and substance abuse to predict HIV/AIDS-risky behaviors among PLWHA. Regression and Pearson's Correlation analysis were used to determine if significant correlations existed between the quantity of alcohol consumed and select risky sexual behaviors. A paired t-test was used to determine if significant differences existed in the prevalence of substance abuse before and after the knowledge of HIV infection status. The McNemar test was used to test the differences between proportions in the matched-pair case.

5.1 Results

Table 1 shows a summary of the demographic characteristics of the respondents.

Table 2 illustrates standardized regression weights for psychosocial factors regarding HIV/AIDS-risky behaviors among PLWHA. The participants who indicated having lost interest in aspects of life that were important before establishing HIV infection status is significantly related to the use of drugs before sex (total effects' standardized regression coefficient = 0.11, p = 0.02); IDU (total effects' standardized regression coefficient = 0.28, p = <0.001); sharing the same syringe/needle with another person(s) to inject him/herself (total effects' standardized regression coefficient = 0.27, p <0.001); number of sexual partners within one year (total effects' standardized regression coefficient = 0.17, p = 0.001); sex with a prostitute(s) (total effects' standardized regression coefficient = 0.16, p = 0.004); and sex with a person(s) who inject drugs intravenously (total effects' standardized regression coefficient = 0.27, p <0.001). Further, Table 2 indicates that depression is strongly correlated with IDU (total effects' standardized regression coefficient = 0.16, p = 0.002); number of sexual partners within one year (total effects' standardized regression coefficient = 0.22, p <0.001); and condom use (total effects' standardized regression coefficient = 0.34, p <0.001).

The regression coefficients for drinking alcohol before sex were also significantly related to all HIV/AIDS-risky behaviors. As indicated in Table 2, drinking alcohol before sex is correlated directly with using drugs before sex (total effects' standardized regression coefficient = 0.44, p <0.001); sharing the same syringe/needle with another person(s) who self-injects (total effects' standardized regression coefficient = 0.14, p <0.001); number of sexual partners within one year (total effects' standardized regression coefficient = 0.25, p <0.001); condom use (total effects' standardized regression coefficient = 0.17 p = 0.001); and sex with a prostitute(s) (total effects' standardized regression coefficient = 0.17, p = 0.003). The results suggest that drinking alcohol leads to promiscuity and then to increased HIV/AIDS-risky behaviors.

Further analysis of the association between psychosocial variables, especially depression, and HIV/AIDS-risky behaviors among PLWHA, shown in Table 3, indicates that IDU, syringe/needle sharing, substance abuse before sex, and sex with injecting drug users are significantly associated with depression. Among those participants reported to have used drugs intravenously, 60% were depressed compared to 40% not depressed. This indicates that PLWHA who experience depression were significantly more likely to report to have used drugs intravenously compared to non-depressed participants (p = 0.005). Results in Table 3 indicate also that depressed participants were more likely report having shared the same syringe/needle with another person to inject him/herself compared to participants who were not depressed (73 % versus 27 %, p <0.001). Depressed participants were significantly more likely to report alcohol consumption before sex compared to non-depressed participants (57 % versus 43 %, p = 0.002). Furthermore, depression is associated with drug use before sexual intercourse (p = 0.006) and sex with injecting drug users (p = 0.01).

Demographic and socioeconomic characteristics		n	%
Sex	Female	136	42
	Male	181	56
	Transgender	4	1
	Transsexual	5	2
Race	African American	208	64
	White (non-Hispanic)	94	29
	Hispanic	10	3
	Other races	14	4
Age group	18-29	53	19
	30-39	86	30
	40-49	104	37
	50-59	34	12
	60 and above	6	2
Marital Status	Single	183	56
	Married	47	15
	Divorced	47	15
	Separated	31	10
	Widow (er)	3	1
	Other	13	4
Employment Status	Employed for wages	122	39
	Unable to work	59	19
	Unemployed	50	16
	Student	25	8
	Homemaker	25	8
	Self-employed	18	6
	Retired	12	4
Level of education	Graduate school	11	3
	College 4 years or more	50	15
	College 1 year to 3 years	85	26
	Grade 12 or GED	126	39
	Grades 9 through 11	40	12
	Grades 1 through 8	11	3
Level of income	$9,999 or under	97	31
	$10,000 to $14,999	45	14
	$15,000 to $19,999	38	12
	$20,000 to $24,999	36	11
	$25,000 to $29,999	23	7
	$30,000 to $49,999	20	6
	$50,000 to $74,999	13	4
	Don't know	46	14

Table 1. Demographic and socioeconomic characteristics of the participants

Variable	Total effects	p-value
The relationship between lost interests in aspects of life and		
Using drugs before sex	0.11	0.02
Injecting drugs intravenously (IDU)	0.28	<0.001
Needle sharing	0.27	<0.001
Number of sexual partners within 1 year	0.17	0.001
Sex with prostitutes	0.16	0.004
Sex with injection drug users	0.27	<0.001
The relationship between depression and		
Injection drug users	0.16	0.002
Number of sexual partners within 1 year	0.22	<0.001
Condom use	0.34	<0.001
The relationship between drinking alcohol before sex and		
Using drugs before sex	0.44	<0.001
Needle sharing	0.14	0.01
Number of sexual partners within 1 year	0.25	<0.001
Condom use	0.17	0.001
Sex with prostitutes	0.17	0.003

Table 2. The relationships between selected psychosocial variables and HIV/AIDS-risky behaviors among PLWHA

HIV/AIDS risky behaviors	Depressed		Not depressed		
	n	%	n	%	*p* value
Used drugs intravenously					0.005
Yes (N=52)	31	60	21	40	
No (N=238)	91	38	147	62	
Shared the same syringe/needle with another person					<0.001
Yes (N=37)	27	73	10	27	
No (N=254)	95	37	159	63	
Drinking alcohol before sexual intercourse					0.002
Yes (N=77)	44	57	33	43	
No (N=205)	76	37	129	63	
Drug use before sexual intercourse					0.006
Yes (N=40)	26	65	14	35	
No (N=210)	82	39	128	61	
Sex with injecting drug users					0.01
Yes (N=43)	27	63	16	37	
No (N=171)	64	37	107	63	

Table 3. Depression by substance abuse and other HIV/AIDS-risky behaviors

Findings about the participants' alcohol consumption, both before and after having established their HIV infection status, are presented in Table 4. The variables selected for analysis were about the consumption of alcoholic beverages and frequency and number of alcoholic beverages consumed before sex. A statistically significant difference (p = .001) was observed in the variable "drinking alcoholic beverages before sex" among the participants before and after establishing their HIV infection status (Table 4). The analysis of the question "Did you drink any alcoholic beverage such as beer, wine, wine coolers, or liquor before you had sexual intercourse the last time?" shows that before establishing their HIV infection status, 35% of the participants had consumed an alcoholic beverage before sex. In comparison, 28% of the participants indicated that they had consumed an alcoholic beverage before sex after establishing their HIV infection status. The difference between drinking alcohol before sexual intercourse - both before and after the knowledge of HIV infection status - among PLWHA is 18.50% with a 95% confidence interval (CI) from 8.07% to 27.07%; this is statistically significant (p = .0001). No significant differences were observed in other measures of HIV/AIDS-risky behaviors. These include frequency and quantity of alcohol consumed before sex, IDU, and sharing the same syringe or needle with another person (Table 4).

Variable	Before the knowledge of HIV infection status	After the knowledge of HIV infection status	A 95% CI and p value for the difference between proportions
Drink any alcoholic beverage before sex	n = 229	n = 229	
Yes	80 (35 %)	65 (28 %)	(CI, 8.07 -27.87%; p = 0.001)
No	149 (65 %)	164 (72 %)	
Frequency of alcohol consumed before sex	n = 175	n = 158	
A few times	101 (58 %)	83 (53 %)	(CI, -6.1 -16 %; p = 0.42)
Half of the time	32 (18 %)	32 (20 %)	(CI, -6.8 -10.9 %; p = 0.75)
Most of the time	20 (11 %)	15 (9 %)	(CI, -5 -8.9 %; p = 0.67)
Every time	22 (13 %)	28 (18 %)	(CI, -3.2 -13.3 %; p = 0.27)
Number of drinks before sex	n = 173	n = 162	
1-2 drinks	99 (57 %)	83 (51%)	(CI, -5.1 -16 %; p = 0.32)
2-4 drinks	39 (23 %)	42 (26 %)	(CI, -6.6 -12.6 %; p = 0.61)
5 or more drinks	35 (20 %)	37 (23 %)	(CI, -6.2 -12.2 %; p = 0.59)
Injecting drug use	13% (n =225)	12% (n =225)	(CI, -6.6 -6.7 %; p = 0.89)
Sharing the same syringe or needle with another person	74% (n =235)	79% (n =235)	(CI, -18.7-27.8%;p = 0.87)

Table 4. The difference between drinking alcohol before and after establishing HIV infection status

6. Discussion

The association between low SES and risk of HIV infection has been well documented in the scientific literature (Hargreaves, 2002; Solorio et al., 2002). The HIV/AIDS pandemic is most severe in the poorest countries, worldwide, and among people of color (UNAIDS, 1999). Similarly, HIV/AIDS prevalence in the U.S. is disproportionately high in poor communities and runs rampant among African Americans. Although HIV/AIDS affects all races in the U.S. there is no single explanation for why HIV/AIDS affects African Americans disproportionately. A combination of biomedical, behavioral, and SES factors, often working together conjointly, seems to be responsible for this health disparity. Poverty, income inequality, and lack of or limited access to appropriate and high-quality health care programs are some of the social determinants that influence the health of PLWHA.

Studies have shown the prevalence of psychosocial problems not only to be common in PLWHA but related to increased high-risk behaviors. These include drug use before sex, sharing the same syringe/needle with another person to inject themselves, and having had multiple sexual partners. The findings suggest that psychosocial problems influence HIV/AIDS-risky behaviors and may contribute to the high probability of HIV infection within high-risk populations. The most plausible explanation for this finding is that psychosocial problems, such as depression, impair both physical and cognitive functioning and can interfere with the decision to practice safe sexual behaviors. Moreover, depression is a barrier to behavior change. Currently, treating depression is the most successful strategy to effectively reduce the risk of acquiring and spreading HIV/AIDS (Paterson et al., 2000).

In this study, results confirmed that psychosocial variables related to HIV/AIDS-risky behaviors are complex. Thus, a detailed understanding of how psychosocial factors impact on HIV/AIDS risk-taking behaviors among PLWHA might be important for prevention and control purposes. Study results demonstrate substance abuse, especially alcohol, is linked to the tendency to have multiple partners and sexual intercourse without condoms. The findings demonstrated the prevalence of depression in PLWHA which occurs concurrently with substance abuse in this population. Participants significantly reduced alcohol intake post-diagnosis - a research finding that highlights the effectiveness of incorporating alcohol-reduction strategies to reduce HIV/AIDS-risky behaviors - however, PLWHA should be advised not to drink excessive amounts of alcohol, which is associated with high-risk sexual and drug injection-related behaviors that increase the likelihood of HIV transmission (Dag, 2008).

The findings of this study also indicate that PLWHA continue to engage in HIV/AIDS risky behaviors after the knowledge of their HIV status. There are several possible explanations for this finding. First, with the advent of HAART in 1996 mortality among PLWHA decreased dramatically (Bouhnik et al., 2007). Most of the PLWHA who get therapeutic benefits from HAART may attain an improved quality of life and functional status with the alleviation of the physiological, social, and psychological consequences of HIV/AIDS. These gains may be accompanied by increases in HIV/AIDS-risky behaviors that include sharing the same syringe/needle with another person. Secondly, PLWHA may have unrealistic beliefs about the impact of HAART on disease transmission rates and therefore may perceive the consequences of transmitting HIV/AIDS as being less serious than in the past. The proven efficacy of HAART in reducing mother-to-child transmission of HIV/AIDS may reinforce these beliefs. PLWHA who have such beliefs may be less likely to use condoms consistently or may have a higher number of sexual partners than those who do not.

Similarly, PLWHA who are using HAART therapy may be less inclined to insist on safer behaviors if they perceive the consequences of HIV infection to be somewhat less terrible because of the availability and efficacy of this antiretroviral therapy. In this era of HAART, addressing the psychosocial health burdens of PLWHA will be an essential component to the development of effective strategies to combat HIV/AIDS.

While the need for effective psychosocial health services for PLWHA is clear, the challenges are equally evident. At least three areas are suggested as high priorities for future research. First, interventions for depression should be developed for PLWHA. Evidence should be gathered on the effectiveness of such interventions not only for improving mental health but also for reducing substance abuse and HIV/AIDS-risky behaviors so as to reduce transmission of HIV/AIDS. Particular attention is warranted for methods or ways to identify PLWHA who are experiencing depression and to understand and address the mechanisms through which these experiences pose barriers to healthy behaviors.

7. Conclusion and recommendations

In this study, an exhaustive review of literature on the epidemiology and determinants of HIV/AIDS transmission has been organized into a repository from which relevant data for building the dynamic epidemiologic models was derived. The results of epidemiologic models can be used to provide important insights into HIV/AIDS transmission dynamics at the macro (human population) level and to evaluate alternative HIV/AIDS prevention and control strategies. Thus, dynamic epidemiologic modelling is an essential research tool that scientists can employ to make prediction estimates of current prevalence and future incidence of HIV/AIDS cases. Computational models can be used to examine alternative strategies for effective interventions that lead to better planning and policy-making for all disease control and prevention efforts.

Despite knowledge of their status, PLWHA are continuing to engage in HIV/AIDS-risky behaviors. Understanding the multiple variables that impact on HIV/AIDS-risky behaviors among PLWHA will be critical in the search for alternatives to the way in which these problems are addressed at the present time. Psychosocial factors and substance abuse variables, which play a significant role in HIV/AIDS-risky behaviors, may contribute to the high probability of HIV/AIDS transmission. Cross-disciplinary research - to include advanced knowledge of basic and applied psychological and social research and the manners in which they interact together - is needed to develop effective HIV/AIDS prevention and control strategies. Scientists interested in HIV/AIDS research can employ these correlation findings to identify factors that covary with behaviors that put people at risk for negative outcomes.

Recognizing that the impact of HIV/AIDS is not only biological but psychosocial in nature, intervention programs, including education and counseling, must be designed holistically to address the complex challenges faced by PLWHA. This population should be offered or provided a comprehensive set of psychosocial interventions at all levels of the health system. In particular, depression-related issues for PLWHA should be addressed and specific psychosocial and psychotherapeutic interventions should be provided to more effectively address associated alcohol and other substance abuse problems. Based on the findings of this study, our recommendations are as follows to identify and create effective strategies to reduce HIV/AIDS and ultimately eliminate this devastating pandemic: 1) Create dynamic epidemiologic models that integrate SES and psychosocial variables as they are required to explore the epidemiology of HIV/AIDS; 2) Use epidemiologic models to address the social determinants of health as these factors are critical to reduce and eliminate HIV/AIDS and other health disparities; 3) Advance research to examine the resistance to behavior change as well as the motivation for behavior change as these factors also are central to the design of effective HIV/AIDS prevention and intervention strategies; 4) Develop cross-disciplinary research that includes advanced knowledge of basic and applied psychological and social research and the ways in which they interact together; and 5) Encourage strong collaborations among researchers, policy-makers, and communities to identify and address biomedical, behavioral, and psychosocial factors that are responsible for the risky sexual behaviors that ultimately result in further transmission of HIV/AIDS.

8. Acknowledgment

This work was supported by a Research Centers in Minority Institutions (RCMI) Award, 2G12RR03059-16, from the National Center for Research Resources and Project EXPORT Award from the National Center on Minority Health and Disparities (NCMHD), National Institutes of Health (NIH), U.S. Department of Health and Human Services (HHS).

9. References

Abderhalden, I. (2007). An increasing major threat to public health. The globalization of alcohol abuse. *Bulletin von Medicus Mundi Schweiz*, 106. 11.16. 2010, Available from http://www.medicusmundi.ch/mms/services/bulletin/bulletin106_2007/chapter2/23.html

Aceijas, C., Stimson, V., Hickman, M., & Rhodes, T. (2004). Global overview of injecting drug use and HIV infection among injecting drug users. *AIDS*, 18, 2295–2303.

Aday, L. A. (2001). *At Risk in America: The Health and Health Care Needs of Vulnerable Populations in the United States*. 2nd ed . San Francisco, CA: Jossey-Bass.

Angelino, F. (2002). Depression and adjustment disorder in patients with HIV disease. *Topics in HIV Medicine*; 10(5): p. 31-35.

Asch, M., Kilbourne, M., & Gifford, L. (2003). Under diagnosis of depression in HIV: who are we missing? *J Gen Intern Med*, 18: 450–60.

Ban Ki-moon op-ed (2008, 6th August). The stigma factor. The Washington Times. 02.18.11, Available from: http://www.washingtontimes.com/news/2008/aug/06/the-stigma-factor

Benotsch, E., S. C. Kalichman, A., & Kelly, J. (1999). Sexual compulsivity and substance use in HIV-seropositive men who have sex with men: prevalence and predictors of high-risk behaviors. *Addictive Behaviors*; 24(6): p. 857-868.

Bing, G., Burnam, A., & Longshore, D. (2001). Psychiatric disorders and drug use among human immunodeficiency virus-infected adults in the United States. *Arch Gen Psychiatry* ;58:721- 8.

Binson, D., Dolcini, M., Pollack, L., & Catania, J. (1993). Multiple sexual partners among young adults in high-risk cities. *Family Planning Perspectives*, 25(6):268–272.

Boarts, M., Sledjeski, M., Bogart, L., & Delahanty, D. (2006) The differential impact of PTSD and depression on HIV disease markers and adherence to HAART among people living with HIV. *AIDS Behav*;10: 253–61.

Bouhnik, D., Preau, M., & Lert, F. (2007). Unsafe sex in regular partnerships among heterosexual persons living with HIV: evidence from a large representative sample of individuals attending outpatients services in France (ANRS-EN12-VESPA Study). *AIDS*;21(Suppl 1):57–62.

Camacho, M., Bartholomew, G., Joe, W., & Cloud, A. (1996). Gender, cocain and during-treatment HIV risk reduction among injection opiod users in methadone maintenance. *Drug and Alcohol Dependence*; 41 (1):1-7.

Centers for Disease Control and Prevention (1982). Update on Kaposi's sarcoma and opportunistic infections in previously healthy persons-United States. *Mortality and Morbidity Weekly Report* ; 31:294.

Centers for Disease Control and Prevention (1996). HIV/AIDS Surveillance Report. *U.S. HIV and AIDS cases reported through December 1996.*

Centers for Disease Control and Prevention (2005). HIV/AIDS Surveillance Report, 2005, Vol. 17. Atlanta, 02.10.11, Available from http://www.cdc.gov/hiv/topics/surveillance/resources/reports/

Centers for Disease Control and Prevention (2007). HIV/AIDS Surveillance Report, Vol. 17, Revised Edition; June 2007, 03.25.11, Available from http://www.cdc.gov/hiv/topics/surveillance/resources/reports/2005report/pdf/2005surveillancereport.pdf

Centers for Disease Control and Prevention (2008). HIV Surveillance Report; vol 20, 02.20.11, Available from http://www.cdc.gov/hiv/surveillance/resources/reports/2008report/

Centers for Disease Control and Prevention (2010). Estimated Lifetime Risk for Diagnosis of HIV Infection among Hispanic/Latinos – 37 States and Puerto Rico, 2007. MMWR, 2010, 59(40)1297-1301, 03. 12.11, Available from http://www.cdc.gov/mmwr/preview/mmwrhtml/mm5940a2.htm

Champion, D., Shain, N., Piper, J., & Perdue, T. (2002). Psychological distress among abused minority women with sexually transmitted diseases. *J Am Acad Nurse Pract* 14:316-24.

Chen, Y., Gibson, S., Katz, M., Klausner, J.M., Dilley, J., Schwarcz, S., Kellogg, T., & McFarland, W. (2002). Continuing increases in sexual risk behavior and sexually transmitted diseases among men who have sex with men: San Francisco, Calif, 1999-2001, U.S.A. *Am J Public Health*; 92(9):1387-8.

Cook, A., Grey, D., & Burke, J. (2004).Depressive symptoms and AIDS-related among a multisite cohort of HIV-positive women. *Am J Public Health*; 94:133-1140.

Dag, E. (2008). Alcohol and HIV/AIDS - possible connections. 11.08.10, Available fromhttp://www.add-resources.org/alcohol-and-hivaids-possible-connections.4451564-76188.html

Dangerfield, B., Fang, Y., & Roberts, C. (2001). Model based scenarios for the epidemiology of HIV/AIDS: the consequences of highly active antiretroviral therapy. *System Dynamics Rev.*;17:119–150.

Desquilbet, L., Deveau, C., Goujard, C., Hubert, J., Derouineau, J., & Meyer, L. (2002). Increase in at-risk sexual behaviour among HIV-1- infected patients followed in the French PRIMO cohort. *AIDS*; 16(17): p. 2329-2333.

Diaz, T., Chu, S., & Buehler, S. (1994). Socioeconomic differences among people with AIDS: results from a multistate surveillance project. *Am I Prey Med*. 1994;10:217-222.

Farinpour, R., Miller, N., & Satz P. (2003). Psychosocial risk factors of HIV morbidity and mortality: Findings from the Multicenter AIDS Cohort Study (MACS). *J Clin Exp Neuropsychol* ;25:654-670).

Fenton, A. (2001). Strategies for improving sexual health in ethnic minorities. *Curr Opin Infect Dis.*;14:63–9.

Forrester, J. W. (1961). *Industrial Dynamics*. Cambridge, Mass: MIT Press.

Forrester, J. W. (1969). *Urban Dynamics*. Cambridge, Mass: MIT Press.

Forrester, J. W. (1971). Counterintuitive behavior of social systems. *Technol Rev.*;73:53–68.

Forrester, J. W. (1980). Information sources for modelling the national economy. *J Am Stat Assoc.* ;75:555–574.

Freeman, M., Nkomo, N., Kafaar, Z., & Kelly, K. (2007). Factors associated with prevalence of mental disorder in people living with HIV/AIDS in South Africa. *AIDS Care*; 19 (10):1201-09.

Galvan, F. Bing, H., Fleishman, G., London, A., Caetano, S., Burnam, R., Longshore, A., Morton, D., Orlando, C., & Shapiro, M. (2002). The prevalence of alcohol consumption and heavy drinking among people with HIV in the United States: Results from the HIV Cost and Services Utilization Study. *Journal of Studies in Alcohol*, 63, 179–186.

Hader, S., Smith, D., Moore, J., & Holmberg, S. (2001). HIV infection in women in the United States: status at the millennium. *JAMA* 20;285:1186–1192.

Hall, I., Song, R., Rhodes, P., Prejean, J., An Q Lee M., Karon, J., Brookmeyer, R., Kaplan, H., & McKenna, T. (2008). Estimation of HIV Incidence in the United States. *JAMA*, August 6, 2008;300(5):520.

Hargreaves, J. R. (2002). Socioeconomic status and risk of HIV infection in an urban population in Kenya. *Trop Med Int Health*. 2002;7:793–802.

Henry, J. Kaiser Family Foundation (2007). An Overview of HIV/AIDS in Black America, 2007., 06.15.2008, Available from www.kff.org/hivaids/ upload/7660.pdf

High Performance Systems (HPS), (2000). *STELLA reference manual*.

Homer, J. B. (1996). Why we iterate: scientific modelling in theory and practice. *System Dynamics Rev.*;12:1–19.

Hu, J., Frey, R., & Costa, J. (1994). Geographic AIDS rates and sociodemographic variables in the Newark, New Jersey, metropolitan area. *AIDS Public Policy* ;9:20-25.

Ickovic, R., Hamburger, E., Vlahov, D., Schoenbaum, E., Schuman, P., Boland, J., & Moore, J. (2001). HIV epidemiology research study group. Mortality, CD4 cell count decline, and depressive symptoms among HIV seropositive women. *JAMA*;285:1466 -74.

Kalichman, C. (1999). Psychological and social correlates among men and women living with HIV/AIDS. *Aids Care*; 11(4): pp. 415-428.

Kalichman, C. (2000). HIV transmission risk behaviors of men and women living with HIV-AIDS: prevalence, predictors, and emerging clinical interventions. *Clinical Psychology: Science Practice*; pp. 32-47.

Kelly, A., Murphy, A., & Bahr, R. (1993). Factors associated with severity of depression and high-risk sexual behavior among persons diagnosed with human immunodeficiency virus (HIV) infection. *Health Psychology* 12:215-19.

Klitzman, L., Kirshenbaum, B., Dodge, B., & Remien, H. (2004). Intricacies and inter-relationships between HIV disclosure and HAART: a qualitative study. *AIDS Care* 16 (628-640).

Kresina, F., Flexner, W., Sindair, J., & Correia, A. (2002). Alcohol use and HIV pharmacology. *AIDS Res Hum Retroviruses;* 18 (757-70).

Leserman, J. (2003). HIV disease progression: depression, stress and possible mechanisms. *Biol Psychiatry;* 54 (295-306).

Lesser, J. (2008). Role of depression, stress, and trauma in HIV disease progression. *Psychosomatic Medicine,* 70, 539-545).

Lowry, R., Holtzman, D.. Truman, B., Kann, I., Collins, L., & Kolbe, L. (1994). Substance use and HIV-related sexual behaviors among U.S. high school students: are they related? *American Journal of Public Health;* 84(7): 1116–1120.

Mahajan, P. (2007). An overview of HIV/AIDS workplace policies and programmes in southern Africa. *AIDS;* 21 (Suppl 3):S31-39.

Martin, L., & Knox, J. (1998). Loneliness and sexual risk behavior in gay men. Psychological Report 24:29-36.

McQuillan, M., B. J. Kottiri, & D. Kruszon-Moran (2006). Prevalence of HIV in the U.S. Household Population: The National Health and Nutrition Examination Surveys, 1988 to 2002. *J Acquir Immune Defic Syndr;*41:651-656

Moore, R.M., Gebo, K.A., Lucas, G.M., & Keruly, J.C. (2008). Rate of Co-morbidities Not Related to HIV infection or AIDS among HIV-Infected Patients, by CD4 Count and HAART Use Status. *Clin Infect Dis;* 47(8):1102-1104.

National Institute of Drug Abuse. (2006, September). ethamphetamine abuse and addiction. 03.23.11, Available from www.nida.nih.gov/PDF/RRMetham.pdf

National Institute on Alcohol Abuse and Alcoholism (NIAAA) of the National Institutes of Health, U.S. Department of Health & Human Services (2008). 02.22.11, Available from http://pubs.niaaa.nih.gov/publications/AA74/AA74.htm

Paterson, L., Swindells S., Mohr J., Brester, M., Vergis, N., Squier, C., Wagener, M., and Singh N (2000). Adherence to protease inhibitor therapy and outcomes in patients with HIV infection. *Ann Intern Med;* 133:21–30

Pence, B. W., Miller, W., Whetten, K., Eron, J. J., Gaynes, B. (2006). N. Prevalence of DSM-IV-defined mood, anxiety, and substance use disorders in an HIV clinic in the Southeastern United States. *J Acquir Immune Defic Syndr* ;42:298 –306.

Pence, B., Reif, S., Whetten, K., Leserman, J., Stangl, D., Swartz, M., Thielman, N., Mugavero, M. (2007b). Minorities, the poor, and survivors of abuse: HIV-infected patients in the U.S. Deep South. *South Med J;*100:1114–22.

Pence, BW, Miller WC, Gaynes BN Eron JJ. (2007a). Psychiatric illness and virologic response in patients initiatiing high active antiretroviral therapy. *Journal of Acquired Immune Deficiency Syndome* 44:159-66.

Pinkerton, S.D. & Abramson, P.R. (1997). Effectiveness of condoms in preventing HIV transmission. *Science & Medicine;*44, 1303-1312.

Preston, D. B., A. R. D'Augelli, and C. D. Kassab (2004). The influence of stigma on the sexual risk behavior of rural men who have sex with men. *AIDS Education and Prevention;*16:291-303.

Ramrakha, S, Capsi A, Dickson N, & Moffitt TE, (2000). Psychiatric disorders and risky sexual behavior in young adulthood: cross sectional study in birth cohort. *BMJ* 321:263-66.

Richardson, G. P. (1991). *Feedback Thought in Social Science and Systems Theory.* Philadelphia, Pa: University of Pennsylvania Press.

Rippeth, J.D., Heaton, R.K., Carey, C.L, Marcotte, T.D., Moore, D.J., Gonzalez, R., & Grant, I. (2004). Methamphetamine dependence increases risk of neuropsychological impairment in HIV infected persons. *Journal of the International Neuropsychological Society*; 10(1), 1-14).

Robins, A. G., M. A. Dew, S. Davidson, L. Penkower, J. T. Becker, & L. Kingsley(1994). Psychosocial factors associated with risky sexual behavior among HIV-seropositive gay men. *AIDS Educ Prev*; 6(6): p. 483-492.

Rogers, G, Curry M, Oddy J, & Pratt N, (2003). Depressive disorders and unprotected casual anal sex among Australian homosexually active men in primary care. *HIV Medicine;* 4:271-75.

Saylors, K., & Daliparthy, N. (2005). Native Women, Violence, Substance Abuse and HIV Risk. *Journal of Psychoactive Drugs;* 37(3), 273-281.

Schiltz, A. & M. Sandfort (2000). HIV-positive people, risk and sexual behaviour. *Social Science & Medicine;* 50: p. 1571-1588.

Simon, P. A, D. J. Hu, T. Diaz, & P. R. Kerndt (1995). Income and AIDS rates in Los Angeles county. *AIDS*;9:281-284.

Solorio, M., R. Asch, S. Globe, & E. Cunningham (2002). The association of access to medical care with regular source of care and sociodemographic characteristics in patients with HIV and tuberculosis. *J Natl Med Assoc.* ;94:581-9.

Spiegel, D., Israelski, D. M., Power, R., Prentiss, D. E., Balmas, G., Muhammad, M., Garcia, P., and Koopman, C. (2003). Acute stress disorder, PTSD, and depression in a clinic-based sample of patients with HIV/AIDS. *J Psychosom Res*;55:128.

Sterman, J. (2001). System dynamics modelling: tools for learning in a complex world. *Calif Manage Rev.*; 43:8-25.

Sterman, J. D. (2000). *Business Dynamics: Systems Thinking and Modelling for a Complex World.* Boston, Mass: Irwin/McGraw-Hill.

Stoskopf, C., Kim, K., Glover, H. (2004). Dual diagnosis: HIV and mental illness, a population-based study. *Community Ment Health J*;37: 469-79.

Strathdee, A., Hogg, S., & Martindale, L. (1998). Determinants of sexual risk-taking among young HIV-negative gay and bisexual men. *AIDS* 19:61-66.

Sun, H., Zhangm, J., & Fu, X. (2007). Psychological status, coping, and social support of people living with HIV/AIDS in Central China. *Public Health Nursing;* 24 (2):132-40.

Sweat, D., O'Reilly R., Schmid, P., & Denison, J. (2004). Cost-efectiveness of nevirapine to prevent mother-to-child HIV transmission in eith African countries. *AIDS;* 18 (1661-1671).

Taylor, L., Burnam, A., & Sherbourne, C. (2004). The relationship between type of mental health provider and met and unmet mental health needs in a nationally representative sample of HIV-positive patients. *J Behav Health Serv Res;* 31: 149-63.

The Antiretroviral Therapy Cohort Collaboration (2008). Life expectancy of individuals on combination antiretroviral therapy in high-income countries: a collaborative analysis of 14 cohort studies. *Lancet;* 20; 372: 293-9.

Todd, C., Patel, E. Simunyu, F., Gwanzura, W., Acuda, M., Winston, & A. Mann (1999). The onset of common mental disorders in primary care attenders in Harare, Zimbabwe. *Psychological Medicine* 29, 97-104.

Tucker, S., Burnam, A., Sherbourne, D., & Kung, Y. (2003). Substance use and mental health correlates of non-adherence to antiretroviral medications in a sample of patients with human immunodeficiency virus infection. *American Journal of Medicine* 114:573-80.

U.S. Bureau of Census (2000). State and County Quick Facts. 05.20.10, Available from http://quickfacts.census.gov/qfd/states/37000.html

U.S. Department of Health and Human Services (2008). Closing The Health Gap. 07.22.10, Available from http://www.healthgap.omhrc.gov/hiv_aids.htm

UNAIDS (1999). Resolution to create and support the partnership. International Partnership against HIV/AIDS in Africa. *Meeting of the UNAIDS Cosponsoring Agencies and Secretariat.* Annapolis, MD, January, 1999.

UNAIDS (2008). Report on the global AIDS epidemic, 2008, 03.15.11, Available from http://www.unaids.org/en/dataanalysis/epidemiology/2008reportontheglobalaidsepidemic/

Vanable, A., Carey, P., Blair, C., & Littlewood, A. (2006). Impact of HIV-related stigma on health behaviors and psychological adjustment among HIV-positive men and women. *AIDS and Behavior*; 10 (5):473-82.

Weller, C. (1993). A meta-analysis of condom effectiveness in reducing sexually transmitted HIV. *Soc. Sci. Med.* 36, pp. 1635–1644.

Whetten, K., Leserman, J., Lowe, K., Stangl, D., Thielman, N., Swartz, M., Hanisch, L., & Van Scoyoc, L. (2006). Prevalence of childhood sexual abuse and physical trauma in a southern HIV positive sample from the Deep South. *Am J Public Health*; 96:970 -3.

Whetten, K., Reif, S. Napravnik, S., Swartz, N., Thielman, J. Eron, K., Lowe, & Toto, T. (2005). Substance Abuse and Symptoms of Mental Illness Among HIVpositive Persons in the Southeast, *Southern Medical Journal*, Volume 98, Number 1, January 2005.

WHO (2005). Effectiveness of drug dependence treatment in preventing HIV among injecting drug users. 02.11.11, Available from http://www.who.int/hiv/pub/idu/idupub/en/

WHO/UNAIDS (2004). Coalition ARVS4IDU (2004, 15th July), Availability of ARV for Injecting Drug Users: Key Facts—2004, XV International AIDS Conference (Satellite meeting), Bangkok.

Wyatt, E., Myers, F., Williams, K., Kitchen, R., Loeb, T., Carmona, J., Wyatt, E., Chin, D., Presley, N. (2002). Does a history of trauma contribute to HIV risk for women of color? Implications for prevention and policy. *Am J Public Health*;92:660–5.

Zablotska, B., Gray, H., Serwadda, D., Nalugoda, F., Kigozi, G., Sewankambo, N., Lutalo, T., Wabwire- Mangen, F., & Wawer, M. (2006). Alcohol use before sex and HIV acquisition: A longitudinal study in Rakai Uganda, *AIDS*, 20, 1191–1196.

9

Growing Up in the Era of AIDS: The Well-Being of Children Affected and Infected by HIV/AIDS in Sub-Saharan Africa

Marguerite Daniel
University of Bergen
Norway

1. Introduction

Children may be affected by HIV/AIDS in numerous ways. When parents fall ill from HIV-related infections, household income falls or is diverted to medical expenses, food insecurity increases and children may have to drop out of school to take on care responsibilities. When parents die, children are orphaned and, besides coping with grief at the loss of their mother or father, they face new care arrangements which may involve separation from siblings and migration to a new location. Most of the children who are orphaned and made vulnerable by HIV/AIDS live in sub-Saharan Africa. UNAIDS (2010, p. 180) estimates that 67.6 percent of people living with HIV globally are found in sub-Saharan Africa, but nearly 90 percent of all children orphaned by AIDS - 12.1 million children - live in sub-Saharan Africa (UNAIDS, 2010, p. 186).

Children may be infected with HIV through mother to child transmission (MTCT) during pregnancy, at birth or through breast milk. Such paediatric AIDS is increasingly being discovered and treated through programmes to prevent MTCT (PMTCT). Adolescents may be living with HIV: they may have been infected by MTCT and survived through childhood or they may have been infected through sexual intercourse, sadly often through being raped. UNICEF et al. (2010, p. 15) call this a "hidden epidemic" because many adolescents living with HIV do not know they are infected, they have never been tested and do not access treatment. UNICEF et al. (2010, p. 41) estimate that in 2009 92 percent of children (under the age of 15) who were living with HIV were in sub-Saharan Africa (nearly 2 million children) and 70 percent of these were found in East and southern Africa. In sub-Saharan Africa in 2009 only 26 percent of children deemed to require antiretroviral treatment (ART) were estimated to receive it (UNICEF, et al., 2010, p. 41).

Sub-Saharan Africa clearly bears a disproportionate burden when it comes to the effects of HIV/AIDS, particularly on children. This chapter gives an overview of the impact of HIV/AIDS on the well-being of affected and infected children, and reviews the responses at community, national and international levels.

2. Children affected by HIV/AIDS

Various terms have been used to describe children who have been affected by HIV/AIDS. Early studies on the social impact of HIV/AIDS used the concept of 'AIDS orphan' defined as a child below the age of 18 who has lost one or both parents to HIV/AIDS. In 2004, UNICEF et al. (2004, pp. 3-4) commented on the fact that there are many ways in which HIV/AIDS can make children vulnerable, for example, children whose parents were ill, but had not yet died, were already vulnerable; hence the term 'orphans and vulnerable children' (OVC) was preferred (Sherr et al., 2008; UNICEF, et al., 2004). However, AIDS is not the only cause of orphaning so the concept of OVC included children orphaned by other causes. Labelling as orphans children who have lost one parent and continue to live with the surviving parent equates their vulnerability with that of double orphans whose lived experience may be very different. Meintjies & Giese (2006) are highly critical of the focus, particularly by international agencies such as UNICEF, on the term 'orphan' when it is used without clear specification of age and the details of which parent(s) died. The term 'children affected by HIV/AIDS' includes children orphaned by AIDS, children who are vulnerable because their parents are ill with HIV/AIDS-related infections or who experience HIV-related poverty, food insecurity or psychosocial challenges. It excludes children orphaned by causes other than HIV/AIDS.

2.1 Caregiving situation

Many children whose parents are HIV positive experience the prolonged illness and eventual death of their parents from AIDS-related infections. Children often take on significant care responsibilities such as preparing food, cleaning, other household chores as well as providing physical and moral support for the ill parent (Bauman et al., 2006). Skovdal and colleagues (2009, 2010) have studied the impact on children's well-being when they care for sick parents and caregivers. Prolonged illness leads to a reduction in household income and food production, depletion of savings due to expenditure on health services (van Blerk & Ansell, 2007) and children are frequently obliged to try and earn some cash and produce food in addition to taking care of their sick parents (Skovdal, 2010; Skovdal & Ogutu, 2009; Skovdal et al., 2009) . When children affected by HIV/AIDS take on productive and reproductive tasks, this often involves dropping out of school. The roll-out of antiretroviral treatment (ART) in the past decade has significantly reduced death from AIDS (Mwagomba et al., 2010; Reniers et al., 2009), but as there is not yet full coverage for all those who need ART, some children continue to experience parental illness and death.

In many parts of Africa it is customary for children to stay for some time with adults other than their biological parents (usually members of the extended family), for example a child from a rural area might live with a relative in an urban area to access a level of schooling unavailable in the rural area. Such 'voluntary' fostering was seen as mutually beneficial: the child would get an education and the foster caregiver would receive agricultural products from the rural area and help with household chores (Madhavan, 2004). AIDS has introduced 'crisis' fostering where adult relatives feel obliged to take on children whose parents have died; such fostering lacks the element of reciprocity and is instead "a normative social obligation" (Goody, 1982, cited in Madhavan, 2004, p. 1444). While many children receive good care from their new caregivers, others may experience varying degrees of injustice and abuse. Several studies document how orphaned children may have to do a disproportionate amount of household chores, and may receive less food and clothing than the children of their new caregiver (M. Daniel, 2005; Madhavan, 2004; van Blerk & Ansell, 2007).

The nature of the kin relationship often affects the experience of the child. A study in Botswana found that when the new caregiver was the maternal grandmother, there was greater stability for the children who had lost parents, while when an aunt or uncle took responsibility the children were more likely to have to migrate (and get used to living in a new place with new neighbours and friends) and they were more likely to suffer physical and psychosocial abuse (M. Daniel, 2005). Van Blerk & Ansell (2007) analyse the experiences of children moving to new homes in terms of the intergenerational contract. Parents invest in their children's education in the expectation that their children will care for them when they are no longer able to work. When HIV/AIDS removes the productive adults from the contract, other productive adults from the extended family have to step in and take on the responsibilities; the contract breaks down completely where the extended family is unable to meet the needs (van Blerk & Ansell, 2007, p. 870).

Orphaned children, in some cases, have no adult who is able to care for them or the adult caregiver is not able to provide adequate care and they live without an adult. Child-headed households (CHHs) may be defined as households headed by a person who is under 18 years of age (Hosegood et al., 2007, p. 331) and Luzze & Ssedyabule (2004) add that it should be recognised by the community as an independent household. Whether or not the AIDS epidemic is contributing to the phenomenon is contested in the literature with some contending that there is an increase in CHHs as a result of parental death and parallel impact on extended family (Evans, 2010; Kipp, Satzinger, Alibhai, & Rubaale, 2010; Luzze, 2002; Luzze & Ssedyabule, 2004) while other authors assert that there is no evidence of an increase in the incidence of CHHs (Hosegood, 2008; Hosegood, et al., 2007; Meintjes, Hall, Marera, & Boulle, 2010; Monasch & Boerma, 2004). Hosegood et al. (2008) point out that it is quantitative studies based on demographic surveys and census material that show low and unchanging incidence while qualitative studies focussed on CHHs find plenty of evidence of their existence. Luzze & Ssedyabule (2004) in a qualitative study of 969 CHHs in one district in Uganda, found that orphans living in CHHs are poorer than other orphans, have lower school attendance and poorer access to social services. Orphans who care for their siblings are no longer classed as children when they turn 18, even though no other circumstances have changed. Evans (2010) notes that rigorous application of age definitions does little to support young caregivers in need; she uses the more inclusive term "sibling headed households" and describes how they often play down their 'adult' roles when negotiating assistance from NGOs or government agencies.

Institutional care is another alternative for orphans when the extended family is unable to meet their needs after the death of their parents. International organisations like UNICEF and UNAIDS, and western researchers view institutional care and orphanages as a last resort and the worst possible alternative. Sherr et al. (2008), for example, state that institutionalised children have poor outcomes and van Blerk &Ansell (2007) mention the inability of orphanages to meet the children's emotional (and sometimes physical) needs. Tolfree (2003) contends that the cost per child of providing institutional care is much greater than community care. In the "Framework for the protection, care and support of OVC living in a world with HIV and AIDS" which was the outcome of the first Global Partners' Forum convened by UNICEF in 2003, five key strategies are outlined (UNICEF, et al., 2004, p. 5). These strategies focus entirely on the family and community, institutions are not even mentioned. More recently the Joint Learning Initiative on Children and HIV/AIDS (JLICA) which concluded its work in 2009, based its learning groups largely on the "Framework" strategies (JLICA, 2011). Publications reflect the lack of interest in institutions, for example, when considering "evidence for changes in children's living and care arrangements" institutions are not even mentioned (Hosegood, 2008, p. 40). However, another JLICA report by Wakhweya et al. (2008, p. 19) describes the difficulty in finding literature on 'family centred' care and they consider this might attributed to 'family' being a Western concept while the extended family or community is more the more usual focus in Africa. Whetten et al. (2009), in a study comparing institutional and community care of orphans and abandoned children in five countries (Ethiopia, Kenya, Tanzania, India & Cambodia) found that children in institutions were no worse off than those in the community in terms of health, emotional and cognitive functioning. They also found that "Many institutions grew out of the community to meet the need of caring for the new wave of orphans and are part of the community in a way that institutions in other regions [...] are not" (Whetten, et al., 2009, p. 9). In very poor communities extended family caregivers may not be able to provide adequate material care and orphans may be better off in institutions (Whetten, et al., 2009). A study in Botswana of a more traditional residential institution found that the children had access to increased resources such as "food security, decent shelter and uninterrupted education" although they felt disconnected to siblings, family and community (Morantz & Heymann, 2010, p. 14). Given the size and growth of the orphan challenge and the indications that the extended family is under stress, institutions should at least be considered; however residential care in Africa is an under-researched area.

2.2 Material well-being

Sickness reduces income earning capacity and ability to produce food leading to a fall in income and an increase in food insecurity. Once parents die, orphans are more likely than non-orphans to lack basic material needs, especially food security. This results in OVC being more likely to be malnourished than non-orphans (Watts et al., 2007).

Households caring for orphans have to spread resources between more people and may therefore experience lower levels of nutrition and health care and a lack of basic needs. A study in Botswana found that even where adults in the household were working, impoverishment increased when orphans were included in a household (Miller et al. 2006) and caregivers had to take unpaid leave from work to care for sick orphans (Heymann et al. 2007).

2.2.1 Access to essential services

Some studies have reported the unequivocal impact of orphanhood on education. Children whose parents were ill were more likely to experience increased absenteeism as they were needed at home for care duties, household chores and food production; as poverty increased, school fees could no longer be afforded and children were forced to drop out; the psychosocial impact of parental illness and death also had an impact on school performance often leading to failure, repetition and drop out (Badcock-Walters, 2002; Bicego et al. 2003; Mishra et al., 2007) . Other studies, however, have had ambivalent results; for example, Bennell (2005) found that there were minimal differences between enrolment rates of orphans and non-orphans, and that there was no correlation between differences in enrolment rates and HIV prevalence. This may be attributed to the introduction of free universal primary education as a result of the Millennium Goals campaign and also targeted aid to orphan households (Bennell, 2005, pp. 480-481). Birdthistle et al. (2009) found little difference between orphans and non-orphans in reasons for drop-out - financial reasons were the main cause for all, irrespective of status - but double orphans were found to have significantly greater absenteeism and lower attainment than non-orphans. However, they found that orphans face a disproportionate risk of acquiring sexual infections like HIV and herpes (Birdthistle, et al., 2009).

HIV/AIDS has had a direct impact on child mortality rates with a rise in infant and under five deaths across sub-Saharan Africa (Miller, 2007) The health of children affected by HIV/AIDS may be impacted in a number of ways. Children living with an ill parent will be more exposed to TB and other opportunistic infections associated with AIDS, orphaned children are more likely to suffer malnutrition and stunting and to have poorer access to health services (Giese, 2002; Miller, 2007). While Miller et al. (2007, p. 2482) found that "orphan status is a critical predictor of poor health", Kidman et al. (2010) - who examine the impact of AIDS in the family and community on child health in Malawi - found that for a range of physical health indicators orphaned children were no worse off than non-orphaned children but children living with ill parents were significantly more likely to suffer serious morbidity. In contrast, in a study in Zimbabwe, Watts et al. (2007) found that OVC were much more likely to suffer malnutrition and ill health than non-orphans and the difference could not be explained by differences in poverty. In the last five years or so, as a result of the introduction of NPAs (see section 2.2.2 below) the most vulnerable children are increasingly being given free access to health services (IATT, 2008).

2.2.2 Social protection

Social protection is "an agenda primarily for reducing vulnerability and risk of low-income households with regard to basic consumption and services" (Sabates Wheeler et al. 2009, p. 109) through 'safety nets' such as food grants or income transfers. In 2001, a year after the UN Millennium Declaration, 50 countries signed the UN General Assembly Special Session (UNGASS) *Declaration of Commitment on HIV/AIDS* agreeing to establish plans for OVC. In 2004, as mentioned above, UNICEF and the Global Partners' Forum established the "Framework for the protection, care and support of OVC living in a world with HIV and AIDS". The five key strategies outlined in the "Framework" form the foundation of the response to children affected by HIV/AIDS which underlie the National Plans of Action (NPAs) (Engle, 2008; Foster, 2008). On the initiative of USAID, UNICEF and UNAIDS, 17 high prevalence countries participated in Rapid Assessment Analysis and Action Planning (RAAAP) followed by NPAs to address the needs of children for basic services. While the exercise raised awareness of children's needs, it has been criticised as a donor-driven, 'emergency' exercise that has not necessarily been integrated into national planning (Engle, 2008). Some of the middle income countries in Southern Africa have social protection systems in place. South Africa for example, has cash transfers for families who care for orphans (IATT, 2008) as well as cash pensions for the elderly who are frequently caregivers to orphans. The Botswana Government provides monthly "food basket" to all registered orphans which often provides food for the whole household where the orphan is staying (M. Daniel, 2005). However, many sub-Saharan African countries are too poor to provide transfers in cash or kind, but since the establishment of NPAs some countries have implemented pilot projects targeting the poorest (IATT, 2008).

2.3 Psychosocial well-being

Children whose parents are very ill and children without parents do not suffer only physically, for example, from lack of basic needs, but they also experience grief at the loss of their parents, and may also have to face stigma and discrimination because of their parents HIV status. Recently the literature has started to explore the psychological impact on HIV/AIDS affected children (see for example Cluver et al., 2007; Cluver & Garner, 2007; Harms et al., 2009).

2.3.1 Cultural silence and children's grief

Cultural silence refers to the cultural taboos against speaking to children about death or about sex (Daniel, 2005; Mdleleni-Bookholane et al., 2004). HIV/AIDS, which in SSA is overwhelmingly spread through heterosexual transmission and which has had a huge impact on mortality rates, has inevitably put a spotlight on these sensitive issues. Many children in southern African countries have been prevented from attending the funerals of their parents, even if they wish to participate. There is a cultural understanding that death is too difficult and traumatic for children to cope with (Mdleleni-Bookholane, et al., 2004; Ndudani, 1998; Rantao, 2002). At an explicit level, culture is frequently used as an explanation for silence: "In our culture we do not talk to children about death, they are too young to understand" (Daniel, 2005, p. 28). Frequently children are not given an explanation about death and if they ask questions about their parents' death they sometimes do not receive answers or the reply does not help them understand the permanence of death, for example they might be told, "She has gone on a journey". Sometimes they are told they will understand when they are older (Daniel, 2005). In East Africa there is also cultural silence, but a different reason is given for not explaining death to children: it is believed that children do not understand and will not be affected by bereavement. Sengendo & Nambi (1997), in a study from Uganda, describe a cultural belief that children do not have emotional problems, while Snipstad et al. (2005, p. 191) in a study from Tanzania, report that adults believe children "have not got the brain yet" to comprehend death. Such beliefs limit children's opportunity to talk about their bereavement and deal with their grief.

Such cultural practices seek to protect children from the "pollution" of death (A. Richter & Müller, 2005, p. 1006) but they may also effectively marginalise "them from the process of grieving" (van der Heijden & Swartz, 2010, p. 45). Van der Heijden & Swartz (2010) stress that it is adults who impose this silence on children, adults reinforce cultural practices that compel children to silence concerning their grief. Cultural silence results in psychosocial problems for bereaved children. Children do understand that something is wrong and they worry about all sorts issues related to HIV/AIDS; such anxieties may hinder adaptive behaviour and the ability to solve problems (Snipstad, et al., 2005). Children also describe ruminating, "thinking too much", about a parent's death and how this can have a negative impact on their ability to concentrate in school with consequences for their attainment level (M. Daniel, 2005).

Only a very few programmes of psychosocial support exist which help children cope with grief and these will be discussed in section 2.4 below.

Another factor that reinforces cultural silence and blocks the processing of grief is AIDS-related stigma (van der Heijden & Swartz, 2010).

2.3.2 Stigma

Goffman (1963, p. 3) defines stigma as "an attribute that is deeply discrediting" and he continues "but it should be seen that the language of relationships, not attributes, is really needed." Frequently only the first part of this definition is quoted and Parker & Aggleton (2003, p. 14) note that this results in "highly individualised analyses" that focus on difference and negative attributes rather than exploring how stigma "devalues relationships". Stigma reinforces existing relations of power and control and perpetuates inequities (Parker & Aggleton, 2003). HIV/AIDS-related stigma is often linked to "immoral" (as judged by the dominant group) behaviour (sex and drug-use) and frequently leads to discrimination (Nyblade et al., 2003). Stigma can also be a reaction to fear of an incurable disease (Ogden & Nyblade, 2005). Stigma and discrimination may manifest as verbal and physical abuse, neglect and isolation, for example, name-calling, separating utensils and denying access to services (Dlamini et al., 2007).

HIV/AIDS affected children experience stigma and discrimination related to HIV/AIDS-related illness and death of their parents. Stigma may exacerbate the effects of bereavement and hinder psychosocial adjustment (Deacon & Stephney, 2007; Makame & Grantham-Mcgregor, 2002). Within households, orphan children may be treated differently to the biological children of the caregiver, made to do more household chores, given less food, and punished more harshly (M. Daniel, 2005; Deacon & Stephney, 2007). They may be denied access to school if they lack full uniform and may experience stigmatising and discriminatory behaviour from other pupils and even from teachers (M. Daniel, 2005; Deacon & Stephney, 2007). Deacon & Stephney (2007, p. 34) also report that stigma affects children's access to health care, for example "health care workers refusing care, or providing inferior care, to children who were HIV positive". In a study on the stigmatisation of AIDS-affected children by other children, Campbell et al. (2010, p. 981) found that "children were often afraid to play with AIDS affected children [...] bullied and ostracised" them as well as stigmatising them through name-calling.

2.4 Responses to OVC

Local communities have responded to the needs of orphans in a range of ways - they may produce food for orphans or provide day care for infants so that older siblings can continue in school (M. Daniel, 2008). Responses are small-scale and disjointed, they often find it difficult to get funding beyond voluntary labour and have little influence on national-level responses to AIDS-affected children (Foster, 2008).

National governments have established National AIDS co-ordinating bodies under the 'Three Ones' agreement (one action framework, one AIDS co-ordinating body, and one country-level monitoring and evaluation system) (Foster, 2008, p. 23). Often programmes and policies to address children are only a small part of these larger programmes. Frequently the response is nominal and inadequate and it is left up to civil society to run programmes and the international institutions such as UNICEF to monitor and co-ordinate. However, civil society is often more aligned with external donors (such as the Global Fund and PEPFAR) than national structures, and international responses are often not in line with national strategies (Foster, 2008, pp. 24-25). Foster (2008, p. 23) terms this "alignment anarchism".

Wallis & Dukay (2009, p. 171) have described the evolution in the response to mass-orphaning as a move from emergency relief aid towards structural integration. Most externally funded programmes targeting orphans tend to provide material aid in the form of uniforms, school fees and food; but very few programmes offer grief counselling or psychosocial support. Material relief aid frequently comes with unintended side-effects like the undermining of social cohesion in the recipient communities, corruption and the exclusion of the most vulnerable (M. Daniel, 2008). Psychosocial support tends to be small-scale and NGO-based, but some regional scale programmes do exist. For example, an organisation called the Regional Psychosocial Support Initiative (REPSSI) is favoured by UNICEF and donors like the Swedish International Development Agency (SIDA). It works with local partners and has emerged as a leading provider of psychosocial services in 13 countries in southern and eastern Africa (Matikanya, James, & Maksud, 2006, p. 7). The "Memory Book" programme, originally developed in the UK to give psychosocial help to immigrant orphans, has also had widespread application in southern and eastern Africa (Witter & Were, 2004).

While some governments provide relief assistance, such as the orphan grant in South Africa and the food basket for registered orphans in Botswana (Kallmann, 2003), it would seem that the Botswana government is the first government to become involved in scaled-up provision of *psychosocial* support to orphans. Since 2006, the Botswana government has been replicating (through 10 of the 16 Regional Councils) a retreat-based programme called "Ark for Children" developed in 2001 by a small local NGO, People and Nature Trust. The approach is culturally appropriate; it revives some customary practices such as age-set group formation as used to be practiced during initiation (M. L. Daniel & Thamuku, 2007). The emphasis in therapy is largely on group work which is effective in a collectivist society, while the use of individual therapy is limited though it effectively helps to breach deep-seated cultural silence.

3. Children infected by HIV

Many children infected at birth or though breast feeding do not survive beyond their second birthday. However increasing numbers of HIV positive children who do survive beyond infancy are now beginning to access anti-retroviral drugs.

3.1 Physical well-being: Illness, diagnosis and treatment

Giese (2002, p. 68) distinguishes between two groups of HIV positive children, namely rapid progressors, and slow progressors. Rapid progressors are "infants who become symptomatic and very sick within a few months of birth and usually die by the age of 2 years" while slow progressors "remain asymptomatic [...] during the first two years" and "generally survive to older childhood" (Giese, 2002, p. 68). Many children live with HIV until they are in early puberty before opportunistic infections begin to emerge. In some cases they are diagnosed with TB or another disease long before their HIV status is diagnosed.

A number of studies have examined the biomedical effects of illness and the implications of their status for their health and quality of life (Brown et al., 2000; Rao et al., 2007). Clinical manifestations of the disease include chronic cough, fevers, nausea and diarrhoea as well as chronic dermatological conditions such as rashes, fungal infections and abscesses (O'Hare et al., 2005). Those on ART may suffer side effects such as rashes, itching all over, a burning sensation in the legs and nausea. If they lack good nutrition they may experience difficulty in swallowing the drugs, nausea and vomiting, sweating and general weakness. Numerous studies have examined factors influencing adherence to ART among children (Bikaako-Kajura et al., 2006; Davies et al., 2008; Polisset et al., 2009; van Griensven et al., 2008; Van Winghem et al., 2008; Vreeman et al., 2008); issues include disclosure, relationship with caregiver, the involvement of health workers and structural issues like poverty.

Studies report that few children are informed of their HIV status and when they are informed, the event is controlled by their caregivers or by health care professionals (Lesch et al., 2007; Vaz et al., 2008). The most frequently given reasons for non-disclosure by caregivers include the associated stigma and discrimination, fear that the child will be unable to keep the secret, parental guilt, and concerns for the child's emotional and mental health, (Brown, et al., 2000; Hejoaka, 2009; Lesch, et al., 2007; Siripong et al., 2007; Vaz, et al., 2008) while disclosure usually occurs because of the need for the child to understand and adhere to their treatment (Brown, et al., 2000; Lesch et al., 2007; Vaz et al., 2008). Disclosure in a way that is appropriate to the child's cognitive development has been found to improve the child's psychological adjustment (Brown, et al., 2000; Lwin & Melvin, 2001).

Access to ART most frequently occurs through NGOs or FBOs rather than through government provided services. In such organisations the children are more likely to receive appropriate counselling and psychosocial support.

3.2 Psychosocial well-being: Secrecy and stigma

The psychosocial experiences of children affected by AIDS have been explored in several studies (Cluver & Gardner, 2007b; Fjermestad et al., 2008; Foster, 2002; Skovdal, 2009), but little research has been done on the psychosocial aspects of the lives of children infected by HIV/AIDS. Many HIV positive children will experience the sickness and, in some cases, the death of their mother and/or their father. Multiple losses may affect the child psychologically, particularly if there is no one to support them in their bereavement (Rao, et al., 2007) or to answer their questions. Secrecy and cultural silence may stimulate feelings of shame and guilt in a child (Brown, et al., 2000; M. Daniel, 2005; Wood, Chase, & Aggleton, 2006). Brown et al. (2000) contend that children more readily adjust to living with HIV when the parent's or caregiver's response is optimistic and this enables them to overcome disease and disability factors. If the mother (or caregiver) is coping well, the child is more likely to respond positively (L. Richter, 2002).

Children living with HIV often have physical symptoms of disease. Even when they start on ART they may have rashes or other visible signs particularly when the dosage is wrong or needs adjusting. This makes it easy for the child to be stigmatised and discriminated against. In addition, the centres where they receive treatment are often associated with HIV/AIDS and a child seen coming and going from such a centre may also be stigmatised. The caregivers of children living with HIV almost always impose secrecy on the child about his/her status. Mothers who are living with HIV feel enormous shame and want their child to keep the secret. This may be extremely difficult when medications have to be taken regularly twice a day and when there are physical symptoms. Children usually comply.

Secrecy involves concealment, either by hiding something from the view or attention of others or by keeping silent about it. In the case of HIV, that which is concealed includes status, ongoing treatment, receipt of medical and material aid and visits to the treatment centre (Hardon et al., 2007). Where children's HIV status is involved, mothers may keep the status secret from the child or co-opt the child into keeping their status secret. Hejoaka (2009, p. 870), in her study on care and secrecy, explores the way in which mothers manage the "tensions between disclosure and concealment" of the HIV status of their children. Mothers have strategies to limit access to their homes but concealment is much harder outside the domestic space, especially when regular hospital visits are required. Mothers hesitated to disclose to their children for fear they would not be able to keep the secret, but where children *were* told, they followed their mother's lead in concealment (Hejaoka, 2009). The issue of secrecy is more about *naming* than about *knowing*: even when children have not been told, they know something is wrong (Nagler et al., 1995) . Once children have the name, they do not necessarily use it, most children will keep the secret as their caregivers and society have taught them (Daniel et al., 2007; Nagler et al., 1995).

What compels to secrecy those who are infected, is the attitudes, beliefs and actions of others in society (Hardon, et al., 2007). Direct stigmatisation and discrimination against some HIV positive people, for example through labelling or exclusion, raises the *fear of stigma* among many others who have not necessarily had severe or direct experience of being stigmatised. This fear of stigma then leads to HIV- affected people adopting coping strategies of secrecy and silence (Ruora, et al., 2009). Shame, another direct cause for secrecy (Duffy, 2005), has its roots in the culture of blame - blame for breaching morality - which is frequently attributed to women (LeClerc-Madlala, 2001). LeClerc-Madlala (2001: 45) contends that this process of blaming women "both reflects and contributes to women's already marginalised and sub-ordinate status in society". The underlying causes of shame are power relations, culture and morality. Cultural norms may be at the root of blame-related stigma and shame when HIV/AIDS is associated with immoral and avoidable behaviour (LeClerc-Madlala, 2001; Ruora, et al., 2009). Social constraints lead to isolation and the secrecy adopted for fear of stigma hinders care (Hejoaka, 2009).

Silence deprives HIV positive children of potential help as they cannot ask neighbours for support without disclosing the reason why. Smith et al. (2008, p. 1268), whose study concerns adults rather than children, note the strong relationship between social support and public openness about HIV status: "people cannot actually receive social support until disclosure occurs. On the other hand, individuals must perceive social support will exist before they make the decision to disclose." Smith et al. (2008) link the fear of stigma-related rejection to limited social networks and low self-esteem; and several studies note that keeping a secret increases stress and anxiety (Duffy, 2005; Smith, et al., 2008). Menon et al (2007: 349) conclude that "interventions to promote disclosure could facilitate access to emotional and peer support". Shame is frequently associated with blame which implies a moral judgement situating the underlying cause within society's culture and morality. Blystad & Moland (2009) show that feelings of guilt and shame lead to isolation, marginalisation, uncertainty and adversity for mothers of HIV positive children, limiting the social support they so desperately need. In order to support and include mothers of HIV positive children it is these underlying causes that should be tackled. Secrecy and silence are the products of shame and the fear of stigma. Both secrecy and silence worsen the experiences of HIV positive children and add to their adversities. Providing ART to HIV positive children is a start and should be seen as part of a much larger process.

4. Conclusion

Children in sub-Saharan Africa are disproportionately affected and infected by HIV/AIDS. Many of them experience physical deprivation such as a lack of basic needs, social disruption when they have to change their living situation and they face psychosocial challenges, particularly cultural silence and stigma. Local, national and international efforts have made some progress in reducing the physical vulnerability of children affected by HIV/AIDS for example by providing food and school uniforms; they have also made progress in providing access to ART for children infected by HIV/AIDS. However, in terms of psychosocial support, particularly in tackling stigma, there is still much to be done.

5. References

Badcock-Walters, P. (2002). Education. In J. Gow & C. Desmond (Eds.), *The HIV/AIDS epidemic and the children of South Africa* (pp. 95-110). Scottsville: University of Natal Press.

Bauman, L. J., Foster, G., Silver, E. J., Berman, R., Gamble, I., & Muchaneta, L. (2006). Children caring for their ill parents with HIV/AIDS. *Vulnerable Children and Youth Studies, 1*(1), 56-70.

Bennell, P. (2005). The impact of the AIDS epidemic on the schooling of orphans and other directly affected children in Sub-Saharan Africa. *Journal of development studies, 41*(3), 467-488. doi:10.1080/0022038042000313336

Bicego, G., Rutstein, S., & Johnson, K. (2003). Dimensions of the emerging orphan crisis in sub-Saharan Africa. *Social Science & Medicine, 56*(6), 1235-1247.

Birdthistle, I., Floyd, S., Nyagadza, A., Mudziwapasi, N., Gregson, S., & Glynn, J. R. (2009). Is education the link between orphanhood and HIV/HSV-2 risk among female adolescents in urban Zimbabwe? *Social Science & Medicine, 68*(10), 1810-1818. doi:10.1016/j.socscimed.2009.02.035

Blystad, A., & Moland, K. M. (2009). Technologies of hope? Motherhood, HIV and infant feeding in eastern Africa. *Anthropology & Medicine, 16*(2), 105-118.

Brown, L. K., Lourie, K. J., & Pao, M. (2000). Children and Adolescents living with HIV and AIDS: a review. *Journal of Child Psychology and Psychiatry, 41*(1), 81-96.

Campbell, C., Skovdal, M., Mupambireyi, Z., & Gregson, S. (2010). Exploring children's stigmatisation of AIDS-affected children in Zimbabwe through drawings and stories. *Social Science & Medicine, 71*(5), 975-985. doi:10.1016/j.socscimed.2010.05.028

Cluver, L., & Gardner, F. (2007a). The mental health of children orphaned by AIDS: a review of international and Southern African research. *Journal of Child and Adolescent Mental Health, 19*, 1-17.

Cluver, L., & Gardner, F. (2007b). Risk and protective factors for psychological well-being of children orphaned by AIDS in Cape Town: a qualitative study of children and caregivers' perspectives. *AIDS Care, 19*(3), 318-325.

Cluver, L., Gardner, F., & Operario, D. (2007). Psychological distress amongst AIDS-orphaned children in urban South Africa. *Journal of Child Psychology and Psychiatry, 48*, 755-763.

Daniel, M. (2005). *Hidden Wounds: orphanhood, expediency and cultural silence in Botswana.* (PhD, School of Development Studies, University of East Anglia), Norwich. Retrieved from http://hdl.handle.net/1956/3294

Daniel, M. (2008). Humanitarian aid to vulnerable children in Makete and Iringa, Tanzania. Bergen: University of Bergen.

Daniel, M., Apila, H. M., Bjørgo, R., & Lie, G. T. (2007). Breaching cultural silence: enhancing resilience among Ugandan orphans. *African Journal of AIDS Research, 6*(2), 109-120.

Daniel, M. L., & Thamuku, M. (2007). The Ark for Children: culturally appropriate psychosocial support for children without parents in Botswana. In E. A. Lothe, M. L. Daniel, M. B. Snipstad & N. Sveaass (Eds.), *Strength in Broken Places: Marginalisation and empowerment*. Oslo: Unipub AS.

Deacon, H., & Stephney, I. (2007). *HIV/AIDS, stigma and children: A literature review.* Cape Town: HSRC press.

Dlamini, P. S., Kohi, T. W., Uys, L. R., Phetlhu, R. D., Chirwa, M. L., Naidoo, J. R., et al. (2007). Verbal and physical abuse and neglect as manifestations of HIV/AIDS stigma in five African countries. *Public Health Nursing, 24*(5), 389-399.

Duffy, L. (2005). Suffering, shame and silence: the stigma of HIV/AIDS. *Journal of the Association of Nurses in AIDS Care, 16*(1), 13-20.

Engle, P. (2008). National plans of action for orphans and vulnerable children in sub-Saharan Africa: Where are the youngest children? Amsterdam: Bernard van Leer Foundation.

Evans, R. (2010). 'We are managing our own lives...': Life transitions and care in sibling headed households affected by AIDS in Tanzania and Uganda. *Area.* doi:10.1111/j.1475-4762.2010.00954.x

Fjermestad, K. W., Kvestad, I., Daniel, M., & Lie, G. T. (2008). "It can save you if you just forget": Closeness and competence as conditions for coping among Ugandan orphans. *Journal of Psychology in Africa, 18*(3), 283-294.

Foster, G. (2002). Beyond Education and Food: Psychosocial Well-being of Orphans in Africa. *Acta Paediatrica, 91*, 502-504.

Foster, G. (2008). Getting in line: coordinating responses of donors, civil society and government for children affected by HIV and AIDS. Nairobi: UNICEF.

Giese, S. (2002). Health. In J. Gow & C. Desmond (Eds.), *The HIV/AIDS epidemic and the children of South Africa* (pp. 59-78). Scottsville: University of Natal Press.

Goffman, E. (1963). *Stigma: Notes on the management of spoiled identity.* New York: Simon & Schuster.

Hardon, A. P., Akurut, D., Comoro, C., Ekezie, C., Irunde, H. F., Gerrits, T., et al. (2007). Hunger, waiting time and transport costs: Time to confront challenges to ART adherence in Africa. *AIDS Care, 19*(5), 658-665.

Harms, S., Kizza, R., Sebunnya, J., & Jack, S. (2009). Conceptions of mental health among Ugandan youth orphaned by AIDS. *African Journal of AIDS Research, 8*(1), 7-16.

Hejoaka, F. (2009). Care and secrecy: Being a mother of children living with HIV in Burkina Faso. *Social Science & Medicine, 69*(6), 869-876.

Heymann, J., Earle, A., Rajaraman, D., Miller, C., & Bogen, K. (2007). Extended family caring for children orphaned by AIDS: balancing essential work and caregiving in a high HIV prevalence nations. *AIDS Care, 19*(3), 337-345.

Hosegood, V. (2008). Demographic evidence of family and household changes in response to the effects of HIV/AIDS in southern Africa: Implications for efforts to strengthen families. *Retrieved April, 14*, 2009.

Hosegood, V., Floyd, S., Marston, M., Hill, C., McGrath, N., Isingo, R., et al. (2007). The effects of high HIV prevalence on orphanhood and living arrangements of children in Malawi, Tanzania, and South Africa. *Population studies, 61*(3), 327-336. doi:10.1080/00324720701524292

IATT. (2008). Expanding social protection for vulnerable children and families: learning from an institutional persective. New York: Inter-Agency Task Team.

JLICA. (2011). Core research areas. Retrieved from http://www.jlica.org/learning-groups/index.php

Kallmann, K. (2003). HIV/AIDS and social assistance in South Africa: a study of social assistance available in South Africa with a comparison to assistance available in Botswana, Namibia, Zambia and Zimbabwe. Johannesburg: Southern African Legal Assistance Network.

Kidman, R., Hanley, J. A., Subramanian, S. V., Foster, G., & Heymann, J. (2010). AIDS in the family and community: The impact on child health in Malawi. *Social Science & Medicine, 71*(5), 966-974.

Kipp, W. E., Satzinger, F., Alibhai, A., & Rubaale, T. (2010). Needs and support for Ugandan child-headed households: results from a qualitative study. *Vulnerable Children and Youth Studies, 5*(4), 297-309. doi:10.1080/17450128.2010.507805

LeClerc-Madlala, S. (2001). Demonising women in the era of AIDS: on the relationship between cultural constructions of both HIV/AIDS and feminity. *Society in Transition, 32*(1), 38-46.

Lesch, A., Swartz, L., Kagee, A., Moodley, K., Kafaar, Z., Myer, L., et al. (2007). Paediatric HIV/AIDS disclosure: towards a developmental and process-oriented approach. *AIDS Care, 19*(6), 811-816.

Luzze, F. (2002). *Survival in child-headed households: a study on the impact of World Vision support on coping strategies of child-headed households in Uganda.* Dept. of Theology, University of Leeds), Leeds.

Luzze, F., & Ssedyabule, D. (2004). The Nature of Child-headed Households in Rakai District, Uganda. Kampala: Lutheran World Federation.

Lwin, R., & Melvin, D. (2001). Annotation: Paediatric HIV infection. *Journal of Child Psychology and Psychiatry, 42*(4), 427-438.

Madhavan, S. (2004). Fosterage patterns in the age of AIDS: continuity and change. *Social Science & Medicine, 58*(7), 1443-1454.

Makame, V., & Grantham-Mcgregor, S. (2002). Psychological well-being of orphans in Dar es Salaam, Tanzania. *Acta Paediatrica, 91*(4), 459-465.

Matikanya, R., James, V., & Maksud, N. (2006). End of programme support evaluation of Regional Psychosocial Support Initiative (REPSSI). Stockholm: SIDA.

Mdleleni-Bookholane, T. N., Schoeman, W. J., & van der Merwe, I. (2004). The development in understanding of the concept of death among black South African learners from the Eastern Cape, South Africa. *Health SA Gesondheid, 9*(4), 3-14.

Meintjes, H., Hall, K., Marera, D. H., & Boulle, A. (2010). Orphans of the AIDS epidemic? The extent, nature and circumstances of child-headed households in South Africa. *AIDS Care, 22*(1), 40-49. doi:10.1080/09540120903033029

Meintjies, H., & Giese, S. (2006). Spinning the epidemic: the making of mythologies of orphanhood in the context of AIDS. *Childhood, 13*(3), 407-430. doi:10.1177/0907568206066359

Menon, A., Glazebroook, C., Campain, N., & Ngoma, M. (2007). Mental health and disclosure of HIV status in Zambian adolescents with HIV infection. *Journal of AIDS, 46*(3), 349-354.

Miller, C. (2007). Children Affected by AIDS: A Review of the Literature on Orphaned and Vulnerable Children.

Miller, C. M., Gruskin, S., Subramanian, S. V., & Heymann, J. (2007). Emerging health disparities in Botswana: examining the situation of orphans during the AIDS epidemic. *Social Science & Medicine, 64*(12), 2476-2486. doi:10.1016/j.socscimed.2007.03.002

Miller, C. M., Gruskin, S., Subramanian, S. V., Rajaraman, D., & Heymann, S. J. (2006). Orphan care in Botswana's working households: growing responsibilities in the absence of adequate support. *American Journal of Public Health, 96*(8), 1429.

Mishra, V., Arnold, F., Otieno, F., Cross, A., & Hong, R. (2007). Education and nutritional status of orphans and children of HIV-infected parents in Kenya. *AIDS Education & Prevention, 19*(5), 383-395.

Monasch, R., & Boerma, T. (2004). Orphanhood and childcare patterns in sub-Saharan Africa: an analysis of national surveys from 40 countries. *AIDS, 18*(Suppl 2), S55-S65. doi:10.1097/01.aids.0000125989.86904.fe

Morantz, G., & Heymann, J. (2010). Life in institutional care: the voices of children in a residential facility in Botswana. *AIDS Care, 22*(1), 10-16. doi:10.1080/09540120903012601

Mwagomba, B., Zachariah, R., Massaquoi, M., Misindi, D., Manzi, M., Mandere, B. C., et al. (2010). Mortality Reduction Associated with HIV/AIDS Care and Antiretroviral Treatment in Rural Malawi: Evidence from Registers, Coffin Sales and Funerals. *PLOS ONE, 5*(5). doi:10.1371/journal.pone.0010452

Nagler, S., Andropoz, J., & Forsyth, B. (1995). Uncertainty, Stigma and Secrecy: Psychological aspects of AIDS for Children and Adolescents. In S. Geballe, J. Greundel & W. Andiman (Eds.), *Forgotten Children of the AIDS Epidemic.* New Haven, NY: Yale University Press.

Ndudani, N. (1998). Accepting Death As Part of Life. *Children First, 2*, 6-7.

Nyambedha, E. O., & Aagaard-Hansen, J. (2010). Educational consequences of orphanhood and poverty in western Kenya. *Educational Studies, 36*(5), 555-567.

Nyblade, L., Pande, R., Mathur, S., MacQuarrie, K., Kidd, R., Banteyerga, H., et al. (2003). Disentangling HIV and AIDS stigma in Ethiopia, Tanzania and Zambia. Lusaka: International Centre for Research on Women (ICRW).

O'Hare, B. A. M., Venables, J., Nalubeg, J. F., Nakakeeto, M., Kilbirige, M., & Southall, D. P. (2005). Home-based care for orphaned children infected with HIV/AIDS in Uganda. *AIDS Care, 17*(4), 443-450.

Ogden, J., & Nyblade, L. (2005). Common at its core: HIV-related stigma across contexts: International Centre for Research on Women.

Parker, R., & Aggleton, P. (2003). HIV and AIDS-related stigma and discrimination: a conceptual framework and implications for action. *Social Science & Medicine, 57*(1), 13-24.

Rantao, P. (2002). How Batswana Handle and Manage Death - Tsamaiso ya Loso mo Setswaneng (Parts I to VI). *Botswana Gazette.*

Rao, R., Sagar, R., Kabra, S. K., & Lodha, R. (2007). Psychiatric morbidity in HIV-infected children. *AIDS Care, 19*(6), 828-833.

Reniers, G., Araya, T., Davey, G., Nagelkerke, N., Berhane, Y., Coutinho, R., et al. (2009). Steep declines in population-level AIDS mortality following the introduction of antiretroviral therapy in Addis Ababa, Ethiopia. *AIDS (London, England), 23*(4), 511. doi:10.1097/QAD.0b013e32832403d0.

Richter, A., & Müller, J. (2005). The forgotten children of Africa: Voicing HIV and AIDS orphans' stories of bereavement: a narrative approach. *HTS Theological Studies, 61*(3), 999-1015.

Richter, L. (2002). Caring for small children: mutual mental health for caregiver and child. *Women's Health Project Review, 42*, 25-27.

Ruora, M., Wringe, A., Busza, J., Nhandi, B., Mbaa, D., Zaba, B., et al. (2009). "Just like a fever": a qualitative study on the impact of antiretroviral provision on the normalisation of HIV in rural Tanzania and its implications for prevention. *BMC International Health and Human Rights, 9*(22), 1-31.

Sabates Wheeler, R., Devereux, S., & Hodges, A. (2009). Taking the Long View: What Does a Child Focus Add to Social Protection? *IDS Bulletin, 40*(1), 109-119.

Sengendo, J., & Nambi, J. (1997). The psychological effect of orphanhood: a study of orphans in Rakai district. *Health TRansition Review, 7*(Supplement), 105-124.

Sherr, L., Varrall, R., Mueller, J., Richter, L., Wakhweya, A., Adato, M., et al. (2008). A systematic review on the meaning of the concept 'AIDS orphan': confusion over definitions and implications for care. *AIDS Care, 20*(5), 527-536. doi:10.1080/09540120701867248

Siripong, A., Bunupuradah, T., Apateerapong, W., Boonrak, P., Pancharoen, C., & Ananworanich, J. (2007). Attitudes of Thai caregivers of children with HIV infection towards HIV disclosure. *Vulnerable Children and Youth Studies, 2*(3), 191-197.

Skovdal, M. (2009). "I washed and fed my mother before going to school": understanding the psychosocial well-being of children providing chronic care for adults affected by HIV/AIDS in Western Kenya. *Globalization and Health, 5*(8).

Skovdal, M. (2010). Children caring for their "caregivers": exploring the caring arrangements in households affected by AIDS in Western Kenya. *AIDS Care, 22*(1), 96-103. doi:10.1080/09540120903016537

Skovdal, M., & Ogutu, V. O. (2009). " I washed and fed my mother before going to school": Understanding the psychosocial well-being of children providing chronic care for adults affected by HIV/AIDS in Western Kenya. *Globalization and Health, 5*(1), 1-10. doi:10.1186/1744-8603-5-8

Skovdal, M., Ogutu, V. O., Aoro, C., & Campbell, C. (2009). Young carers as social actors: Coping strategies of children caring for ailing or ageing guardians in Western Kenya. *Social Science & Medicine, 69*(4), 587-595. doi:10.1016/j.socscimed.2009.06.016

Smith, R., Rossetto, K., & Peterson, B. (2008). A meta-analysis of disclosure of one's HIV positive status, stigma and social support. *AIDS Care, 20*(10), 1266-1275.

Snipstad, M. B., Lie, G. T., & Winje, D. (2005). What do Tanzanian children worry about? *African Journal for AIDS Research, 4*(3), 183-193.

Tolfree, D. K. (2003). Community based care for separated children. Stockholm: Save the Children, Sweden.

UNAIDS. (2010). UNAIDS report on the global AIDS epidemic 2010. Geneva: UNAIDS.

UNICEF, UNAIDS, & USAID. (2004). Children on the Brink 2004: A Joint Report of New Orphan Estimates and a Framework for Action. New York: UNICEF.

UNICEF, UNAIDS, WHO, & UNFPA. (2010). Children and AIDS: Fifth stocktaking report, 2010. New York: UNICEF.

van Blerk, L., & Ansell, N. (2007). Alternative care giving in the context of AIDS in southern Africa: complex strategies for care. *Journal of International Development, 19*(7), 865-884. doi:10.1002/jid.1328

van der Heijden, I., & Swartz, S. (2010). Bereavement, silence and culture within a peer-led HIV/AIDS-prevention strategy for vulnerable children in South Africa. *African Journal of AIDS Research, 9*(1), 41-50.

Vaz, L., Corneli, A., Dulyx, J., Rennie, S., Omba, S., Kitetele, F., et al. (2008). The process of HIV status disclosure to HIV-positive youth in Kinshasa, Democratic Republic of the Congo. *AIDS Care, 99999*(1), 1-11.

Wakhweya, A., Dirks, R., & Yeboah, K. (2008). Children thrive in families: Family-centred models of care and support for orphans and other vulnerable children affected by HIV and AIDS. *AIDS JLICA*.

Wallis, A., & Dukay, V. (2009). Learning how to measure the well-being fo OVC in a maturing HIV/AIDS crisis. *Journal of Health Care for the Poor and Undeserved, 20*(4), 170-184.

Watts, H., Gregson, S., Saito, S., Lopman, B., Beasley, M., & Monasch, R. (2007). Poorer health and nutritional outcomes in orphans and vulnerable young children not explained by greater exposure to extreme poverty in Zimbabwe. *Tropical medicine & international health, 12*(5), 584-593.

Whetten, K., Ostermann, J., Whetten, R. A., Pence, B. W., O'Donnell, K., Messer, L. C., et al. (2009). A comparison of the wellbeing of orphans and abandoned children ages 6–12 in institutional and community-based care settings in 5 less wealthy nations. *PLOS ONE, 4*(12), e8169. doi:10.1371/journal.pone.0008169

Witter, S., & Were, B. (2004). Breaking the silence: using memory books as a counselling and succession-planning tool with HIV-affected households in Uganda. *African Journal for AIDS Research, 3*(2), 139-143.

Wood, K., Chase, E., & Aggleton, P. (2006). `Telling the truth is the best thing': Teenage orphans' experiences of parental AIDS-related illness and bereavement in Zimbabwe. *Social Science & Medicine, 63*(7), 1923-1933.

10

Psychosocial Aspects of People Living with HIV/AIDS

Lenka Fabianova
Trnava University, Faculty of Health Care and Social Work, Trnava
Slovakia

1. Introduction

The chapter reports on psycho-social aspects of people living with HIV/AIDS and their responses. Besides identifying particular issues like fear, loss, grief, hopelessness and helplessness syndrome, guilt and self-esteem, anxiety and depression, denial, anger, aggression and suicide attempts are also identified. The objective is also to analyse the spiritual needs, discrimination and stigmatization of HIV positive people. Special remark is directed towards children, as a most vulnerable group, especially in the situation when they are orphaned and need to cope with the dead and dying.

Discussion on HIV/AIDS is in many third-world countries still accompanied by taboo, misunderstandings, shame, guilt and rejection. Culturally conditioned silence about sexuality, sexual behaviour conceals risky sexual behaviour and sexual abuse and especially sexual abuse of children. Due to cultural, religious and legal aspects of the topic is HIV/AIDS, death, sexuality, the discussion is led only by a small group of experts. Rejection or lack of awareness about HIV/AIDS significantly limits the ability of effective and decent care for HIV-positive people and their families. It is very important to speak about HIV/AIDS loudly, to speak about the feelings and reactions of people living with HIV/AIDS.

The research study rivets at psycho-social aspects of HIV/AIDS people living in Nairobi, in Kenya, who received voluntary counselling and testing services.

2. Psychosocial responses

People living with HIV/AIDS (PLWHA) feel uncertainty and they have to cope with the situation. Feelings of insecurity have its origin in the fear from the upcoming future and the people focus on their families and their fob. They feel even more uncertain and are more concerned because of the quality of life and life expectancy as well the treatment´s outcome and the reaction of the society. All concerns are unpredictable, and therefore they should be discussed. Above all, positive thinking and faith of is recommended.

The situation is very special for children, who have lost their family and home. The HIV positive child must react to this uncertainty and make several decisions to adapt to the current situation. Even if it seems, that the child does not react at all, it can be the very adaptation to the illness by denying it. People begin their adaptation process from the day they learnt about it. Their daily life reflects the tension between uncertainty and coping with the situation. It is the tension, which raises a lot of *psychosocial responses* of bigger and smaller intensity.

2.1 Fear and loss

Fear of HIV/AIDS is closely associated with fear of our own death, which belongs to the most basic of fears. It is the fear which most of us are trying to fight with by constantly running away from the idea of self-termination or by inventing a series of comforting ideas. Escape and rationalization will help only to cultivate the fear of death. Above all, people have to be settled with self-extinction, with own death and thus perhaps would help those who just need help in the process of dying.

In countries with high rate of infected people are found amongst doctors and other health-care staff. PLWHVA are pushed to the margins of the society, and are isolated. They are forced to leave their job, they, lose their homes, often their family and friends. They are not given adequate health care and by the provided health care they are confronted with rejection. All of this happens because of an illness which cannot be transmitted by common contact. This attitude of professionals who are unable to overcome prejudices and refuse to provide health care is a deep misunderstanding of their mission. The reasons for this kind of handling is fear of being infected with HIV and, ultimately, fear from death itself. (Frensman, 2000)

Another aspect associated with HIV/AIDS is *a loss*. People in the developed stage of AIDS are worried because of the loss of their life, their ambitions, physical performance and potency, sexual relations, loss of their position in the society, financial stability and independence. With the increasing essential need of systematic tendency they lose their sense of privacy and control over their lives. Perhaps the most problematic issue is the loss of confidence. It may affect the future, anxiety originating from a relationship with a loved one or caregiver and negative reactions from the society.

For many people finding out about their HIV/AIDS status it is the first opportunity, to realize their mortality and psychological vulnerability. They face social isolation due to the inability to perform all daily activities which they used to do. Relationships within the family change more frequently, one loses their colleagues and the attitude of acquaintances and friends changes frequently as well. Many are afraid of the loss of memory, their concentration and ability to make decisions.

Death of a relative, who dies of a deadly disease, presents an extreme burden for each human being. He tends to surrender the pressure of the situation, which seems to be insolvable. Mental failure is accompanied by significant behaviour, changes in physiological and psychological processes in the body, which have sometimes permanent effects on health. This persistent extreme burden leads to disruption of relationships with the social environment.

2.2 Grief, hopelessness and helplessness syndrome

Grief is another strong emotion that is closely linked to the loss. The HIV/AIDS positive patients often dive into sadness because of their loss they experienced or the one they expect. Natural sadness results from unfulfilled dreams and plans and from the nearness of an inevitable end. The patient may lose the sense for relationship with parents, children, friends or life partner, as well as with other people. In connection with the impending death of a loved one there is mentioned a so called "anticipate grief", which occurs by the closest relatives of people with long-term illness, in terms of expected death. HIV/AIDS is a fatal disease. Some people survive ten years, another few months from diagnosis. As the disease gets hold of their body, they lose control over their life. PLWHA tend not to care anymore about things which made them happy, they submit to their fate, they do not see any hope and wait for the death to come.

Hopelessness and *helplessness syndrome* includes elements of giving up and leaving. The survival mechanism includes the following:

- Painful feeling of helplessness and hopelessness face to face to the situation,
- The subjective feeling of reduced ability to deal with the situation ("it is beyond my strength"),
- Feeling of danger and decreased satisfaction from relationships with others,
- Loss of continuity of the past and future, a reduced ability to hope and trust,
- Tendency to revive and re-construct former deprivations and failures. (Simek, 1993 as cited in Bastecky, 1993)

Small children, since most of them do not know about their diagnosis, experience their state very differently. They still have a bit of life joy. In their ignorance, purity and their nativity they can spend a nice childhood, in the case, if somebody takes care of them and provides them with their basic needs as well as health care.

2.3 Guilt and self-esteem

Diagnosis of HIV/AIDS infection often brings feelings of *guilt* from the possibility of infecting the other people or from the previous way of life which led to the infection There is also a feeling of culpability of what disease brings to people in one´s own family, especially children. Previous events that caused pain or sadness of others remained unresolved; they can reoccur and cause the patient even greater feelings of wrongdoing.

People living with HIV/AIDS, who have to cope with their complicated destiny, very often lose rapidly their *self-esteem.* Rejection of colleagues, relatives and loved ones and often people can very quickly lead to loss of self-esteem and social identity, which leads to the feeling of one´s own worthlessness. This condition can be enhanced by worsening of symptoms accompanying the disease, e.g. facial disfigurement, deteriorating body, loss of strength as well as loss of control over one's body.

Self-esteem is an ability to appreciate oneself and treat oneself with dignity and love. Anyone who is loved is willing to change. Human beings can grow and change throughout their life." The behaviour is the result of managing well. Coping is the expression of the level of self-evaluation. In coping the way how a person perceives oneself is reflected and one´s own relationship. The problem is not the problem itself, but how one handles it. It can be deduced from that fact that the increase of one´s self-esteem and self-evaluation can lead to well managing the life´s situation of these children.

2.4 Anxiety disorder and depression

Feelings of anxiety in PLHWA can be detected very soon which reflects the continuous uncertainty associated with the disease. This state results from:

- short and long-term prognosis,
- risk of infection with other diseases,
- risk of infecting other people
- social, professional, familiar and sexual rejection,

- separation, isolation and physical pain,
- fear from degradation,
- fear of undignified dying and dying in pain,
- inability to change the circumstances and consequences of HIV infection
- the inability to ensure optimal health condition,
- failure of the one´s close relatives to deal with the situation,
- unavailability of appropriate therapeutic procedures,
- loss of privacy and fear of disclosure of information,
- future social and sexual rejection
- sequential failure of vital functions,
- loss of physical and financial independence. (Satir, 2006)

Anxiety disorders are often accompanied by characteristic somatic, physiological, and autonomic, biochemical, endocrinal and behavioural changes. The fact is that so far there is no possibility to cure HIV infection, leading to the feeling of helplessness, loss of personal control, which may be associated with a resulting depression.

Depression can have many causes. An affected person may get the feeling that the virus takes control over his body. Just the fact that a close person died of AIDS, together with not existing the possibility of planning one owns long-term future has a negative impact on one´s psychic condition.

In connection with the depressive syndrome there are several types of depression, i.e. exogenous, endogenous or neurotic depression. By the *exogenous depression* there have been reported such problems as the experience a sudden loss caused by the death of a loved one. There is expected an internal biological ability, which causes depressive psychopathology regardless of external circumstances by the so-called *endogenous depression*. By the *neurotic* depression there is an expected effect of long-term stress and frustration. This form is present in the condition of most HIV/AIDS positive orphans. The symptoms of depression are present in neurotic and anxiety disorders such as mixed anxiety depressive disorder and the disorder of adaptation. Depressive behavioural disorder is often diagnosed especially, in the childhood, within a mixed behavioural and emotional disorder. (Koutek & Kocourkova, 2003)

The prevalence of depressive disorders rates up to 40 to 55% by orphans with HIV up to the age of 10, up to 50 to 75% of adolescents who were given professional help. (Rubinstein, 2001)

Depressive syndrome in these children is associated with an extremely sad mood, slowing of psychomotor speed, sleep disturbance and suicidal thoughts. A typical symptom is presented by increased irritability, behavioural problems with elements of aggression.

2.5 Denial, anger, aggression and suicide attempts

Some people react to news about their HIV/AIDS status by denying it. For some of them, such refusal may present a constructive way to handle the shock of the diagnosis. However, if this condition persists, the denial can become unproductive, because these people refuse also the social responsibility associated with HIV positivity. This reaction is typical for children, in the case of the death on a parent.

Anger and aggression are typical aspects which accompany people in situations of bereavement. Some individuals become angry and aggressive. They are often very upset about their fate. They continuously have the feeling, that they are not treated decently and tactfully enough. Anger can sometimes escalate into self-destruction: suicide. Aggression is one of the most frequently reported reactions in frustrating situations. In the frustrating situations, an individual may focus his anger, remorse, indignation, outrage, hostility on other people that are considered as suitable object. There is another possibility, presented by the concept of self-accusation, which the aggressive reaction are aimed at oneself. (Bratska, 2001)

There is an increased risk of *suicidal attempts* for HIV positive people. They may see the suicide as a way out from pain and difficult situation, out of their shame and grief for their loved ones.

Suicide may be active (e. g, causing a fatal injury) or passive (planning or preparation of such a situation, which could result in fatal complications of HIV/AIDS). (Yelding, 1990)

HIV positivity presents a risk factor, particularly amongst adolescents. There are significant complications in the development of personality in adolescence age and it can be perceived as an unacceptable problem. Suicidal behaviour is associated with a wide range of mental disorders, HIV positive children and adolescents suffer primarily from depression.

3. Spiritual aspects

A situation in which one must face loneliness, loss of control and death, can lead to *spiritual questions* and seeking assistance in the faith. Concepts such as sin, guilt, forgiveness, reconciliation and tackle, may become subjects of spiritual and religious discussions. Similar moments become topical for many HIV positive patients. The cause of many emotional and psychic problems is presented by various infections, difficult situations and difficult periods of exhaustion. Even greater impact on the HIV positive person, however, presents the rejection of one´s own family or friends and one is separated from the society and pushed aside.

Many people believe that only religious people have spiritual needs. But non-believers begin to deal with questions about the meaning of one´s own life exactly during their illness and when they suffer. Everybody needs to find out, that the life has had had and still have some meaning. Everybody needs to deal with things, which are hard for him and which are unchangeable.

Sometimes the suffering radically changes the actual life and it often affects moral values of people. (Dobrikova, 2005)

When talking about the spirituality of children, many may argue that children´s ability of abstract thinking needed for understanding of religion is not developed and that they cannot understand the concept of God Despite the developmental perspective that generally criticizes the view of children's spirituality, we must acknowledge the fact that children are the pilgrims, who are trying to the meaning of world and the meaning of their own life.

Of course, the initial views of spiritual values and experiences children may experience in different ways, depending on whether they are raised in religious families, if they regularly experience religious rituals and to what extend are they raised in a religious way. Every child explains these events introspectively to oneself. It is perhaps not so important, at what age, the child begins to understand and express spirituality, but it is important to create room for a child´s questions and to supply her or him with the answers. (Dane & Levine, 2002)

Any death, especially death of a parent brings many spiritual issues. The child asks: "Why did he / she die?" "Why is this happening to me?" "Who will take care of me?" All these

questions imply the spiritual dimension. These questions are very real for children whose parents died of AIDS but they are suppressed from fear and because of the stigma associated with HIV positivity.
The child can have trouble finding help and support from peers and adults because there is a mysterious silence about everything, no one wants to talk about the death of his close relative or what so more, to talk about HIV / AIDS. The child feels fear and shame to share his feelings with others, or it makes the situation deteriorate. If somebody belongs to the Christian faith, who perceives AIDS as a consequence of the moral bankruptcy of the individual, it does not make the situation easier. While the church preaches to love sinners, at the same time it condemns the sin. From this perspective, PLHWA are responsible for their conditions, but they deserve compassion and assistance. The child could eventually find their harbour in the church, even if it offers a very mixed or negative image of people with HIV / AIDS. This point of view complicates the child´s spiritual interpretation. All life situations the child had already had to go through, such as the death of a parent, poverty, deprivation, sniffing the glue, violence, make the spiritual survival complicated and they burden his purity. HIV positivity present chaos, uncertainty, unpredictability to the child, it causes lot of problems and on-going struggle. (Shorter & Onyancha, 1998)
The spirituality and religion can present a complicated issue. It is necessary to have the child explained his own responsibility for loss, death, disease, so that the child does not perceive these as his own sins. It is necessary to give them room, time and assistance in this direction. Religious rituals, in which the child can take part, can help and be one of the most significant is at the funeral. The child itself has to make the decision, whether he wants to be part of it or nor. Memorial mass, private rituals, lightning the candles, prayer, all of that can be a part of the therapy for the child.

4. Discrimination and stigmatization

Article 1 of the Universal Declaration of Human Rights speaks of the equality of all people. Right for health, which is enshrined in the status of WHO, i.e. the highest level of physical, mental and social well-being, reminds us all that HIV-infected people have the same right for equal treatment as well as the right to protect their civil, political, economic, social and cultural rights as all other members of human society do. The issue of human rights is given a priority position in the programs of such institutions as Council of Europe, UNICEF and many others. The next evidence of this priority is presented by the creation of the United Nations Program for the Fight against HIV/AIDS (UNAIDS), by a combination of powers and funding of six institutions of UNO.
The most inexorable form of discrimination against people with HIV/AIDS is that of popular or institutionalized retribution. This can go for mere avoidance to the refusal of medical treatment, imprisonment, ostracization or even physical assault against high-risk groups, such as gay people, commercial sex-workers, and intravenous drug users. All these forms of discrimination have been recorded in different parts of the world. A frequent prejudice is that people living with HIV/AIDS should be subject to legal controls or quarantined in order to stop the spread groups should be compulsorily tested for HIV. Such beliefs have influenced the enacting of laws, especially those relating to immigration and emigration. Such laws have, in turn, helped to define public attitudes towards those living with AIDS. (Shorter & Onyancha 1998)

In the current phase of the unstoppable progress of HIV/AIDS pandemic and development of the fight against HIV/AIDS, is a systematic effort needed more than ever. Effort, which could counteract with the spreading of infection from the position of respecting human rights, in particular in these areas:

- Wide access to modern medicines and clarifying of their correct application. Treatment success depends on a motivated and diligent cooperation with the physician. As a broad and comprehensive approach a wide-spread, not-discriminating use of drug prophylaxis is understood and is indicated in cooperation with health insurance,
- Extension of expert advising, testing and other activities related to prevention,
- Informational and educational campaigns which lead to increased tolerance of the society towards the affected population and to elimination of the constant re-occurring social stigma,
- Improvement of legislation protecting privacy and preventing discrimination. (Mayer, 1999)

HIV/AIDS positive individuals have the same right to protect their rights as other members of the society. They have the right to work, have a job, right to obtain education, the right to attend a school, right for the social security and assistance, right for the protection against inhuman or degrading treatment or punishment. The most important and recognized principle is, that people or groups of people, who are at a higher risk of getting infected, in particular those, who are already infected or those who develop AIDS will not be discriminated.

Probably the most common reason for the discrimination is an irrational fear of and fear from contact with people infected by HIV/AIDS, fear from infection and from, the possible consequences of the disease, suffering and death. Based on ignorance, all of these factors cause discrimination tendency. It is also subconscious, but irrational. A significant percentage of discriminatory attitudes of the population are related to the fundamental ignorance, about HIV transmission routes. That is another reason for the necessary repetition of targeted informational and educational campaigns.

Another reason for discrimination is usually called *pre-existing discrimination,* i.e. disagreement or disapproval with the existence of certain opposition groups. Only few common people are aware that in this case, the discrimination itself presents a risk of further spreading infection. It is necessary to combat the discrimination as such, in all its forms and manifestations. Frequently, the reasons for this are certain social manifestations originating from certain professional attitudes. They usually manifest themselves in condemning people with certain lifestyle or still uncertain attitudes of some churches, based on intolerance. Daily preventive practice is therefore necessary, so that new social and other moments can be steadily implemented into plans of prevention to weaken the mentioned attitudes. (Mayer, 1999)

One group which has experienced overriding forms of discrimination is that of women. All over the world there is evidence that women have been coerced or pressured to have abortions or be sterilized because they are HIV-positive. Doctors have even exaggerated the rate of perinatal transmission of HIV to infants in order to convince women to terminate a pregnancy. Others have refused outright to offer reproductive health services to such women. In health care, there are reports of a refusal to treat HIV-positive patients and of discrimination against health workers who are HIV-positive. Health workers are also compromised because of their physical closeness to AIDS patients. Discrimination has occurred in the provision of funeral services. This includes the refusal to handle bodies of

people known or suspected to be HIV-positive, the imposition of an extra fee, etc. (Shorter & Onyancha 1998)
The most common forms of discrimination experienced by people living with HIV/AIDS, we could include:

- condemnation, isolation,
- ignoring or avoiding people with HIV/AIDS, because a person does not know how to handle an unpleasant situation during the meeting,
- refusal of care,
- unwillingness to disclose HIV status to someone other because of the fear from discrimination,
- inability to discuss the sexual behaviour, personal preferences and desires, as these topics are accompanied by unpleasant feelings of shame or guilt,
- refusal or neglecting of discussion about the guidance by the risk behaviour and HIV prevention,
- inability and unwillingness to accept a person with AIDS and their families with understanding and without prejudices,

One apparent consequence of discrimination for people living with AIDS is the break-up of families. On learning that their wives are HIV-positive, many husbands desert tem and marry other women. His not only deprives women of the love and care due from their spouses, but also promotes the spread of the disease via their husbands. Another shocking phenomenon is the extent to which infants who are HIV-positive are abandoned in hospitals by their parents. Parents, who cannot face up to the dilemma which the epidemic poses for their children, often abandon their parental responsibility altogether. Various organizations have been set up to deal with the problem, but the battle is still far from being won. Most foster homes are reluctant to take HIV-positive children, claiming that thy do not have the resources to care for them. In some cases, even members of extended families are reluctant to care for HIV/AIDS members for fear of being infected. In such cases, these people are left lonely and desperate. ((Shorter & Onyancha 1998)
Discrimination is closely linked with the concept of *stigma.* Stigma can be distinguished into two basic types. The first category is called *felt stigma,* which distinguishes the individual sensitivity to the potential of negative attitudes and fear of discrimination based on HIV status. Repeated or *enacted stigma* presents a real discrimination experience based on HIV status. For example, an individual may intentionally avoids a HIV test because of the fear that the community would react negatively to any disclosure of its positivity. Should his positivity be disclosed, the patient fears that he would be rejected from the community by his family as well.

5. Children as the most vulnerable group

Children infected with HIV live almost their whole life with some fear. Many of them first experience fear from loss of their parents. Many of them have to watch by, as one or both parents suffer from the AIDS, and they take care of them and spend time with them during the process of dying. After death of one of the parents many of the children must deal with other fears and concerns. In many cases the children guess, that they are sick themselves, too and this fact results in other further concerns. They are constantly confronted with the burden of evidence, which they carry with them for the rest of their life. Some of them will experience a hospitalization associated with many changes, which have to be adapted. If they happen to realize, that their life will not last very long, they are confronted with the fear from their own death.

Children, in particular, suffer from grief after losing their parents, when confronted with the fact that one becomes an orphan. Many of them never experienced, what it means to have a family. They may also suffer from grief, which is transmitted to them from their loved ones, family members and friends. People, who take care of these children and provide them with daily support and assistance, can observe a continual comedown of these children.

Children lose their hope when they have to deal with the loss of their parents, siblings or other relatives. And these are the greatest wounds none of which are ever healed.

If their status becomes known to others e.g. peers, family members and the community it can have a very bad impact on the further development of a child. The child often gets isolated; he or she is excluded by the classmates, in many cases even by their own family members. It is therefore necessary to talk about HIV / AIDS in all its aspects and not make it a taboo topic. It has to be discussed among at all the groups of the society and HIV positive people have to be showed, how to live with this disease.

Many children blame themselves from causing the disease of their parents and dying. They feel responsible for events that occurred. They blame themselves of not being caring enough, that they were evil and that is the reason for their parents´ death. They feel very guilty.

The feeling of guilt, anxiety and their fears can be so strong, which can lead to depression. It happens very seldom, but still, that a child may attempts to commit a suicide. An attempt to commit a suicide can be according to Spitz affected by several elements, such as:

- The concept of death is usually corresponds with age and mental maturity of a child. Even a seven-year old child is able to express the wish that it would rather like to be dead, since his life is meaningless,
- The perception of oneself, the consciousness of one´s own value. Feelings of guilt, lack of adequate self-appreciation, excessive underestimation from the others, unfavourable comparisons with others - lead to the idea of making an end to all of it. Feelings and expressions of depression begin to appear, such as, loss of social interest, feelings of sadness and emptiness, eating and sleep disorders, decreased activity, feelings of loneliness, stubbornness.
- Familiar environment of the child has great impact on him, the idea of a complete family, the fact of experiencing the death of the parents; all of this plays a significant role,
- Form of discrimination is the child experiencing, if it is stigmatized and isolated, what are the social ties. (Spitze, 1991 as cited in Brabec, 1991)

A specific situation is on in which children living with HIV/AIDS are a most vulnerable group. There are some specific psycho-social issues, counsellors have to deal with. Most of them are experiencing fear, anxiety, lethargy and quietude. Some children are segregated by the guardians, who fear their children might also contract the virus when they will play together, sleep together or eating together by sharing the utensils. Some parents have feared to send their children to school; they don't go to school, as some schools don't allow them to play with the rest. There is also high risk, possibility of dropping from school due to ill health. They don't get well balanced food; there is poor access to medication. Some HIV/AIDS positive children already lost their parents; some older children take on the roles of the parents.

They are experiencing stigma and discrimination as well as the adults, even more. Counselling psychologists believe that the age when a child can know the HIV status varies. What is important is the amount of build-up activities related to the disclosure either of the child's status or of a very close relative. The older the child the better and easier it is thought, but this doesn't guarantee easiness with status disclosure.

The care of HIV/AIDS suffering children requires high quality synchronisation and combination of health and social services with taking account on special needs these children. The mail goal is to lengthen and to improve children live and life of their families. (Botek et al., 2005)

Every child is unique in his own way and has special attributes that must be honoured, respected and used carefully. They need help to create the necessary support they need to live with the reality about disclosure of their or other significant people's status in their lives. They are encouraged through their parents/guardians to join support groups that help to reduce the impact of the shocks they receive.

5.1 Psycho-social aspect of children living in developing country, whose parents died due to HIV/AIDS

Organizations such as WHO and UNICEF had assumed that the number of orphans will double every 6 to 9 months and in many developing countries it happened. Many of them stay on the street and they become victims of discrimination. Orphans, who live on the street, so called "street-children„ become often victims of sexual abuse, and in the case, they did not get infected, it can happen very quickly.

The majority of them suffer from lack of proper care and supervision. Most of them live with their relatives or grandparents, who themselves suffer from a lack of income and have a problem and take care of themselves. Some of them start to run their own household and take care of their younger siblings. For example 1996 in Kenya, up to 58% of all orphans who survive were aged from 10 to 14 years, 19% are 15 or more. Up to 58% of orphans are dependent on their relatives or on the community to be able to survive. 32% of the orphans depend on the sale of vegetables, roasted corn or collection of paper, and iron for living and 10% survive only thanks to begging. (Shorter & Onyancha, 1998)

In the research study from Nairobi in Kenya in 2008 shows, that nearly 20% of street children were complete orphans, 10% had only their fathers and 59% only their mothers alive. These survey results show that most street children have single parents, predominantly the mother. (Fabianova et.al, 2010)

Children whose parents died of AIDS are discriminated against, the society often treats them as potential carriers of HIV virus and they are expected to lead a promiscuous life following the way of life of their parents. These children live in real poverty, in an extraordinary situation including the lack of basic resources and lack of access to services, which would help them to resolve the difficult situation. The wider family usually takes care of orphans, but the rapid increase of the number of orphans needing care requires extended possibility apart from family. In many cases, the orphans are taken care of by their grandparents, sometimes elder children take care of their younger siblings, and surprisingly, their age is about 10 to 12. In some cases, children live completely outside of the family structure and very often on the street.

The death of one or of both parents, who died of AIDS triggers many sociological, economic and psychological changes for the orphaned child. Orphans are exposed to a large number of problems, such as malnutrition which is associated with a lack of food or poor position to

occupy in the familiar environment. Their educational opportunities are limited due to domestic responsibilities, or lack of funds to purchase books and uniforms. Suffer physical and psychological support and protection, as well as lack of parental attention and their absence. Orphans - girls are more vulnerable because of sexual abuse and are at greater risk of HIV transmission and continuing spreading of infection. Sometimes orphaned boys are rejected more often than their sisters because the girls are more useful in the household.
The situation gets worse, when the orphans have to live on the street and they are exposed to the danger of abuse. Street-girls in their early adolescent age were tested for a small study of Undugu association, and the outcome showed, that more than one quarter is HIV positive. Some of the tested girls suffered from syphilis, gonorrhoea or some other infections. (Guest, 2001)
The social situation of each orphaned child is always difficult and it can have long-lasting and traumatic effects. The situation of AIDS orphans presents some more specific problems which are specific only for this type of group of children, It is necessary to eliminate and to get to know, the stigma associated with AIDS which interfered with the lives of many orphans and it is necessary to satisfy the basic needs of children using the practical interventional programs. There are slight socio-economic differences amongst the orphans in Kenya, even though the majority of them live in extreme poverty. HIV/AIDS, combined with the problem of poverty presents a significant stress for the traditional structure of assistance, as well as for the complete set-up of the household. Satisfaction of all the demands of the family plays a priority role for the orphans despite of significant limitation of financial resources. It is very difficult to discuss the long-term consequences of pandemics, but it is clear, that adaptability, power and the survival of a Kenyan family is seriously threatened in the social system.
In the developing counties the services for HIV/AIDS children are often provided by professionals coming from western countries. Most of the approaches, used in Europe, are based on local traditions, religion, and mentality and so on. Using of these approaches in other parts of the world can cause problems, or, can cause their non-efficiency. There is strong necessity to adapt the European standards of care to local standards and search for appropriate range of services. An adaptation of educational and therapeutic approaches is necessary due to significant differences, in upbringing, such as the use of punishments, and so on. (Botek & Kovalcikova, 2008)

5.1.1 Psycho-social aspects of children living in developing country, who have lost their father due to HIV/AIDS

A majority of men, who are also fathers become infected and die before their wives. Along with the death of the father, who presents the male element of the family, the family loses the social and physical protection associated with male authority. A woman as a head of the family in the developing countries does not have any right of property inheritance, because the relationships to her husband's family are weakened. The mother has to manage her time to be a parent and to satisfy the needs of the family. Children usually help to run the household. In rural areas children work on family farms in order to help the family to survive.
These households often bear an additional burden, the commitment to pay for the treatment and care of the dead father; the family must deal with the loss of income, which was supplied by him. Children usually stop going to school and are forced to look for a job, which is depressing for them. They are exposed to abuse as workers, who work for the

minimum wage and it does not cover their basic need at all. This fact strengthens the difficult situation and the family sinks into poverty.

In the developing countries in the majority of families, in which the father dies, the widow after the funeral rites returns from the countryside, where he was buried, to the city. These Kenyan widows, if not previously employed, often begin with to sell smuggled good, such as illegal alcohol to keep their household supplied with needed stuff. The children usually help or try to help in other ways to replace the father. In some cases they are forced to sell their body, because the income of the mother is insufficient. In such cases children stay with their grandparents from the mother´s side in the country, while she tries to make some money in the city. Women leave their children primarily because of economic reasons. If the mother comes from a monogamous relationship, children usually stay with their grandparents from her husband's side. If a widow comes from a polygamous relationship, children are often taken care of by the first wife, who usually becomes head of the family after the death of her husband. In Kenya children living with grandparents from the father's side suffer from lack of care, and so they tend to find the grandparents of the mother's side. It is still difficult for the children to live with the uncle, because they are often perceived by their relatives as a potential candidate for the property inheritance and they are abused mainly for work. But reality shows that orphans are traditionally excluded from old-parental inheritance.

The impact of negative living conditions is significant and influences the child's mental state. We can talk of *psychological deprivation* if the child does not have sufficient amount of stimuli and such living conditions, which are necessary for its satisfaction of basic needs and healthy emotional development.

We can thus conclude that a child who has lost his father experiences this situation to its full extent. The amount of stressful situations increases and they often overlap. Death of a parent is a frustrating situation for each child and threatens its existence. It becomes a long-term stress factor in his life. The loss of the mother is equally stressing for the child.

5.1.2 Psycho-social aspect of children living in developing country, who have lost their mother due to HIV/AIDS

Men, who have lost their wives get, married as soon as possible which is reasoned by wanting the best for their children. Most children, however, do not perceive this fact as favourable, on the contrary, father's protection and support decreases with the arrival of a step-mother. These new circumstances cause a tense situation and relationships at home, the children miss the attention they used to get from their mother. It happens sometimes, that the step-mother is the same age as the children and is unable to take care of them, which makes the family situation even worse.

Children are rarely able to re-create the same emotional connection to the new mother. It is often an unsecure, uncertain and chaotic relationship of the child to its step-mother and it is filled with ambivalent feelings. With the arrival of the step - mother many children experience regular physical attacks and unbearable punishment. Many of them must follow strict rules regarding the access to food; they are discriminated in comparison to her children, who are preferred by her for the food supply. The children do not get enough of protection from their father and they are forced to seek shelter at their dead mother´s family. Men, widowers who have not had the chance to marry after the death of the wife yet, are trying in the majority of cases to do so as quickly as possible. Only in few cases, stays the father with his children alone. Spreading epidemics may cause problems for a widower to find a partner in many third-world countries. They sometimes must handle the fact that they have to raise their children alone, which presents a new created phenomenon and is a significant deviation from a traditional family life for the majority of men.

Children are social beings since the early stages of development. The tendency of social handling is not learnt, but it is probably a part of the biological equipment of a man. A strong primary motivation to be as close to the mother as possible for the child is natural. The mother presents a fundamental source of security for a child and she is a source of future relations to peers and partners, as demonstrated in recent years in long-term studies. Mother - child relationship are characterized by a strong emotional relationship, trying to be each other as much close as possible in the intimate contact. This condition it is not static, but it is a constant interaction of mother and child, it is performed repeatedly many times a day, it constantly changes, improves and strengthens weakens, depending on the proper/improper approach, which means life security and safety for the child. It is the basis for individual orientation and in the environment and getting to know the surroundings approximately from the second year of age of a child.

The close relationship of mother and child develops instantly after the birth and has a wide variety of forms. It is initiated by the mother – intimate contact, smile, voice signals and some games and by an overall positive and joyful relationship. Sensitivity to the needs of the child is expected. Interaction dynamics between mother and child has several phases for a small child:

- feeling of security in the presence of the mother,
- child leaves the mother to play or to get to know the environment,
- there is a growing sense of insecurity in the absence of mother,
- the child looks for its mother and also the safety and security,
- reunion with the mother is associated with satisfaction. (Dunovsky, 1999)

The whole cycle repeats constantly, the child goes on to discover the environment, comes back again and so on.

A number of studies showed, that children, who develop a strong attachment to their mother, develops much better emotionally, socially and in the cognitive area. This is obvious in the early years, but also in the age of 6 years and more. It is the same relationship, when the child is stressed when the mother leaves, but it calms down, when she returns and makes lively contact with her. There is a clear difference in response to the mother and foreign persons. Relationship created in such a way is beneficial for the child and in most cases it is associated with the next development of other positive stages in its development. (Dunovsky, 1999)

A number of situations and life circumstances undermine and weaken the bonding process. We distinguish two basic situations:

- Privacy: meaning living conditions in which no bonding could be created, because after the birth the child and the mother were separated, or the mother is unable to take care of the child. The damage of the development is usually significant which mostly causing irreparable changes in the development.
- Deprivation meaning the conditions in which the relationship was being built, but they were interrupted by a negative interference. It can be primarily a disease of a mother, or child's long-term hospitalization.

The impact of similar situations might not be so critical if a solution were found, which is good for the life of a child.

Other negative moments and deviations from normal development ("turning points" as they are called in evolutionary psychology) can be:

- *Long-term or repeated hospitalization of a child* without a mother (during this period of time an anxiety connection or substitution connection to some other person is often created, for example a sensitive nurse),
- *Changes in the child´s environment*: mother's long-term illness, change of environment, loss of a loved one, death of someone in the family, associated with a strong child's grief and so on.

Bratska states that the worst impact is caused by a long-term hospitalization of children within 7-12 months of age. In the case, that during this period the child lacks an emotional contact with his mother, the proper relationship to his mother cannot be created, which gives basis for the social relationships of the child. (Bratska, 2001)

In a later child´s and also of adults' development, significant turning points appear which are watched by the developmental psychology, focused on the length of life (life history). They can be presented by a series of events for the child, which modifies his life. These include: experience with violence, an accident, illness, serious moments associated with the maturity process of the child in various stages of its development, experience with the start of puberty and first sexual partner or relationship.

5.1.3 Children who lost both parents due to HIV/AIDS

Most of the children whose parents died of AIDS find their new place in their wider family network. But even if someone gives them a shelter, they usually do not have the feeling that they had a real home. The decision of someone from their wider family to take care of the orphan is not just an economic issue. It usually happens that the richer family is very rarely in contact with the orphans; on the contrary, the orphans are taken care of by the family, which lives in poverty.

The new family that decides to take care of those children has to deal with many reactions and their own emotions. Many family members show and feel compassion; they show the children their sympathy and understanding. But for many of them it is also a shock situation, which is filled with fear. Some families tend to blame the deceased parents, blame them for irresponsibility and children have to listen to wide variety of remorse. In such households, these children are often excluded from equal distribution of family resources. The substitute family expects and counts on the fact, that the orphans will work themselves for their living. Many of these children state that they do not have the same rights in the foster family; they have limited food supply, because they may eat after the other family members have finished their meals.

Most of the orphans prefer therefore to stay at their own home, even without an adult member. In these cases, the oldest child tends to adopt the role of head of the family, regardless of the gender. Girls take over the role of mother, trying to provide food for other children. When there is not enough food, they are the ones that eat as the last, if their mother did so. They are responsible for the household with all the things that are associated with it.

These young girls grow up without parental assistance and they gain knowledge about the world, the family, about sex from their peers, who are also low educated and are discovering the world only by them. Most of them have minimal education, they are starting too early with the intimate life and soon after that they usually have to take care of their own child. They miss the premature loss of parental love and they seek emotional support; they are an easy victim of sexual abuse. They would like to be married, but younger siblings are often an obstacle for a potential husband. In a situation, when a brother takes care of younger siblings, his role is of the man in the family. This role is associated with the enforcement of the authority and leading positions often by the use of physical violence. He tries to provide an income and to keep the household running. Usually he avoids doing the so-called "female" work, such as preparation of food; such activities are to be done by younger sisters.

Perhaps the children of prostitutes find themselves in the most difficult situation. After the death of their mother, they are left alone, with a huge psychological trauma. Most of these orphans stay temporarily with their grandparents, who live often in extreme poverty; those children do not usually have any possibility to attend school. What happens to children after the death of grandparents is questionable, but it is clear that they are exposed to many risks. Most of them are neglected and face hostility from all people. The girls are sometimes taken care of by other family members with the intent to have somebody for house work or marry the girl to anybody, who would bring them some profit. Some of the girls make the same mistake as their mother did and they sell their body almost for nothing, which provides them some income for their living. Many of them are from 12 to 16 years of the age, presuming that they are not HIV positive.

5.2 When a child survives the death of his parents

The death of a parent means in particular a relational loss. It means the end of all opportunities to be in contact, to communicate, to have common experiences, to love, or have in some way the emotional and physical presence of the mother or father. The fact that this is a permanent loss is particularly difficult.

The death is probably the most significant loss, which may affect a person's life. It is therefore normal that the child feels profound grief, the child feels abandoned, desperate and helpless. This is a real and deep crisis for them. Mourning after the death of a parent in many aspects resembles some kind of an illness; it is in fact not an illness, but a natural way of processing a loss. It presents a complex of psychological, social and somatic reactions to the loss.

The children react to death and to the loss of a loved one with strong emotions, which often remain hidden. Around the age of 7 to 9 years appears more realistic understanding of the death and reaction of children may appear as those of the adults. Around the age of 10 a child starts to understand the death in its social and biological context. In the first years of life the loss of a parent has the biggest potential impact on the pathological personality development, but can serve as the basis of psychiatric problems in the later years. For children in the age from 3 to 4 years of age, his death of a parent of the same gender is the most critical. The overall behaviour of younger children may seem incomprehensible and unbounded to the tragic event. It is definitely necessary to know, that the child at this time in its life will have a new surge of emotions. (Vizinova & Preiss, 1999)

The following outlines the most common demonstrations of emotion in children losing their parents:

- Sadness, grief and sorrow,
- Concerns that may be caused by insecurity. The child asks questions like ("What is going to happen to me? What am I supposed to do all alone?"), but also questions about the meaning of life, they are confronted with the own mortality, especially with the fear of its own death,

- Anger, wrath and aggression, these negative emotions can be addressed to all the other, e.g. the medical staff ("Why could the doctors not help my parent somehow? Why couldn´t he is saved?") Or these emotions can be addressed to the deceased ("How could he/she done that to me? Why did he/she leave me here alone?"), but also to themselves ("Why didn´t I do something? Why was I so bad?"), and so on.
- Feelings of guilt, arising from the own survival ("Why didn´t I die instead?")
- Feeling of loneliness the children experience, when they are left by the other parent and they are left all alone or with their siblings.
- Feeling of relief especially if the child watched the parent suffer, the idea that the parent does not suffer anymore is comforting for the child
- Somatic problems of children are demonstrated in particular, by exhaustion, fatigue, anorexia and by an overall weakness of the organism.
- Disorganization of daily life and daily routines, the child is excluded from activities that he or she used to do and life of the child has stopped to run as it usually did.
- Impulsive, chaotic handling. These are common symptoms caused by stress and fear that the child is experiencing.
- The child is having imaginings/fantasies about the deceased parent, the child may imagine, they see, hear and feel the deceased parent.
- The child identifies himself or herself with the deceased parent. The children may take over certain behavioural models and patterns of deceased parent, they use his/her words, gestures, and ways of speaking and so on.
- Avoidance of social contact, the child has the feeling that nobody understands him. It can often cause irritability and hostility, especially in the presence of strangers.

It is perfectly natural and normal that a child experiences such a combination of emotions and reactions. It is important for the child to have the opportunity to express and to talk about what the child is going through and it is also very important that the child has someone, who would help him to overcome this difficult and traumatic situation.

5.2.1 The process of mourning of children: The stages of handling the death of a parent

Mourning is a consequence of the loss, which the individual realizes. It is considered a natural, normal and necessary mechanism for handling the loss in life. To what extent is this process successful depends on how one handles the tasks of mourning.

Between the mourning steps we can include: acceptance of loss of life, acute mourning, adaptation to the environment without the lost object, redirecting power to the second object, overcoming fear of change, finding new and the meaning of life. Signs of mourning can be seen in the following areas:

- Emotional (grief, anger, feelings of guilt, anxiety, helplessness, indifference).
- Vegetative (tension, sensitivity to noise and light, shortness of breath, dry mouth, asthenia).
- Cognitive (mistrust, confusion, obsessive deal with memories of lost object, forgetfulness, disorders in new memory, hallucinations, difficulty in concentrating attention).
- Lifestyle and behaviour disorders (sleep disorder, loss of appetite, secretiveness', keep oneself to oneself, out from society, scary dreams).

Even if all the processing of grief and death is unique and individual, it is possible to distinguish several phases that are not always in the same order but they stand side by side and often can be repeated.

The process of mourning is described by different authors, for example. Kubler-Ross divided the period of 5 phases:

1. Stage of shock, denial and negation of death,
2. Stage of anger and aggression,
3. Stage of negotiations
4. Stage of depression
5. Stage of acceptance and reconciliation with death. (Kubler-Ross, 2003)

These phases often overlap; they can last a different period of time and can happen parallel or do not exist at all. There is some specificity identified for children´s experience when handling this situation.

Kubickova talks about 4 phases experienced by children: (Kubickova 2001)

1. **Phase of shock, denial and isolation**. Immediately after the loss of a parent, the child, responds by feeling confused numb, stunned and shocked. He usually denies the whole situation, does not want to believe that it had happened. ("No, it cannot be true! I don´t believe it!") Children convince themselves, that it is not possible. They reject and deny the reality, which is actually a psychological defensive reaction. They attenuate the effects of negative news. They try not to face the fact. At the same time, they show that they still do not handle their own pain and the child seems emotionally overloaded. Some children tend to play various games, e.g. they are being cruel to animals to express the sadness and pain.

2. **Self-control phase**, which is a pretence that lasts until the evening of the funeral day. Preparation and organization of the burial ceremony makes it impossible for the surviving family to fully succumb to the grief. After the mourners have left, the surviving family are able to surrender and feel the pain of their loss to its full extent. This process may be experienced in some other way by the children, since they usually are not involved in organizing of the funeral, the shock phase may be extended to a longer period of time. Some children idealize the deceased parent at this phase of the mourning process. For some children everything that reminds them of the death parent becomes important. Objects reminding children of the dead mother or father reminds them of having a nice time that they had together. The younger children sometimes show strong desire to amalgamate with the deceased parent. Some children might to wear clothes of the deceased parent or to have the same job. At this stage of the process, children without stable identity are in danger, that the development of their own „self" will be negatively influenced.

3. **Regression phase**, which may take from one to three months. The lamentation and mourning phase takes often the most extended period of time. The mourning child often cries, elements of regression can be found in his behaviour, these children are apathetic, closed up into his own inner world, they are anxious and desperate. The disorganizing of behaviour is obvious; the surviving family is not able to function normally in everyday life. They are unable to get their life back and they retreat from their social contacts. Many children may suffer from sleeping disorders and lack of appetite. The children sometimes switch from their idealizing of the deceased parent to his/her disparaging. Their pain is mixed with anger and rage that they have been left alone. Negative evaluation of the deceased parent is an attempt of child to let go. If the idealization of the deceased partner happens too soon, there is a danger for the child not to be able to let go. Only a realistic

picture of the deceased, accepting of all sides of his/her personality can become basis for the child to converge to his deceased partner on other level.
4. **Adaptation phase**. It usually takes up to one year, depending on the next development of the situation after the death of a parent. This is a period of reconciliation with past events, the child does not forget, but starts getting used to the absence of the parent. We must not overlook, that the process of handling grief is a long, painful process and it needs a lot of energy. Therefore a child needs time without sadness and when it rejects the sadness, when it wishes the deceased parent to be alive again. The last period of mourning is called a phase of a new relationship to children themselves and to the world, which reflects the fact that something new starts, something totally different from what the child has been accustomed to.
The time course of the mourning process cannot be predicted. At its end stands rapprochement to the deceased parent on a qualitatively new level. Mourning ends, but is not completed yet. The child is usually able to find a more mature relationship to the deceased parent. The deceased father or deceased mother are not physically present, but tend to be very clearly present "spiritually". The children may still feel sorrow and pain. The scars remain. The loss cannot be erased. The adult can show the children, how to treat these wounds and how to live with them.
It would be ideal if we could provide each child, whose the parent died with the following:

- Relevant information adequate their age,
- Open communication about the death,
- Supported expressing of their feelings,
- Provision of basic needs,
- As stable and safe environment as possible,
- Support and relief in the pleasant memories of the deceased parent,
- Involvement of the child in the preparations of the funeral rites,
- Respect for the needs of the child to maintain the connection to the deceased parent (Dane & Levine, 2002)

There are various different types of care for orphaned and abandoned children, which differ from country to county. In many third-world countries the concept of "adoption" does not exist in the same sense as in Europe. Orphans are taken care of by some relatives in order to avoid a total disappearance of a father´s household.
In Kenya, for example, each household belonging to the given tribe is valuable and therefore it should be protected by the tribe. Although the desire to survive as a family is very strong, poor economic and social circumstances lead to the separation of some orphans. Four categories of households with orphaned children can be distinguished according to practice:

- Foster families: children are taken care of by some relative from the father´s family, mostly an aunt or uncle.
- Caretakers of the third generation: presented by the grandparents
- Orphans leading their own household: when there is nobody, who could take care of those children, they usually stay alone. This forces immature children to start an adult life with full responsibility for their lives and lives of their younger siblings. Many orphans - girls become mothers in their teenage years.
- Households employing orphans: some families employ children - orphans as cheap hand in the household.

6. Forms of defence and adaptation mechanisms

In stressful situations, each person reacts differently. Each has his own defence mechanisms which help to reduce tension and anxiety. These mechanisms function on the subconscious level and they deny or distort the reality. The most common defence mechanisms occurring in different types of situations, which are stressful for the child, such as HIV / AIDS thus frustrating in situations, include the following: (Bratska, 2001)

- **Repression -** according to S. Freud repression is one of the most important defence mechanisms. During displacement memories or impulses are causing stress (pain, anxiety, guilt) and thus pushed out of consciousness.
- **Suppression** - is presented by purposeful self-control, during which a person controls his impulses and desires or temporarily removes all painful memories, especially when he needs to concentrate the effort on a particular activity.
- **Projection** - requires looking for causes of their own failures in other people, accrediting their own unacceptable impulses to another person.
- **Reactive creation** - presents acquiring attitudes and behaviour that are the very opposite of the actual thoughts and feelings.
- **Fixation** - is presented by persistence and focus on areas, which are typical for certain period of development for long time after the person should move to the next level or phase.
- **Regression** - a return to the ways of behaviour, that were adequate to an earlier developmental stages.
- **Inversion** - shows a sort of "reverse behaviour. The person in crisis reacts exactly in the opposite way one would expect. "
- **The types of rationalization** - a person reasons and apologizes for the motives for original handling by rational argument to keep self-confidence and good judgement of him. In these mechanisms can be included: is one of belittlement, which reduces and disparages the value, the aim one did not reach and the next mechanism is relativization, which rationalizes the worries comparing them to previous worries one was able to solve successfully. Another form of relativisation is the acquisition of overview; comparison with the future ("what is this in comparison with what is ahead").
- **Substitution and compensation**- the original object, who satisfied one´s needs is replaced for an analogic one by substitution and substitution by compensation.
- **Identification** - when a person agrees with the behaviour of others.

Defence mechanisms are often used by adults, but almost by all children. An acceptable level of use is considered normal. Only when it becomes the predominant way of response, when the child uses this mechanism electively, it signalizes a bad adaptation. The reason for that is because: they prevent the child in dealing with the world in a realistic way. They waste energy that could be used more efficiently. When they fail, the resulting anxiety can present for the child serious difficulties.

Coping with difficult life situations, describes various coping strategies. Unlike defence mechanisms, which falsify the reality, coping strategies - respect the reality. We can define "coping" as behavioural, cognitive or social response of an individual whose aim is to control internal or external pressures stemming from the individual interactions with the environment. We can distinguish two basic coping strategies:

- *Focus on self-development* - reflects the natural self-centeredness. Individual focuses on his or her own person and on their own emotions. He tries to reduce uncomfortable tension by using of the escape mechanisms - escape into fantasy, to the memories and the like.
- *Focus on your problem* - involves efforts to influence the environment and to change it. An individual seeks adequate information, to reformulate and redefine the problem and find other alternative ways of coping with the situation.

Choice of coping strategy depends on the previous experience and subjective evaluations of the event. Optimal coping strategies include an estimation of the significance of the critical events and consideration of the risks of the subsequent acts or, conversely, the risk of interruption of activity. In some emergency situations it is necessary to respond immediately, while in others it is better to stop the activity. It is a very difficult period for children and it is necessary for them to get help, whether from close relatives, friends, acquaintances or institutions in the form of emotional support, practical help, advice and information. Social support has a direct impact on reducing stress; or rather it acts as a buffer or blocking in dampening the impact of a crisis. It is also an important determinant of mental health and subjective well-being. When a system of social support is lacking, it leads to a reduction in the child's mental endurance and the possibility to deal with the crisis.

7. Process of counselling

Counselling in HIV/AIDS is a core element of the holistic approach to health care. During the process of counselling psychological aspects are recognised. Counselling enables frank discussion of sensitive issues in the client's life. People may suffer from great psychosocial and psychological stresses through a fear of rejection, disease progression, social stigma and the uncertainties associated with future.

Laboratory diagnosis of HIV infection for evidence of the specific antibody or HIV is a serious step in the life of an individual; it should be accompanied by an interview/counselling session before and after the examination. And this is especially important by diagnose of children.

In Kenya, VTC (Voluntary Counselling and Testing Centres) were created for free diagnosis and advice across the whole country. They provide services for all residents by professionally trained counsellors. The counsellors discuss a lot of psychosocial issues which people diagnosed with HIV/AIDS face in their everyday life.

Probably the most important service being offered to people living with AIDS is counselling. This is carried out by individuals and by groups. The common objectives of counselling are firstly to win the confidence of people with AIDS, so that they return for continued help. Then, people have to be helped to grow and develop, so that they can decide what they want and live valuable lives regardless of their HIV status. People who have been tested must be helped to get through the initial period of crisis. Infected people must be shown how to keep from spreading AIDS and how to take preventive steps. They must be encouraged to talk with their family members. (Shorter & Onyancha, 1998)

Because we have no cure for HIV/AIDS, we have to focus our interventions on caring for the physical as well as the psychological welfare of the HIV positive individual and his or her significant others. The aims of counselling should always be based on the needs of the client. The purpose of counselling could be as follows:

- to assist clients manage their problems more effectively and develop unused opportunities to cope more fully,
- to empower clients to become more effective self-helpers in the future

Counselling should be about constructive change and about making a substantive difference in the life of the client. However only the client can make that difference, the counsellor is merely an instrument to facilitate that process of change.

7.1 Counselling before and after testing HIV/AIDS

The counselling before and after testing HIV/AIDS has phenomenal emotional, practical, psychological and social implications for each client. This type of counselling has some specifications:

- HIV testing never is done without thorough pre-test counselling.
- Pre-test counselling that is done in a proper and comprehensive way prepares the client and counsellor for more effective post test counselling.
- Clients are often too relieved or shocked to take much information in during post-test counselling. The counsellor should make use of the educational opportunities offered by pre-test counselling.
- Counsellors are trained to do pre- and post-test counselling in a professional way and to keep all information confidential. It is also a right of client to sty anonymous.
- Nobody may be tested for HIV without informed consent and without proper pre-HIV test counselling.

The counselling before the examination is focused on providing information regarding the technical side of screening, but also the possible personal, medical, social, psychological and legal implications of diagnosis, whether it is positive or negative. Information should be given in an appropriate form and must be based on actual information. The process of child counselling has specific differences. It is necessary to explain to them every act of procedure that will reduce the initial fear.

Interview before the inquiry should focus on two main areas:

- Personal history of the client and risks that they were or are exposed to,
- Consideration of whether the client understands the HIV / AIDS issue, as well as his previous experience in crisis management.

The initial interview should include discussion and assessment of the client's attitude, appraisal of psycho-social factors and knowledge about HIV/AIDS issues.

People who have been confirmed as being infected with HIV must be informed about it as soon as possible. The first interview should be confidential and the client should get some time to deal with this report. After that, he should be very clearly and factually informed about the importance of the diagnosis. At this time, devoid of different speculations about the forecast or consideration of how much time remains the affected person has to live. It is a time period, when a person has to deal with the new reality and overcome the *shock*. It's also time to provide security support and assistance. It is a time of hope for resolving personal and practical problems that may arise. If there are real possibilities of such support, it is appropriate to talk about possible ways of therapy in case of some HIV / AIDS symptoms, as well as the effectiveness of treatment.

Whether the client will or will not accept the diagnosis is usually determined by the following factors: (Bar, 2000)

- Current state of health. Persons, who are already sick, may have a prolonged reaction time. Their actual response occurs, only when they are physically stronger.

- Readiness to accept the situation. People, who are not ready, may respond differently than those who expect such a result. Unexpected reactions may appear even if the individual is prepared for the situation.
- Real or potential support of the environment. Factors such as satisfaction at work, harmonic family cohesion, as well as opportunities for recreation and sexual relations, may act as very positive support mechanisms. Conversely, those, who are socially isolated, have little money, scant employment perspective, poor family support and inadequate housing, react much worse. HIV positive parent, who learns that his child is infected, usually accepts the news very badly. An HIV positive parent knows his own situation and knows about the chances the child may wait.
- Personality of tested before testing and the psychological health. If there was any mental stress before the test, the response may be more or less complicated and require a different strategy compared with those who did not have such problems. Management after such information should take into account personal psychological or psychiatric problems of clients. The stress of possible HIV positivity may cause a recurrence of previous conditions. In some cases, information about HIV positivity may unearth some unresolved issues and concerns. These often complicate the process of coping with the diagnosis. Therefore, this situation is to be handled very sensitively and carefully as soon as possible.
- Cultural and spiritual values related to disease and death. In many cultures people believe in an afterlife or fatality, so they receive the report of their HIV infection in a much calmer way. On the other hand, there may be a region where AIDS is seen as a punishment for antisocial and immoral behaviour, and therefore it is associated with feelings of guilt and resistance. Counselling and support are very important when reporting the news about the disease. Some reactions can be initially very turbulent. One has to realize, however, that this is a normal reaction to the report, which for the individual represents life threatening condition and that they often do not want to admit it.
- Although the post-HIV test counselling interview is separate from the pre-test counselling interview, both are inextricably linked. The pre-test counselling interview should have given the client a glimpse of what to expect in post-test counselling.

Pre- and post-test counselling should preferably be done by the same person because the established relationship between the client and counsellor provides a sense of continuity for the client. The counsellor will also have a better idea of how to approach the post-test counselling because of what he or she experienced in the pre-test counselling. The counsellor should always ask the client if he or she is prepared to receive the results. In the case of the rapid HIV antibody test - where the results are available within minutes - the client should be asked if he/she is ready to receive the results immediately. Some clients need time to prepare for the results. For both the client and the counsellor, a negative HIV result is a tremendous relief. A negative test result could however give someone, who is frequently involved in high-risk behaviour, a false sense of security. It is therefore extremely important for the counsellor to counsel HIV-negative clients in order to reduce the chances of future infection. Advice about risk reduction and safer sex must therefore be emphasised. The possibility that the client is in the "window period" or that the negative test result may be a false negative should also be pointed out. If there is concern about the HIV status of the person, he or she should return for a repeat test after about three months and ensure that appropriate precautions are taken in the meanwhile. To communicate a positive test result to a client is a huge responsibility. The way people react to test results depends to a large extent on how thoroughly the counsellor has educated and prepared them both before and after the test.

Clients' responses to the news usually vary from one person to another. Reactions may include shock, crying, agitation, stress, guilt, withdrawal, anger and outrage - some clients may even respond with relief. The counsellor should allow clients to deal with the news in their own way and give them the opportunity to express their feelings. The counsellor should show empathy, warmth and caring, maintain neutrality and respond professionally to outbursts. Because the loss of health is equated with bereavement, it manifests with all the components of denial, anger, bargaining, depression and acceptance. The counsellor must respect the personal nature of an individual's feelings.

People's needs, when they receive an HIV positive test result, vary, and the counsellor has to determine what those needs are and deal with them accordingly. Fear of pain and death are often the most serious and immediate problems and these can be dealt with in various ways. Talking to clients about their fears for the future is one of the most important therapeutic interventions that the counsellor can make. Often it is enough for the counsellor just to be "there" for the client and to listen to him or her. One of the major concerns for HIV positive people is whom to tell about their condition and how to break the news. It is often helpful to use role-play situations in which the client can practise communicating the news to others. In responding to a client's needs, an attitude of non-judgmental and empathic attentiveness is more important than doing or saying specific things. Listening is more important than talking; being with the person more important than doing some specific action.

Crisis intervention is often necessary after an HIV positive test result is given. The counsellor must be sure that the person has support after he or she leaves the office. A person in crisis should never be left alone: he or she should have somebody with whom to share the burden. If the client shows any suicidal tendencies, emergency hospitalisation should be arranged if a friend or family member cannot be with the client. Follow-up visits are therefore necessary to give clients the opportunity to ask questions, talk about their fears and the various problems that they encounter. Significant others, such as a partner, spouse or other members of the family may be included in the session. During the follow-up visits, clients should be offered a choice concerning their treatment.

If health care professionals are not in a position to do follow-up counselling, information about relevant health services should be given. If there is a concern that the person might not return for follow-up counselling, information about available medical treatments such as anti-retroviral therapy, treatment of opportunistic infections, and social services for financial and on-going emotional support should be given.

The counsellor should inform the client about support systems such as the "buddy system" that is usually available at the nearest Aids centre or from the offices of non-governmental organisations who work in the community.

It is necessary to convey information about safer sex, infection control, health care in general and measures to strengthen the immune system. It is very important also to encourage clients to go for regular medical check-ups to the health clinic. Infections and opportunistic diseases can be prevented if treated in time.

8. Research study, objectives, methodology

The *main goal* is to analyse the psycho-social aspects of people coming to the Voluntary Counselling and Testing Centre in Nairobi, Kenya. The study is realized in order to acquire feedback information about psycho - social aspects in practices. The *main objectives* are follows:

- To discover the percentage of clients in VCT, who have certain behavioural features (anger, fear, anxiety, distress, shock and so on)
- To analyse the psycho-social factors that affect PLWHA in Nairobi,
- To identify the sources of stigmatization and discrimination of PLWHA in Nairobi,
- To analyse the most problematic social issues of PLWHA,
- To discover whether or not clients of VCT are able to speak about spiritual issues,
- To analyse the meaning of regular counselling session in order to change the behaviour of PLWHA.

The target group and place of research study.

Counsellors of VCT collected the data in the years from 2005 to 2009. They have provided counselling to 12 685 clients altogether; out of them 1165 were tested positive, which were included into the research study.

The clients were mostly from Mukuru slums, South B, South C, Nairobi West, Mugoya and from the industrial area in Nairobi. The VCT centre has a total staff included of six trained VCT counsellors, who have background trainings in public health (degree level) and psychological counselling (degree level) with vast experiences since the centre was started (2003) VCT for Mukuru slums was initiated with the aim to raise awareness about the spread of HIV/AIDS and to prevent the spread within the Mukuru population and its environment.

Being the entry point to HIV/AIDS prevention and care, the service has the specific objectives to achieve: to offer voluntary counselling and testing to the clients for HIV positivity; to provide information and education about HIV/AIDS ; to offer referral services for further management to designated referral points; to increase couple counselling and testing of VCT.

Any testing at the site must be accompanied by pre-test information and post-counselling information as prescribed in the National HIV counselling and testing guidelines. 70% of clients of VCT are coming to VCT based their own decision; this means they are not sent by doctors or nurses from any clinic or hospital.

Year	2005		2006		2007		2008		2009		Total	
	tested	positive	tested	positive	tested	positive	tested	positive	tested	positive	tested	positive
Male	1079	93	1128	82	1218	94	1367	59	1672	62	6464	390
Female	1011	208	1056	162	1132	145	1264	145	1758	115	6221	775
Total	2090	301	2184	244	2350	239	2631	204	3430	177	12685	1165

Table 1. Number of clients at Mary Immaculate VCT Nairobi, Kenya by gender (Okoth & Namulanda, 2010)

Table shows clients in Voluntary Counselling and Testing Centre at Mary Immaculate Clinic in Nairobi, in Kenya. Out of 12 685 tested clients were 1165 positive. From the total number 775 were female and 390 male.

Age	15-19	20-24	25-29	30-34	34-39	40-44	45-49	50-54	55+	Total
Male	2	24	64	103	88	62	31	7	9	390
Female	27	149	216	162	118	47	39	7	10	775
Total	29	173	280	265	206	109	70	14	19	1165

Table 2. Number of HIV positive clients at Mary Immaculate VCT Nairobi, Kenya in years 2005 to 2009 by age and gender (Okoth & Namulanda, 2010)

Methodology and realization of the research study

An exploratory qualitative research study using in-depth interviews was conducted by the 6 counsellors in voluntary counselling and testing centre in Nairobi, Kenya. The interviews were carried out using semi-structured questions, open and closed questions. The counsellors collected data from their client´s record for the last 5 years (2005-2009). Data were assessed using content analysis, the study of the documentation of clients, observation, comparison and interview.

8.1 Summary of results from research study

The first objective is to discover the typical reactions of clients to their HIV/AIDS positivity. Based on the research study 60% of clients felt *fear, anxiety,* 30% of them *anger,* 25% of them indicated *distress,* 15% *cried.* Clients spoke about *grief,* feelings of sadness of loss they experienced, or are expecting. Obviously, almost all, clients confirmed positive for HIV felt *sadness* because of their status (89%). Many clients feel this way when referring to close relatives, who had suffered and died of HIV/AIDS. Only clients who are confirmed negative of HIV feel free to continue talking of this *topic-(grief).*

Identification of clients' way of feeling´ *anger and aggression* after being tested differs according to gender. We came to conclusion, that many male clients who are tested positive openly show anger, disbelief, as opposed to their female counterparts. Some became aggressive (5%) towards a counsellor and demanded a repetition of the tests. The female clients tested positive for HIV tended to cry, go into shock, swallowed big lumps of air, saliva subconsciously, shook both their hand in refusal and blame the others almost immediately.

The results, if clients were to speak with counsellors were with regard to the *loss,* loss of life, their ambition, physical performance and potency, sexual relations, position in society, financial stability and independence are still challenging area for counsellors, 89% of clients are not ready to discuss the issue of loss. What they want to hear is the assurance that there is treatment, that they will live as long as any other person, or curing miracles happen and therefore one day they will be cured and be able to lead a normal life like others. It is very evident in most sessions that the magnitude associated with this status is depends on how well prepared a client is during a pre-test session. Very few clients talk about the loss of sexual relations (2%). Most of the clients register fears relating to loss of position in the society.

Another psycho-social issue that was discovered by the clients is a *hopelessness and helplessness* syndrome. It includes elements of giving up and leaving. It is interesting, that in years 2005 to 2007, many clients felt hopeless because of the lack of immediate elaborate support structures or mechanisms.

However as time has passed, the level of awareness increased, and the level of stigma decreased. These facts were expressed in the faces of most clients, who feel hope. Information on the availability of subsequent services (comprehensive care) has boosted the morale and thus an increase in VCT service uptake. Most of the clients responded to the following question "How would you accept the fact, if you turned out to be positive for HIV" with more confidence. "There are available drugs nowadays, many people take them, and so I will be able to join the support groups, start my medication and move on with my life".

By the analysis of issues, many of these were related to *guilt*. Very few people would feel guilty about the way, in which they were infected with HIV - they got infected because of their lifestyle. The majority would blame their partners or the environment, because most of them claim to have been true to their partners. (62%).In a stable relationship (marriage) the individual will feel guilt with regard to infecting the spouse. But in instable relationships (not married), the culprit will not feel guilt, so they are both guilty.

Almost all clients seeking voluntary HIV testing services have a reason for their visit, based on some form of one´s own or partner's failure, accidental happenings or poor health background and work/professional related commitments. More than half of these blame themselves subconsciously whilst up to 30% do it consciously. This is then transformed into guilt, though it is not easy to point it out openly or state it in sessions. We ask a direct question to help the client address guilt and help him accept guilt, when necessary, for example: "Do you know the direct impacts of your actions on your health when you engage yourself in unprotected sexual relationships with somebody whose state of health you do not know? "

Based on results of the research study HIV positive clients are exposed to *stigmatization* and *discrimination* which is communicated by their spouse, family members, friends, colleagues, employers, medical staff and the church. There is the complicated situation in some churches, as it is still believed, that HIV can only be spread via promiscuous way of life and they spread this message in information when preaching. The situation is really difficult, when the people living with HI/AIDS wants to get married; some religious leaders in Kenya still have a lot to say against it.

Back in 2005 to 2007 incidents of stigmatisation were higher in comparison to recent years in Kenya. 5% of women have been sent away from the husband's homestead, after his death. This was done in the belief that only women can spread HIV virus. This situation seems to be gender biased, as most of complainers were women. Some of them were helping out in houses; they were discriminated against by their employers. Mostly women from rural areas experienced discrimination from the husband's relatives.

Only a few discrimination cases are reported because it could be perceived as an offence according to some legal matters changed in Kenya and it is punishable by both jail and a fine. Clients were made redundant by an employer, who believed, that HIV positive people can become an insurance-liability issue for the company. Some companies revoked the insurance of particular employers, because they feared of overrunning of annual medical insurance costs based on misuse or on continuous illnesses treatment. It can be concluded, that stigma fades slowly away from Kenya.

The people living with HIV/AIDS themselves suffer from self-stigma, which presents an obstacle in the progress of acceptance and the consequence is low *self-esteem*.

The best way how to support PLWHA is to ask him to join *self-help support groups*. The clients who agree to join support groups and work within these groups develop internal relationships. This shows the importance of supporting one another. They have access to up-to-date information; they can discuss issues like prevention, getting infected with HIV, how to stop spreading HIV, and where to seek appropriate medical and psychological assistance and access to appropriate home based care. The self-support groups are often the instrument within which to accept the status and accept the comprehensive care services.

It is also rare, to see the "AIDS picture" in public, thanks to the devoted involvement of ARVs, the HIV issue starts to be discussed more in families, at workplaces and in the media. A lot of PLWHA in Kenya wish to fight the stigma and to give HIV positive people hope and to encourage those who have not been tested yet to get tested and get the treatment.

As a result of self-help support groups and better edification of the public, less and less *depressive* cases seem to be recorded in VCT. In the study less than 1% of clients have tried to commit suicide. There were clients, who came get tested for HIV positivity already decided, that if confirmed positive, they would commit suicide, however with the help of counselling they changed their decision. In one case the client brought poison in VCT, just in case, he would be confirmed positive, and so he would be able to commit the suicide.

A situation in which one must face loneliness, loss of control and subsequently the inevitability of death, can lead to *spiritual questions* and seeking assistance in faith. Concepts of sin, guilt, forgiveness and reconciliation may be the subject of spiritual and religious discussions. There are a number of similar moments in life for the HIV positive patient. 35% of clients wish to discuss these spiritual issues. In their prayers they often express a wish for a so called miraculous curing. The counsellors have never seen even one client with a negative approach after so called miracle healing. The strong belief in God helps them to hope that God can heal at his own time, using his own ways and for his own reasons. In Kenya, especially in the slums, there are a great number of people living with HIV/AIDS communities seeking divine healing. This fact was of significant meaning for greedy pastors, who misuse the faith of believers and make them, in their hope for healing, to deliver offerings, tithing and to plant the seed of healing in the church. So people sell their properties, go and plant the seed of healing in the church (church business).The counsellors discourage client from dropping or even stopping the use of ARVs after "prayers" and remind them that it is not all right, when they are asked for money for a "prayer". They try politely without wanting to influence one´s spirituality and make clients understand, that the love of God is the same to all people, whether positive or negative, Muslim or Christian, one tribe or another.

The issues of *grief bereavement* and issues related to *death and dying* found to be taboo issues during counselling for a large number of clients. Based on our results, only 5% felt free to speak openly about these matters. The clients, who come to be tested for HIV, do not know whether the result is going to be positive or negative. In this case should the result of the test be confirmed as negative, they state their plan to change their behaviour to reduce risk of getting infected.

If the result is confirmed to be positive, most of the clients perceive themselves as if they were already dead (walking corpses). They imagine their funeral and its realization and they visualise their grave. People regret their failures and they are not ready to discuss such an issue as the death. Most clients tend to avoid this topic. It takes a lot of encouragement and assurance form the counsellor to help them open up and to talk about these matters.

The counsellors need to encourage the clients to understand that the dying process either their own or the one of someone they know, for a HIV positive person or with some other comparable disease or sickness, is an issue that can be openly discussed.

The following outlines the *most problematic social issues* of people living with HIV/AIDS in Mukuru slums, Kenya want to discuss with counsellors in VCT:

- Financial instability,
- Lack of support and understanding from close relatives and community members,
- Follow up of adherence and compliance of drug usage in public, during working hours/in church/while travelling, and so on.
- The big challenge of disclosure and the subsequent steps,
- The issue of having a child / children. ("Will the new-born child be HIV negative?")
- Will there be some partner of the same status to marry?
- The challenges of getting a job despite HIV positivity, (Will they be accepted as any other person?)
- In situations where the spouse is negative (the discordant couples) the positive spouse is worried if she/ he will be accepted in that relationship or will be chased away.
- Another question is, if the partner accepts him/her? Will family members of the negative partner bless that marriage?
- Relatives start to handle the property of the HIV positive person as if the was already dead.
- Recognition, HIV positive people are human beings and they should be treated with respect,
- They should be offered quality health care services.

The clients of VCT mentioned also some other issues, which they face, for example poor supplies of ARVs; how the available treatment is not available for all; corruption, which allows receiving treatment only in the case of some acquaintances and contacts with higher positioned staff in rural clinics. Clients have also financial problems. Some of them have a long way to travel from home to the treatment centres.

The service providers, who always seem to have "permanent issues" with anybody who has HIV/AIDS constantly breach confidentiality. Some clients start to drink alcohol and turn into heavy drinkers / drug users in order to avoid stress.

On the side of counsellors in VCT the challenging issues are often linked with the poor level of education of the clients and strong traditional beliefs. There is usually a high level of conflict that some clients find themselves in, for example conflict between religious beliefs and traditional African beliefs.

Another issue is the high expectation referring to the dependency syndrome, depending too much on guidance and not being able to be self-dependant or self-sufficient. There is an increase of the threshold for starting ARVs by the government from CD4 counts of below 250 to CD4 counts of below 350. This is very important and positive for a third-world country; it is not only practical but also realistic. It easily caused a shift of half a million people to be immediately put on ARVs yet the stock, stores, staff, infrastructure, expertise and counselling staff were not present and available.

9. Conclusion

The main determinants of HIV/AIDS that have a great impact on the psycho-social life of HIV positive people could be divided in four main groups: biology, behaviour, microenvironment and macro environment determinants. From the biology determinants the most affecting ones are: virus subtypes, stage of the infection, other health complications, circumstances, and so on. From the behavioural determinants the most

influential belong to issue pertaining to sexual practices, rate of partner change, prevalence of partners, condom usage and so on.
On the micro environmental level there are determinants as urbanization, mobility, access to health-care services, and status of women, violence issues, stigmatization and discrimination and so on.
The macro environment determinants influencing the daily life of people living with HIV are culture, religion, governance, income distribution as well as wealth.
All these aspects should be taken into account by analysing the psychological and social living of HIV positive people. Psychological mechanisms such as denial, avoidance, grief, discrimination, etc. are encouraged by practices and gender-dominant relationships in the African culture, which increases women's and children vulnerability to HIV infection. It is very important to create a positive environment and positive mind-set for people living with HIV/AIDS.
The stigma can be minimized through campaigning, so that people can continue to lead a life, which is productive and full-valued. For a wider outreach of actions, programs cannot be restricted to massive information diffusion but the psycho-educational strategies need to be applied on a small number of target groups. There is the need, not only to increase the medical knowledge but also to enhance the awareness about HIV/AIDS in general.
Culture, values, traditional norms and taboos are lost as a consequence of too many HIV/AIDS deaths. The support groups seem to be a very positive way in supporting people how to cope with the situation. The services provided to the families are needed very much and also the wider family should be well–informed and educated in order to provide basic emotional and psycho-social support.
A great amount of special care must be given to HIV positive children and children, who became orphaned due to HIV/AIDS. Education and support is the most effective tool that helps people living with HIV/AIDS to live a psychologically well-balanced life. Proper support will also help people with HIV/AIDS to move through the appropriate stages and to reach the acceptance of their status and to cope with all the psycho-social issues in their lives.
HIV positive people can use the educational activities to learn the way of how in order to be in charge of their own medical care, and how to protect themselves as well as those around them. They can also disseminate this education to others and help to reduce the stigma within their communities. Through the many changes and challenges, it the support of family, friends, communities, and health care professionals which are essential to overall well-being.

10. References

Bar R. et.al. (2000). *Counselling in Health Care Settings,* Casell, ISBN 0-304-33986-5, London, England

Bastecky, J. et al. (1993). *Psychosomatic medicine,* Grada Avicenum, Praha, Czech Republic

Botek, O., Zakova, M. & Docze, A. (2005). *Palliative care of HIV/AIDS suffering children in Cambodia.* In: Collection contributions of the 3rd International conference on Hospice and Palliative Care, Faculty of Health Care and Social Work, Trnava University, ISBN 80-88949-84-x, Trnava, Slovakia

Botek, O. & Kovalcikova, N. (2008). *Particularities of building institutional services for HIV/AIDS suffering children in South-Eastern Asia,* In: Assessing the "Evidence-base"

of Intervention for vulnerable children and their families, Fondazione Emanuela Zancan, ISBN 88-88843-24-8. - S. 424-425, Padova, Italy
Brabec, L. (2001). *Christian thanatology*, Gemma, Praha, Czech Republic
Bratska, M..(2001). *Zisky a straty v zatazovych situaciach*. Praca, ISBN 80-7094-292-4, Bratislava, Slovakia
Dane, O.B. & Levine, C. (2002). *AIDS and the New Orphans – Coping with Death*, Auburn House, ISBN 0-86569-249-1, Westport, USA
Dobrikova-Porubcanova, P. (2005). *The incurable sick on the present. The meaning of palliative care*, Spolok sväteho Vojtecha, ISBN 80-7162-581-7, Trnava, Slovakia
Dunovsky, J. (1999). *Social paediatrics*, Grada Publishing, ISBN 80-7169-254-9, Praha, Czech Republic
Frensman, D. & Mc Culloch, M. et al. (2000). *Doctors attitudes to the care of children with HIV in South Africa*, AIDS Care, South Africa
Fabianova, L., Pechacova, D. & Alumbasi, B. (2010). *Quality of life of street children in Africa*, In: Health and Quality of Life, Faculty of Health Care and Social Work, Trnava University, ISNB 978-80-8082-274-8, Trnava, Slovakia
Guest, E. (2001). *Children of AIDS. Africa´s Orphan Crisis*, Pluto P-ress, ISBN 0-7453-1769-3, European Union by TJ International, Padstow, England
Koutek, J. & Kocourkova, J. (2003). *Suicidal behaviour*, Portal, ISBN 80-7178-732-9 Praha, Czech Republic
Kubickova, N. (2001). *Zarmutek a pomoc pozustalym*, Nakladatelstvi ISV, Praha, Czech Republic
Kubler-Ross, E. (2003) *About children and dying*, Ermat, ISBN 80-903086-1-9, Praha, Czech Republic
Mayer, V. (1999) *AIDS. Uvod do patogenezy ochorenia, klinickeho obrazu a liecby. Infekcia HIV pri drogovej zavislosti. Prevencia a profylaxia*. SAP, *ISBN* 80-88908-39-6, Bratislava, Slovakia
Rubinstein, A. (2001). *Children with AIDS*, English Press Limited, Nairobi, Kenya
Satir, V. (2006). *Book about family*, Prah, Bratislava, Slovakia
Shorter, A. & Onyancha, E. (1998) *The church and AIDS in Africa. A Case Study: Nairobi City*, Paulines Publications Africa, ISBN 9966-21-384-x, Limuru, Kenya
Vizinova, D. & Preiss, M. (1999). *Psychological trauma and therapy*, Portal, ISBN 80-7178-284-x, Praha, Czech Republic
Yelding, D. (1990). *Caring for someone with AIDS*, Research Institute for Consumer affairs and Disabilities Study Unit, ISBN 0-34-52678-5, Great Britain

Part 3

The Impact of Social and Psychological Factors on HIV/AIDS and Related Behaviours

11

Societal Beliefs and Reactions About People Living with HIV/AIDS

Ngozi C. Mbonu, Bart Van Den Borne and Nanne K. De Vries
School of Public Health and Primary Care (CAPHRI)
Faculty of Health Medicine and Life Sciences, Maastricht University
The Netherlands

1. Introduction

Although the overall growth of the global AIDS epidemic appears to have stabilized, still, Sub-Saharan Africa has the majority of new infections with 1.8 million (1.6 million- 2.0 million) people becoming infected in 2009 (UNAIDS, 2010). Sub-Saharan Africa remains the region most heavily affected by HIV/AIDS, accounting for 68% of all people living with HIV/AIDS (PLWHA) and for 72% of AIDS related deaths in 2009 (UNAIDS, 2010). In West Africa, Nigeria has the largest epidemic in absolute numbers (UNAIDS, 2008) with 2.98 million people living with HIV and 192,000 adults and child deaths from AIDS in 2009 (UNAIDS, 2010). The HIV/AIDS prevalence rate in Nigeria remains uneven across different states (Utulu & Lawoyin, 2007; UNAIDS, 2010). A retrospective study carried out between 2000 and 2004 among 10,032 pregnant women attending the antenatal clinic at the Braithwaite Memorial Hospital, Port Harcourt Nigeria showed that 5.93% of the women were HIV- positive patients (Obi et al., 2007). Another study carried out in the university teaching hospital at Port Harcourt Nigeria between 1999 and 2004 showed a paediatric prevalence rate of 25.8% (Alikor & Erhabor, 2005). More recently, HIV prevalence among pregnant women attending antenatal clinic in Rivers State is 7.3% in 2008 (UNAIDS, 2010) making Rivers state one of the states with high HIVprevalence among pregnant women in Nigeria.

One of the many challenges associated with HIV/AIDS is stigma. Stigma is generally recognized as an 'attribute that is deeply discrediting' that reduces the bearer 'from a whole and usual person to a tainted, discounted one' (Goffman, 1974). Herek (2002) describes stigma as an enduring condition, status, or attribute that is negatively valued by a society and whose possession consequently discredits and disadvantages an individual (Herek, 2002). Steward and colleagues noted further that stigma is very much about the socially constructed meanings associated with the attribute or characteristic (Steward et al., 2008). Because AIDS or HIV infection is an enduring condition or characteristic that is negatively valued (Herek, 2002), AIDS-related stigma continues to be a barrier to caring for, and supporting, people whose HIV status is known in society (Campbell et al., 2007).

Stigma arises and stigmatization takes shape in specific contexts of culture and power (Parker & Aggleton, 2003). Stigma is especially significant in many developing countries, such as those in Africa, where social networks and, therefore, societal values, are relatively strong (Greeff et al., 2008). The family and the community constitute vital aspects of the social structure that normally offers strength and support during times of need and crisis (Ajuwon et al., 1998; Hilhorst et al., 2006; Kipp et al., 2007). In this communal and social network, contact with someone afflicted with a disease regarded as a mysterious threat, inevitably, feels like trespassing or, worse, as violation of a taboo (Sontag, 1989).

Stigma influences all phases in prevention, detection and care for PLWHA. It decreases turn-up for facilities for voluntary counselling and testing in hospitals (Weiser et al., 2006). Anticipated stigmatizing societal reactions may also decrease the tendency to disclose sero-status to the immediate social environment and, more importantly, to sexual partners. Specifically, a study carried out in Port Harcourt, Nigeria, showed that 77% of PLWHA had disclosed their HIV sero-status to one or more others, of which 22.3% disclosed their condition to their parents, 9.7% to their siblings, 27.8% to pastors, 6.3% to friends, 10.4% to their family members and 23.6% to their sexual partners (Akani & Erhabor, 2006). Other studies has also documented selective disclosure patterns among PLWHA. (Gari et al., 2010; Anglewicz, et al., 2011; Stutterheim et al., 2011).

In a previous study, we reviewed behavioral problems of PLWHA in Sub-Saharan Africa in seeking care, and argued that this is partly due to stigmatizing responses to PLWHA from health care professionals and society at large (Mbonu, Van den Borne, & De Vries, 2009). Given the negative impact of stigma on care seeking and the selective disclosure of a positive HIV-sero-status to close and trusted people, it is important to understand why HIV/AIDS attracts such a degree of negative reaction in society. In the present study, we focus further on a description and analysis of public beliefs and reactions towards PLWHA in a multi-street study located in Port Harcourt Nigeria, to understand why and what makes society stigmatize PLWHA. The paper concludes with recommendations that may help reduce the negative reaction towards PLWHA.

2. Methodology

A descriptive qualitative research design, using a convenient multi-venue street-intercept interview technique was used to explore public beliefs and reactions towards PLWHA. The street-intercept methodology provides access to segments of the urban population that are hard to reach and has a high degree of validity and reliability (Green, 1995; Miller et al., 1997; Baseman et al., 1999; Rotheram-Borus et al., 2001; Fortenberry et al., 2007). It is also used frequently in studies of sensitive topics, such as drug use and sexual behavior (Hidaka et al., 2008). In our study, due to the sensitivity of the topic, and in order to get remarks about PLWHA, we talked not only about individual processes but also at a meta-level about social processes. Furthermore, participants sometimes gave examples of processes or perceptions based on hearsay while in other parts they talked about themselves and their own experiences, perceptions and thoughts.

Participants were recruited between January and April 2006. Eligibility requirements included being an adult older than 18 years and residence or employment in Port Harcourt. Streets were selected from the Obio Akpor local government area of Port Harcourt. We recruited 40 participants for the interviews. Self- reported PLWHA were excluded. Port-Harcourt city is located in the Southern part of Nigeria specifically in the Eastern Niger Delta. The area is particularly rich in crude oil. Families have a median of 5 persons per household (Akpogomeh & Atemie, 2002).

2.1 Recruitment and consent of participants

A convenience sample was used in this study. Interviewees were approached at the recruitment venues and interviews were held in workplaces, offices, restaurants, shops or on the street. An introductory sentence informed participants that the interviews were covering stigma towards PLWHA. Verbal consent was obtained from participants and total anonymity was guaranteed. Forty-one persons were approached, of whom 40 agreed to participate in the interviews (See Table 1). The one person who refused was too busy to grant an interview. No compensation was offered to participants. Interviews were conducted throughout the week. Interviews were conducted in the English language and were face to face. The interviews lasted between an hour and one and half hour. Basic demographic data about participants were gathered before the interviews. Interviews continued until no new information emerged. All interviews were audio-taped and transcribed verbatim.

2.2 Data analysis

Nvivo (QRS release 2.0), a computer-assisted qualitative data analysis system, was used to aid analysis and reporting. The analysis of the interviews enabled us to identify causal relationships and, therefore, come up with a causal structure. Field notes and information from the literature review were also used during the analysis. Emerging issues were examined to identify related concepts. Different factors were formed from the emerging themes. A model was built to explore important relationships between concepts. Attributes were formed to include important characteristics such as gender and work category, which were subsequently imported into Nvivo.

2.3 Validity

An independent researcher coded a random selection of data to look for new concepts. The independent researcher compared emerging themes with the coding by the authors. New meanings and discrepancies were checked by re-reading the transcripts and fine-tuning interpretations until unambiguous categories and themes were agreed. No important discrepancies were found.

3. Results

Demographic characteristics are presented in Table 1. Twenty four persons were female and 21 persons were married. An explanatory model was organized in a causal structure based on the combined responses of the interviewees (Figure 1). The model shows stigma by society as being affected by 10 different determining factors, all of which relate to processes and conditions that allow a manifestation of the stigma. These determining factors are degree of knowledge, association with promiscuity, blame, societal reaction to care givers, media, poverty, fear, religion, gender, and government role. Blame functions both as a determining factor that creates stigma, as well as manifestations of stigma. Other manifestations of stigma are abandonment, isolation, and harassment.

The views of both men and women are combined. The described findings and interpretations offer a general insight, illustrated with verbatim excerpts. In the following sections, the various determining factors are presented. Subsequently, we describe different manifestations of stigma. Thirdly, the conditions of care will be described, and finally, we discuss how these processes and condition interrelate in the explanatory model.

Participant	Gender	Marital Status	Types Of Work	Tribe
1	Female	Single	Company Worker	Efik
2	Male	Married	Police Officer	Kalabari
3	Female	Married	Legal Practitioner	Efik
4	Female	Married	Legal Practitioner	Ibo
5	Female	Married	Sales Woman	Ibo
6	Female	Married	Teacher	Yoruba
7	Female	Married	Teacher	Ibo
8	Male	Single	Company Worker	Yoruba
9	Female	Single	Motor Company	Ibo
10	Male	Married	Manager	Yoruba
11	Female	Single	Manager	Efik
12	Male	Married	Supervisor	Ibo
13	Male	Single	Manager	Efik
14	Female	Single	Office Secretary	Ibo
15	Female	Single	Hair Dresser	Ibo
16	Male	Single	Company Worker	Efik
17	Female	Single	Company Worker	Efik
18	Female	Single	Company Worker	Ibo
19	Female	Single	Company Worker	Ibo
20	Male	Single	Company Worker	Ibo
21	Female	Married	Company Worker	Ibo
22	Male	Married	Police Officer	Efik
23	Female	Married	Legal Practitioner	Efik
24	Female	Married	Manager	Yoruba
25	Female	Married	Teacher	Ibibio
26	Male	Married	Businessman	Ibo
27	Male	Married	Manager	Yoruba
28	Female	Single	Computer Analyst	Yoruba
29	Female	Married	Shop Owner	Ibo
30	Male	Married	Government Worker	Ibo
31	Male	Married	Company Worker	Efik
32	Male	Single	Restaurant Worker	Efik
33	Male	Single	Company Worker	Ibo
34	Female	Married	Insurance Worker	Ibo
35	Female	Married	Motor Company Worker	Ibo
36	Female	Single	Student	Ibo
37	Female	Single	Student	Efik
38	Male	Single	Student	Efik
39	Male	Single	Student	Ibo
40	Female	Married	Surveyor	Yoruba

Table 1. shows the information about the participants

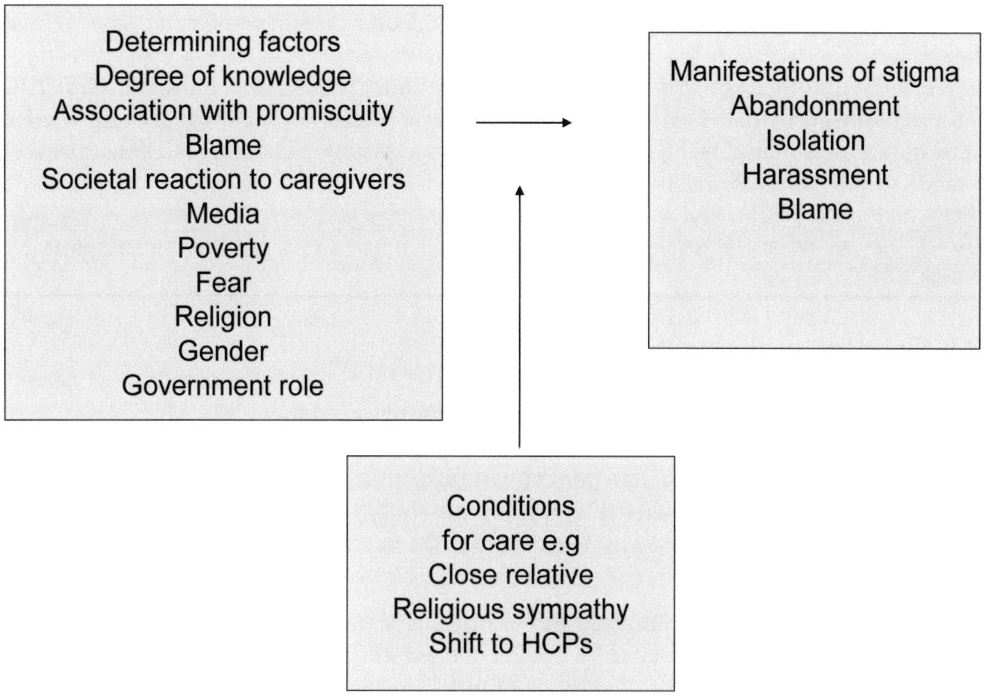

Fig. 1. shows determining factors, conditions of care And manifestations of stigma

3.1 Determining factors

We distinguished many factors, such as degree of knowledge, association with promiscuity, blame, reactions to care givers, media, poverty, fear, religion, gender, and government role.

3.1.1 Degree of knowledge

We found that inadequate knowledge about transmission and about HIV/AIDS can influence how people react to PLWHA. Although information on different ways of transmission of HIV may be increasing, still many people are not aware of accurate means of transmission of HIV virus. To some of the participants, people's lack of knowledge about HIV/AIDS infection and the routes of transmission contributes to reluctance to care for PLWHA, as the following quote illustrates:

'Reaction depends on the education of the person involved, the mentality. Many people think if they touch the HIV person they will get it.' (Male, single)

PLWHA are especially ostracized when they show signs and symptoms of AIDS. Many participants based a judgment about HIV status on appearance, rather than on information, and a person's looks may determine how negative the reaction he or she receives. For instance, if a person with HIV is heavy weighted, people around may not believe that the person has HIV. When the person has an appearance widely associated with HIV, people begin to react negatively to the person, even if they are wrong about the diagnosis. Participants in our study described the appearance of a HIV-positive person as slim with skin rashes. They frequently mentioned loss of weight and being sick for a long time, as elaborated on in the following quote:

'The hair of people with HIV starts falling out with boils all over the skin and they are slim.' (Female, single)

People felt confirmed in this judgment strategy, and looked for outward HIV/AIDS features. Some participants, without knowing the exact illness of a person, assume the HIV status of that person and feel they are right if they see prototypical HIV/AIDS features. For instance, in the words of one interviewee:

'I know someone has HIV when someone is real lean and before you know it the person is sick. When they take the person to the hospital the doctor will examine and find out that the person is HIV positive.' (Male, single)

3.1.2 Association with promiscuity

According to the participants, people associate HIV/AIDS with promiscuity and perceive this as a barrier to caring for PLWHA. Many of them reported that HIV/AIDS is contracted from unprotected sexual intercourse. The general impression among our participants is that HIV/AIDS is acquired when the person has had much sexual activity with different persons. It was common for the participants in this study to depersonalize themselves from the belief of associating promiscuity with HIV/AIDS by shifting the belief to other people, for instance:

'Most people believe HIV is contracted through sexual transmission so immediately they see someone with HIV they automatically believe the person is promiscuous and goes around sleeping around but it can be got from different ways like blood transfusion.' (Male, married)

3.1.3 Blame

According to our respondents, a person with HIV/AIDS in society is frequently an object of blame. When people blame PLWHA for contracting the illness, it makes them stigmatize those people. Many of the participants said that society expects people to stick to their steady or wedded partners, as that is the way of avoiding contracting HIV/AIDS; infected people deserved to be blamed, in their view for instance:

'I think people blame HIV persons. Some people feel HIV persons get HIV because they are prostitutes or go about having sexual intercourse with men or flirting about. So if people find out someone has HIV, people will see the person as somebody who is not responsible. The society feels if the person has not been going from person to person sexually, why should they come in contact with such illness?' (Male, single)

Another participant put it this way:

If you are married to somebody, you are not supposed to go to another woman. You should stick to your wife. Then the single person has to be careful with their movement. People with HIV/AIDS should be blamed because they met someone; that is why they got HIV/AIDS.' (Male, single)

3.1.4 Societal reaction to caregivers

There was a consensus among participants that the reactions to people who care for PLWHA originate from their immediate environment, such as communal reactions, neighbors' influence and spousal reactions or from healthcare professionals. A participant expressed the idea that people care for one another with the expectation of reciprocity, that is, that they themselves may have a need for the care of another person in the future. Unfortunately, caring for a person with HIV/AIDS may not fit into this method of care because they are regarded as people who will die soon. Many of the participants were also concerned about the way other people will react to them when caring for a person with HIV/AIDS. A female participant described what happened when she went to hospital to learn the result of a HIV/AIDS test of a relative visiting her, which turned out to be positive. She received this response in the hospital:

Laboratory worker: 'Oh madam, how long has this HIV person been staying with you in your house?
Woman: She has been staying for three months
Laboratory worker: You have to bring all your children for a HIV test. No, No, infact any help you want to give her let it be from a distance. She should be sent packing [sic] (sent away) from your house.' (Female, married)

This exchange indicates the extent of stigmatizing reactions even from health care professionals. In some cases, people fear that neighbors might spread the word that a family is caring for a person with HIV/AIDS, thereby affecting the possibilities of family marriage. One of the common procedures in marriage is that the family of the groom asks around for information about a potential bride before going into marriage. This implies that neighbors' judgments can be significant. Some participants felt that their desire for marriage and to have children overrides caring for a person with HIV/AIDS. This concern was shown vividly in the following comment:

'Of course, caring for a person with HIV matters to me, because people around me can know about it or how else do people get husbands? They (potential suitors) can ask questions around about me where I live. I will not care for a person with HIV/AIDS even if she is my twin sister. Do you want me to get AIDS? I do mind as long as it is HIV/AIDS or do you want me to die young. You know it is a very serious disease that has no cure. You can see I am not married. I am a single girl. I do not want anything that will stain my image.' (Female, single)

3.1.5 Media

According to some participants, the media have created an image that HIV/AIDS is contracted by people who have sex with multiple partners, or who visit sex workers. One participant had the following to say:

'People react to a person with HIV in the same way, no matter how you get it. The reason why it is like that is that the first awareness of HIV publicity said HIV was for people sleeping around. The media always said stick to one partner, use a condom. This made people feel that once people stick to one partner, they will not get HIV, not realizing that it is possible the one partner already has HIV.' (Female, married)

Participants said that the information people get from radio and television is that HIV/AIDS can be guarded against. This helps in fuelling the negative public reaction people give to PLWHA by shifting the responsibility to the individual. The next participant was concerned by the way media send HIV/AIDS messages to the public using words as for instance "obirinajocha" (means you end up in the white sand underground), which can contribute to how people respond to HIV/AIDS:

'What is being chumed out in the media is also an issue. One begins to wonder whether they are out to create an undesired effect because we hear all over the media that this is an incurable disease and people should better not attempt by any means to pick it up. The media create an atmosphere of helplessness for HIV positive people, as well as their care givers'. (Male, married)

3.1.6 Poverty

Poverty is seen as an underlying factor in preventing care for people suffering from HIV/AIDS. Poor people are often looked down upon in the society. Thus, HIV/AIDS only contributes further to stigmatization of such people. Economic difficulties complicate the situation for persons with HIV or for people who may be willing to care for them. Sometimes, even when relatives provide PLWHA with money for drugs, people caring for the person with HIV/AIDS can divert the money for personal use or for burial because they feel the person is dying anyway, in addition to trying to avoid caring for the person. They regard it is a waste of scarce resources, as one interviewee noted:

'...when the HIV person was sick, his elder brother was given money by people to take care of the person with HIV for drugs but he spent the money on him self. He believed his brother was going to die so there was no need of giving him that money for care.' (Female, single)

3.1.7 Fear

Many of the participants had a fear of HIV/AIDS infection, and felt they could make mistakes when caring for such a person. People feel that PLWHA are close to death and since people are afraid of death, they try to avoid anything that reminds them of their own mortality, for instance:

'People who know someone with HIV, the relationship with the person will change somehow because people are scared. Nobody wants to die. When we see someone (HIV person) like that we need to know how to deal with them.' (Male, single)

3.1.8 Religion

Our data revealed that religion may play both a detrimental and a supportive role. It is an important factor in the stigma of PLWHA with some of the participants placing religion above the medical treatment, causing much conflict in caring for PLWHA. Some of the participants believed it was possible to heal HIV/AIDS because there is nothing God cannot do. This merely reflects the notion that, if they contract HIV/AIDS, they may likely seek care in faith healing houses. This affects care-seeking behavior and, especially may cause treatment delay. This participant was convinced that, in her church, HIV/AIDS can be cured:

'Many people with HIV/AIDS will fear to tell their pastor that they have AIDS so it is a problem because I know in my church they heal HIV/AIDS.' (Female, married)

However, another participant felt that the way the church goes about HIV/AIDS is wrong. In the church, where people look up to pastors and hope to get comfort, clergy may misuse the power they have over people, as demonstrated by the following comment:

'There is segregation in the church. The church counselors give a paper to new couples to go for compulsory HIV screening and when the results turn positive, they give them back seats in the church. The church committee gossip around and people who have heard are not comfortable with the persons with HIV so they feel segregated.' (Female, married)

Giving them back seats is possible because they are able to use their power to give them whichever seat position they wish. Information about who has HIV also travels very fast in the church, as one participant noted:

'I heard about the HIV couple in the church I attend. I did not know until people found out and started telling others. It was the pastor who found out through spiritual means and called them out. He asked them whether they are HIV positive and they said yes.' (Female, single)

Openly asking for persons with HIV/AIDS to come out in public has added implications because the whole church will become aware of the HIV status of those involved.

3.1.9 Gender

Our data show that women living with HIV experience more problems because their position is often marginal and inferior. Many of the participants expressed the concern that women encounter more problems because they are largely dependent on their husbands in almost every aspect: financially, emotionally, and in decision-making. Many of the participants said some women may be willing to care for a person with HIV/AIDS, but they need the approval of their husbands before they can go ahead. Chastity are also expected from women so when they contract HIV/AIDS, they are blamed to a larger extent, which may affect the willingness to care for them. The following illustrates a classic example of gender difference in blame:

'The person I know living with HIV is a girl. It will be different for a man because people will not think immediately of sex as a cause of the HIV. They will think he got it from barbing salon.' (Female, single)

When a woman is infected with HIV, she is easily labeled a prostitute, as one participant observed:

'Women seem to suffer in everything. You find out that when a lady is HIV positive, nobody wants to hear anything apart from the fact that she has been fornicating and moving from place to place. They say she deserves what happened to her.....but if it is a male it is different.' (Female, single)

This male participant showed concern that women have a possibility of spreading HIV/AIDS more purposively than men, as the following illustrates:

'It is better to tell government to take away a person with HIV especially females because if one does not take care she can spread it to other male people. Some of them know they will die one day so they start flirting about.' (Male, single)

3.1.10 Government role

Many of the participants felt that government has a major role in providing care for PLWHA and increasing the knowledge of people about HIV/AIDS. Take the following quote, for example:

'Government should continue with public information. People are still not educated very well. Some people think that if you share toilet with a HIV person you will get HIV.' (Female, married)

Participants also felt government should be involved in the care of persons with HIV, as shown by the following quotes:

'Government should make antiretroviral therapy within the limit of individuals. Some should be helped if they cannot afford it because I read in the newspapers that ART is very expensive.' (Female, married)

3.2 Manifestations of stigma

As a result of these factors, there are changes in the relationship between the general public and PLWHA. The various manifestations of external stigmas, such as abandonment, isolation, harassment and blame will be discussed.

3.2.1 Abandonment

Participants in this study reported knowing PLWHA that are abandoned or would advocate abandoning PLWHA. People are suspicious that people with HIV/AIDS can purposely share household sharp objects or start flirting because they know they will die. Because of that, some participants wanted the government to restrict the movement of PLWHA. Other people felt that persons with HIV/AIDS have to accept their fate and need to learn to live

with the fact that people will stigmatize them. Another participant preferred to shift the responsibility of care to health care professionals:
'Why must a HIV person come to the house? They should stay back in the hospital.' (Female, married)

3.2.2 Isolation
Participants described how their relationship will change upon realizing that a person with HIV/AIDS, or a caregiver of such a person, is around. People avoid people with HIV/AIDS. This explains why PLWHA are reluctant and selective in disclosure as a way of coping with HIV/AIDS stigma. People also feared that, once they care for someone with HIV/AIDS, word will spread around and from there on, people will isolate them. This participant talks about her experience of how PLWHA are cared for:
'Sometimes people with HIV/AIDS are locked up in the room and the care givers pass a hole through which they give them food so that the caregivers do not come in contact with the person. Sometimes the caregivers do not even give the person food so that the person can die.' (Female, single)
A participant shared what happened when a person with HIV/AIDS living close to her came back home from hospital:
'They try to isolate the woman who is caring for her daughter. When she was discharged and came home to their house, people started peeping at them through the window. People will not want to go to the kitchen when she is cooking and they will not want to go near the bathroom until they finish using the bathroom. Everybody wants to keep away. People look at the care giver as someone who is not reasonable anymore.' (Female, single)

3.2.3 Harassment
We also found that harassment can be a manifestation of stigmatisation and can be shown in any form of unwelcome behavior. According to this participant, who tried to describe what will happen to someone caring for a person with HIV/AIDS:
'The care givers of HIV persons will have a problem because it will be the talk of the area. People will say there is a person with HIV/AIDS in that area. Some will not be relating to them because they are afraid.' (Male, single)
In addition, people gossip in the community. This participant gave an account of a person she knows and has HIV/AIDS:
'People were running away, they always say they don't want to be involved, wherever she passes people will point at her and say look at that person with HIV. Nobody wants to visit her. The ones that go just want to gossip.' (Female, single)

3.2.4 Blame
Our findings indicate that the society frequently assigns blame to PLWHA. Blame is another way used by the people to stigmatize persons with HIV, for example:
'People blame them because they feel a responsible person is supposed to live a rightful life so they cannot contact the disease.' (Male, married)
Consider also the following point:
'You know, here in Nigeria, if you have such sickness, people will start blaming the person with HIV. They will tell her all sorts of things. They do not care how she got it. They will say the person got it from sexual intercourse.' (Female, single)
Despite these various effect factors manifesting as stigma, some participants set conditions for care, which will be discussed in the next section.

3.3 Conditions for care

The extent to which a person with HIV is discriminated against can, sometimes, depend on the closeness of the person who is rendering the care. Some of our participants felt that they will only care for a close person with HIV, as in the following instance:

'Caring for a HIV person depends on how close the person is. If it is my brother or sister I can manage but if it is my house help I will be afraid.' (Female, single)

Due to sympathy on religious grounds, some participants felt some people will still care for persons with HIV/AIDS when they have no other option:

'People will run away though it may not be everybody. Some people because of fear of God, will like to encourage that HIV person because there is no other way to do it. One cannot poison a person with HIV to die. One will prefer to take care of the person until God wants him or her.' (Male, single)

The way people discriminate home caretakers of a person with HIV/AIDS can be different from the way they react to healthcare professionals. Many of the participants in our study mentioned that the public may not react to healthcare professionals in the way they react to home care givers, because they feel they may have a need for a healthcare professional themselves. They are generally expected to be doing their work and their duty, which includes caring for PLWHA in a protective way. One participant, when asked whether healthcare professionals caring for PLWHA will be stigmatized like home caregivers, responded by saying that their profession makes them different from home care givers:

'Look at the name you called them, professionals. Healthcare professionals know how to take care of themselves.' (Female, single)

The various factors, conditions and processes that give rise to external stigma, and the way they relate, will be discussed below.

4. Discussion

This study offers a description and exploration of the various factors, conditions and processes that allows stigma to manifest in Port Harcourt Nigeria. Our study indicates that people are still not very knowledgeable about HIV/AIDS, its mode of transmission and treatment possibilities. People react negatively towards PLWHA because they know little about the disease. Hence, they cannot handle PLWHA even when it is a close relative (Hilhorst et al., 2006). Lear (1998) argued that the problem of behavioural change is compounded by the persistence of myths concerning HIV/AIDS. Furthermore, as long as diseases such as HIV/AIDS are not well understood in an era in which medicine's central premise is that all diseases can be cured (Sontag, 1989), it will continue to evoke reactions from the society. Apart from our present data which show that society has negative reactions towards PLWHA, other studies in Sub-Saharan Africa, (Hilhorst et al., 2006; Campbell et al., 2007; Greeff et al., 2008; Demmer, 2011; Singh et al., 2011) have also shown that those who care for PLWHA receive negative reactions, putting the entire family at risk, making HIV/AIDS a societal problem. Moreover, 2010 UNAIDS report also shows that PLWHA have experienced different stigmatization reactions ranging from verbal abuse, physical harrassment to denial of health care (UNAIDS, 2010).

Our data show that not only that people stigmatize people diagnosed with HIV/AIDS, they also preoccupy themselves with the health diagnosis of other people through creating ideas about special features and body structures associated with certain illnesses such as HIV/AIDS. People not only live in a society that is structured by communal interaction (Wood & Lambert, 2008) but is also intertwined with gossip and rumors. HIV/AIDS inspires much gossip, rumor and speculation. The images and the ideas associated with PLWHA are an expression of their concern for social order and of a sense of dissatisfaction from within society (Sontag, 1989). This has significant implications for PLWHA. It increases self-stigmatization, in addition to the stigmatization from society when they have body features that are widely believed to indicate HIV/AIDS. It is perhaps not surprising that our study shows that PLWHA who are heavy weighted may be exonerated because people do not believe they can be heavy weighted and at the same time have HIV/AIDS, especially when they are on antiretroviral therapy (ART) and have less need for frequent hospitalization. This aspect of body politics was also reported by Greeff and colleagues (Greeff et al., 2008).

Our data emphasize that people link HIV/AIDS to promiscuity, which makes people stigmatize PLWHA because they are regarded as people who have gone against the societal values by having indiscriminate sex. Society has strong morals and values that guide it (Campbell et al., 2007) and sex is considered a highly private issue not to be discussed in the open (Ajuwon et al., 1998; Stewart & Richter, 1998). HIV/AIDS is also seen as a disease that flushes out an identity of a certain "risk group", a community of pariahs that might have remained hidden from neighbours, colleagues, family and friends because HIV/AIDS is considered as a calamity brought about by oneself (Sontag, 1989). Our data shows that the association with promiscuity is what causes blame because of the assumed bad behavior. The linking of blame to immoral behaviour was also similarly reported in a multi-country study of Zimbabwe, South Africa, Tanzania and Thailand, in which participants from Tanzania and Zimbabwe felt that PLWHA deserved what they got in terms of being punished for their reckless behavior (Maman et al., 2009). In our study, participants often assigned blame to PLWHA without bothering to find out the cause of infection with HIV/AIDS of the person. It is noteworthy that our findings show that blame is both a cause of stigma and a manifestation of stigma. First, society acts as a social watchdog for people by linking moral judgments to people's assumed behavior. Secondly, the judgment meted to PLWHA affects the willingness to give care; society is not ready to help someone whose illness arose from wilful social misbehavior thereby stigmatizing PLWHA. Moreover, due to societal judgment, PLWHA and the family care givers may find it difficult to justify for any financial help since many people do not have health insurance. This finding, taken together with another study carried out in Nigeria, confirms the likelihood of people needing financial help in Nigeria (Hilhorst et al., 2006). The probability of being helped is worsened by the principle of reciprocity in society, which is of particular concern. Hilhorst and colleagues (2006) went on to say that social capital implies reciprocity that has to be built and maintained requiring investments and resources which PLWHA may not be able to meet with such obligations. Furthermore, society is a death-denying one, where the prospect of no future or the loss of independence is an abomination (Chateauvert, 1993). Our data show that, while some people may be willing to assist PLWHA because they feel they can end up in the same situation in the future, others stigmatize PLWHA by expecting government to take them away or keeping them back at the hospital. Those who choose to care for PLWHA often prefer to keep that a secret so that the stigma does not spread to the rest of the family. This is particularly significant in Nigeria, because when people find out someone close to them is HIV-positive, it can jeopardize the chance of marriage because of the high value of marriage and pregnancy (Ajuwon & Shokunbi, 1998).

Findings from our study have shown that the churches do help PLWHA, but sometimes they make their situation very difficult. People are often obedient to the pastors and in the church, and the pastors were very influential, making their actions very crucial. Aholou and colleagues further noted that the churches have strengths, credibility and are well grounded in communities (Aholou et al., 2009). Many PLWHA regard church as one of the places of protection from negative reaction from society, but they end up being stigmatized by their fellow worshippers. Our data show that a positive HIV test result from premarital HIV screening means that the information may leak to other members of the church and the continuity of the marriage maybe jeopardized since there is no standard guideline regarding the privacy and confidentiality of people. Premarital HIV screening is also quickly becoming a prerequisite for marriage to be contracted in many churches (Uneke, Alo & Ogbu, 2007) and since marriage is very important in society, many people end up knowing their status by necessity while ill prepared for the negative reactions from the society. Sontag (1989) argues that any disease that is considered a mystery and acutely enough to be feared will be felt to be morally, if not literally, contagious, in addition to the notion that cleanliness is next to godliness; thus, stigmatization is not unexpected for PLWHA even in the church. Lear (1998) shows that some Roman Catholic churches in Kenya and Uganda have used words such as "Love faithfully to avoid AIDS" to discourage usage of condoms. Other recent studies (e.g., Iwelunmor et al., 2006; Campbell et al., 2007; Neville & Rubin, 2007) also reported both supportive and detrimental roles. The belief in faith healing and miracles was also found in our study, which means that many who know of their status may choose faith healing as a first choice of care, or combine it with care from a health institution.

With all these negative reactions towards PLWHA in general, our study also shows that societal reactions can be different depending on the person's gender. Society is constructed in such a way that it is a man's world because decisions and actions are often dependent on men (Ajuwon & Shokunbi, 1998). Society exonerates men with multiple partners (Ankra, 1994; Ajuwon et al., 1998; Hartwig et al., 2006; Utulu & Lawoyin, 2007) as it reflect male virility. The sexual norm in Nigeria promotes sexual liberty for men and sexual purity for women (Ajuwon & Shokunbi, 1998). Yet, our study shows that, when a man contracts HIV/AIDS, he may be regarded a victim and attracts more sympathy. This is in keeping with studies carried out in Nigeria, which show that male PLWHA are more accepted than female ones (Hilhorst et al., 2006; Babalola et al., 2009). A man is also often able to hide his HIV-positive status if he chooses, and may end up spreading the infection because he is the breadwinner and may have money to care for himself. A woman, on the other hand, is mostly, financially dependent (Ajuwon et al., 1998; Hilhorst et al., 2006; Strebel et al., 2006), often finding it difficult to hide her status. Their maginal position also means they will not be able to seek appropriate care since they are mostly embarrassed if seen in a sexually transmitted infection (STI) clinic, making them resort to traditional healers or patent medicine dealers (Ajuwon & Shokunbi).

Our data point out that, even when money is given for the care of PLWHA, family members may decide not to use it, since the person is regarded as dying and they may want to save it for the burial. This finding, taken together with other studies carried out in Sub-Saharan Africa (Plummer et al., 2006; Campbell et al., 2007; Amuri et al., 2011) shows that poverty creates an additional burden to PLWHA and their carers. Corpses are valued and cost money to be buried, with people more willing to offer help during funerals than during the period of actual illness (Hilhorst et al., 2006).

Our study also shows that the media contributed to stigmatization because of the way they portrayed information about HIV/AIDS earlier in the epidemic. For example, in a Nigerian news paper in October 19, 1987, HIV/AIDS was typified as "a self-inflicted scourge caused by reckless sexual extravaganza, and the person must be prepared to bear the consequence of their lustful discretion" (Lear, 1998). Such images in the media flourish and take time to be reversed.

5. Limitations of the study

A major weakness of this study is that the data cannot be generalized. We can also conclude that these results are not representative of Port Harcourt city or the community, but the study aims to gather a broad perspective on stigma and societal reactions to PLWHA. The study was carried out in the city where people from different tribes live and reflects only the ideas or culture of the people interviewed.

Another weakness of the present study relied on verbal reports of participants. It was difficult for participants to admit to stigmatizing HIV persons because of social desirability, but when indirectly asked about others or spontaneously describing other's reactions, many of them expressed the view that stigmatization is still strong in society. Despite these limitations, this study illustrates the importance of not only knowing that stigma is still very much present, but also calls for more research in this area.

6. Conclusion and recommendations

The findings of our study may be valuable for developing interventions on stigma. The societal image of PLWHA can fuel the spread of HIV/AIDS because people continue to have unprotected sex based on their personal judgment on physical features associated with HIV/AIDS, because they believe a person with HIV/AIDS is supposed to be emaciated, without knowing that a well-cared-for person with HIV/AIDS can have a normal weight. Sometimes, the long-term nature of illness of someone can fuel suspicion from people, especially when the person is moved from one hospital to another or from the hospital in the city to the village. Participants placed great emphasis on faith-healing power when the pastor prays, which may influence the way they care for PLWHA. At the same time, some other participants felt the church should use their position to teach people how to care for sufferers of HIV/AIDS. The church should also use their position to protect the rights of PLWHA. Almost all the participants were of the opinion that care givers of people with HIV/AIDS should continue to care for them, mainly because they felt that they may find themselves in that position, as can anyone. Government should play a more active role in supporting PLWHA financially especially the vulnerable ones, such as women and children, to help cover the basic needs and accessing HIV/AIDS programmes. When people are knowledgeable about HIV/AIDS they know the steps they may take to protect themselves. Government should also create policies that protect PLWHA in important areas, such as the workplace. HIV/AIDS is likely to stay for many years, and so society may benefit from learning to live with it and not discriminating against PLWHA. Emphasis on the proactive role by media and faith-based institutions should be encouraged by government.

Problems associated with HIV/AIDS are very real in society. The government needs to educate the entire population through radio, television, markets, churches and everywhere there is a possibility of people listening. Continuous education of people about HIV/AIDS, modes of transmission, and how people can protect themselves when caring for HIV/AIDS is important. People should fully be aware that caring for a person with HIV/AIDS can be done without necessarily running a risk of contracting HIV/AIDS. A significant proportion of people in society have heard about HIV/AIDS and the kind of aggression with which the media initially provided information on HIV/AIDS, which enhanced discrimination, should now be turned towards giving HIV/AIDS a human face.

7. Acknowledgments

The authors wish to thank Dr Anja Krumeich for her help in the design of the questionnaires.

8. References

Aholou, T.M., Gale, J.E., & Slater, L.M. (2009). African American clergy share perspectives on addressing sexual health and HIV prevention in premarital counseling: A pilot study. *Journal of Religion and health,* PMID: 19495984.

Ajuwon, A.J., Oladepo, O., Adeniyi, J.D., & Brieger, W.R. (1998). Sexual practices that may favor the transmission of HIV in a rural community in Nigeria, In D. Buchanan and G Cernada (eds), Progress in preventing AIDS? Dogma, Dissent and Innovation, Global perspectives (pp21-33), Amityville, New York: Baywood publishing Company, Inc.

Ajuwon, A.J., & Shokunbi, W. (1998). Women and the risk of HIV infection in Nigeria: Implications for control programs, In D. Buchanan and G Cernada (eds) (pp21-33), Progress in preventing AIDS? Dogma, Dissent and Innovation, Global perspectives, Amityville, New York: Baywood publishing Company, Inc.

Akani, C.I., & Erhabor, O. (2006). Rate, pattern and barriers of HIV serostatus disclosure in a resource limited setting in the Niger delta of Nigeria. *Tropical Doctor,* 36 (2), 87-89.

Akpogomeh, O.S., & Atemie, J.D. (2002). Population profile in: The land and people of Rivers State, Eastern Niger Delta. Edited by Alagoa and Derefaka. A.A. Onyoma Research Publications, PortHarcourt, Nigeria.

Alikor, D.E., & Erhabor, N.O. (2006). Trend of HIV- seropositivity among children in a tertiary health institution in the Niger Delta region of Nigeria. *African Journal of Health Sciences,* 13 (1-2), 80-85.

Amuri, M., Mitchell, S., Cockcroft, A., & Anderson, N (2011). Socio-economic status and HIV/AIDS stigma in Tanzania. AIDS Care, 23 (3): 378-382.

Anglewicz, P & Chintsanya, J (2011). Disclosure of HIV status between spouses in rural Malawi, *AIDS Care,* 9, 1-8.

Ankrah, E. M., & Henry, K. (1994). Empowering women may retard HIV. *Network* 15, 20-21.

Babalola, S., Fatusi, A., & Anyanti, J. (2009). Media saturation, communication exposure and HIV stigma in Nigeria, *Social Science and Medicine,* 68 (8), 1513-1520.

Baseman, J., Ross, M., & Williams, M. (1999). Sale of sex for drugs and drugs for sex: An economic context of sexual risk behaviour for STDs. *Sexually Transmitted Diseases,* 26 (8), 444-449.

Campbell, C., Nair, Y., Maimane, S., & Nicholson, J. (2007). Dying twice: a multi-level model of the roots of AIDS stigma in two South African communities. *Journal of Health Psychology,* 12 (3), 403-416.

Chateauvert, M. (1993).AIDS related stress in Canadian healthcare workers. In H. Van Dis and E Van Dongen, Burnout in HIV/AIDS Health Care and Support: Impact for professional and Volunteers, Amsterdam: University Press, Amsterdam.

Demmer, C (2011). Experiences of families caring for an HIV-infectedchild in KwaZulu-Natal, South Africa: an exploratory study, *AIDS Care*, PMID: 21400305

Epidemiological fact sheet (2008). Retrieved 5 May 2009 from WHO website: www://apps.who.int/globalatlas/predefinedreports/efs2008/full/efs2008_ngpdf.

Fortenberry, J.D., Mcfarlane, M.M., Hennessy, M., Bull, S.S., Grimley, D.M., Lawrence, J, St Lawrence, Stone, B.P., & Van Devanter, N. (2007). Relation of health literacy to gonorrhea related care. *Sexually Transmitted Infection online,* DOI: 10.1136/STI.77.3.206.

Gari, T., Habte, D., Markos, E (2010). HIV positive status disclosure among women attending ART clinic at Hawassa university referral hospital, South Ethiopia, *East African Journal of Public Health*, 7 (1), 87-91.

Goffman, E. (1974). Stigma: Notes on the Management of Spoiled Identity. New York: Jason Aronson.

Greeff, M., Phetlhu, R., Makoae, L.N., Dlamini, P.S., Holzemer, W.L., Naidoo, J.R., Kohl, T.W, Uys, L.R., & Chirwa, M.L. (2008). Disclosure of HIV status: experiences and perceptions of persons living with HIV/AIDS and nurses involved in their care in Africa. *Qualitative Health Research*, 18 (3), 311-324.

Green, G. (1995). Attitudes towards people with HIV: Are they as stigmatizing as people with HIV perceive them to be? *Social Science and Medicine*, 41 (4), 557.

Hartwig, K.A., Kissioki, S., & Hartwig, C.D. (2006). Church leaders comfort HIV/AIDS and stigma: A case study from Tanzania. *Journal of Community and Applied Social Psychology*, 16, 492-497.

Herek, G. M. (2002). Thinking about AIDS and stigma: a psychologist's perspective. *Journal of Law, Medicine and Ethics*, 30(4), 594-607.

Hidaka, Y., Operario, D., Takenaka, M., Omori, S., Ichikawa, S., & Shirasaka, T. (2008). Attempted suicide and associated risk factors among youth in urban Japan. *Social Psychiatry and Psychiatric Epidemiology*, 43 (9), 752-757.

Hilhorst, T., Van Liere, M.J., Ode, A.V., & de Koning, K. (2006). Impact of AIDS on rural livelihoods in Benue state, Nigeria. *Journal of Social Aspect of HIV/AIDS Research Alliance (SAHARA)*, 3(1), 382-393.

Iwelunmor, J., Airhihenbuwa, C.O., Okoror, T, A., Brown, D.C., & Belue, R. (2006). Family systems and HIV/AIDS in South Africa. *International Quarterly of Community Health Education*, 27 (4), 321-325.

Kipp, W., Tindyebwa D., Rubaale, T., Karamagi, E., & Bajenja E. (2007). Family caregivers in rural Uganda: the hidden reality. *Health Care for Women International*, 28 (10), 856-71.

Lear, D. (1998). AIDS in the African press. In D. Buchanan and G Cernada (eds) (pp. 215-226). Progress in preventing AIDS? Dogma, Dissent and Innovation, Global perspectives, Amityville, New York: Baywood publishing Company, Inc.

Maman, S., Abler, L., Parker, L., Lane, T., Chirowodza, A, Ntogwisangu, J., Srirak, N., Modiba, P., Murima, O., & Fritz, K. (2009). A comparison of HIV stigma and discrimination in five international sites: The influence of care and treatment resources in high prevalence settings, *Social Science and Medicine,* DOI: 10.1016/J.socscimed.2009.04.002.

Mbonu, N.C., Van Den Borne, B., & De Vries, N.K. (2009). A model for understanding the relationship between stigma and health care-seeking behaviour among people living with HIV/AIDS in Sub-Saharan Africa. *African Journal of AIDS Research (AJAR),* 8 (2), 201-212.

Miller, K.W., Wilder, L.B., Stillman, F.A., & Becker, D.M. (1997). The feasibility of a street intercept survey method in an African-American community. *American Journal of Public Health,* 87 (4), 655-658.

Neville, M.A., & Rubin, D.L. (2007). Factors leading to self-disclosure of a positive HIV diagnosis in Nairobi, Kenya: people living with HIV/AIDS in the Sub-Sahara. *Qualitative Health Research,* 17 (5), 586-98.

Obi, R.K., Iroagba, I.I., & Orjiakor, O.A. (2007). Prevalence of human immunodeficiency virus (HIV) infection among pregnant women in an antenatal clinic in Port Harcourt, Nigeria. *African Journal of Biotechnology,* 6 (3), 263-266.

Parker, R., & Aggleton, P. (2003). HIV and AIDS-related stigma and discrimination: a conceptual framework and implications for action. *Social Science and Medicine,* 57 (1), 13-24.

Plummer, M.L., Mshana, G., Wamoyi, J., Shigongo, Z.S., Hayes, R.J., Ross, D.A., & Wright, D. (2006). 'The man who believed he had AIDS was cured': AIDS and sexually transmitted infection treatment-seeking behaviour in rural Mwanza, Tanzania. *AIDS Care,* 18(5), 460-466.

Rotheram-Borus, M.J., Mann, T, Newman, P.A., Grusky, O., Frerichs, R.R., Wight, R.G., & Kuklinski, M. (2001). A street intercept survey to assess HIV- testing attitudes and behaviors. *Aids Education and Prevention,* 13 (3), 229-238.

Singh D., Chandoir, S.R., Escobar, M.C., Kalichman, S. (2011). Stigma, burden, social support and willingness to care among caregivers of PLWHA in home-based care in Soth Africa, PMID: 21400316.

Sontag, S. (1989). Illness as metaphor and AIDS and its metaphors. New York: Doubleday publishers.

Steward, W.T., Herek, G.M., Ramakrishna, J., Bharat, S., Chandry, S., Wrubel, J., & Ekstrand, M.L. (2008). HIV-related stigma: adapting a theoretical framework for use in India. *Social Science and Medicine,* 68 (8), 1225-1235.

Stewart, T.J. & Richter, D.L. (1998). Perceived barriers to HIV prevention among University students in Sierra Leone, West Africa. In D. Buchanan and G Cernada (eds) (pp 35-46), Progress in preventing AIDS? Dogma, Dissent and Innovation, Global perspectives, Amityville, New York: Baywood publishing Company, Inc.

Strebel, A., Crawford, M., Shefer, T., Cloete, A., Henda, N., Kaufman, M., Simbayi, L., Magome, K., & Kalichman, S. (2006). Social construction of gender roles, gender based violence and HIV/AIDS in two communities of the Western Cape, South Africa. *Journal of Social Aspects of HIV/AIDS Research Alliance (SAHARA),* 3 (3), 516-528.

Stutterheim, S.E., Shiripinda, I., Bos, A.E., Pryor, J.B., De Bruin, M., Nellen, J.F., Kok, G., Prins, J.M., Schaalma, H.P (2011). HIV status disclosure among HIV-positive African and Afro Caribean people in the Netherlands. *AIDS Care,* 23 (2), 195-205.

The Joint United Nations Programme on HIV/AIDS (UNAIDS) (2008). Retrieved 5 May 2009 from UNAIDS website:

www://data.unaids.org/pub/report/2008/jc1526_epibriefs_subsaharanafrica_en.pdf.
The Joint United Nations Programme on HIV/AIDS (UNAIDS) (2010). The Global Report. Retrieved 10 March 2011 from UNAIDS website: http://www.unaids.org/globalreport/documents/20101123_GlobalReport_full_en.pdf.
The Joint United Nations Programme on HIV/AIDS (UNAIDS), 2010 country progress report. Retrieved 17 March 2011 from UNAIDS website: http://www.unaids.org/en/dataanalysis/monitoringcountryprogress/2010progressreportssubmittedbycountries/nigeria_2010_country_progress_report_en.pdf.
Uneke, C.J., Alo, M., & Ogbu, O. (2007). Mandatory premarital HIV testing in Nigeria: The public health and social implications. *AIDS Care,* 19 (1), 116-121.
Utulu, S.N., & Lawoyin, T.O. (2007). Epidemiological features of HIV infection among pregnant women in makurdi, Benue state, Nigeria. *Journal of Biosocial Science,* 39 (3), 397-408.
Weiser, S.D., Heisler, M., Leiter, K., Percy-de Korte, F., Tlou, S., De Monner, S., Phaladze, N., Bangsberg, D.R., & Lacopino, V. (2006). Routine HIV testing in Botswana: a population-based study on attitudes, practices and human rights concerns. *PLoS Medicine,* 3 (7), e261.
Wood, K., & Lambert, H. (2008). Coded talk, scripted omissions: the micropolitics of AIDS talk in an affected community in South Africa. *Medical Anthropology Quarterly,* 22, 213-233.

12

Trends and Levels of HIV/AIDS-Related Stigma and Discriminatory Attitudes: Insights from Botswana AIDS Impact Surveys

Gobopamang Letamo
University of Botswana
Botswana

1. Introduction

For a very long time now, people living HIV and AIDS have been stigmatized and discriminated against and these negative attitudes have been observed to deter people from seeking health care services such as participating in voluntary counselling and testing and prevention of mother-to-child transmission (Nyblade and Field, 2002). UNAIDS (2007) argued that in many countries and communities, the stigma associated with HIV and the resulting discrimination can be as devastating as the illness itself: abandonment by spouse and/or family, social ostracism, job and property loss, school expulsion, denial of medical services, lack of care and support, and violence. It found that these consequences, or fear of them, mean that people are less likely to come in for HIV testing, disclose their HIV status to others, adopt HIV preventive behaviour, or access treatment, care and support. If they do, they could lose everything. Previous research (for example, Alonzo and Reynolds, 1995) has found that HIV-related stigma originates from several sources. First, HIV and AIDS are associated with the deviant behaviour that is suspected to have caused the HIV-positive status. Second, that the individual was irresponsible to have contracted HIV. Third, that it is the individual's immoral behaviour that caused HIV and AIDS. Finally, that HIV and AIDS are contagious and threatening to the community.

One of the major challenges for studying HIV/AIDS-related stigma discrimination is how to best measure the concept of "stigma". At the moment, as USAID (2006) rightly stated: "...measures that can both describe an existing environment, and evaluate and compare interventions, are lacking" (p.2). A wide range of questions are used to measure stigma. There is a need to correctly measure stigma for a variety of reasons. USAID (2006) has summarized why there is a need to measure stigma and the reasons are summarized below. One such reason is the fact that anti-stigma interventions that have been designed and implemented need to be evaluated to determine if the intervention is effective or not. Another equally important reason for measuring stigma is to identify effective models and take them to scale. Measurement of stigma allows researchers to test the hypothesis that stigma would decline if antiretroviral drugs were more widely available. These are some of the reasons for developing a tested and validated measure of stigma.

In responding to the HIV/AIDS epidemic, the Government of Botswana embarked on various strategies to fight the disease, including HIV/AIDS-related stigma and discrimination. The National Strategic Framework (NSF) for HIV/AIDS 2003-2009 had as some of its key goals psycho-social and economic impact mitigation and the provision of a strengthened legal and ethical environment. It also had as one of its objectives the minimization of the impact of the epidemic on those infected and/or affected and creation of a supportive, ethical, legal and human rights-based environment conforming to international standards for the implementation of the national response (Republic of Botswana, 2002b). The NSF also identified stigma and denial as creating an environment maintaining the potential for increased infection as well as limiting the ability of people to live positively and responsibly with HIV and AIDS. The provision of voluntary counselling and testing was expected to enable people living with HIV and AIDS to go public with their serostatus.

In reviewing previous efforts before the NSF to address HIV and AIDS in the country, Government observed that important gaps existed. One such gap was that support groups for people living with HIV/AIDS (PLWHA) needed to be expanded in order to increase coverage and further assist in the breakdown of stigma and denial around HIV/AIDS. Another important gap identified was that the legal, ethical and human rights environment required strengthening to enable and support an effective national response (Republic of Botswana, 2002b).

The Government of Botswana has assumed that as voluntary counselling and testing becomes easily accessible and people know their status, it will bring down stigma and discrimination. It is argued that in countries such as Uganda, Cuba and others where HIV status is openly discussed, stigma surrounding HIV and AIDS has been dramatically reduced, if not completely eliminated (Republic of Botswana, 2002b:31)

On the basis of the foregoing, the key objective of this paper is to assess progress made in reducing the prevalence of HIV-related stigma and discriminatory attitudes in Botswana which was and continues to be a key objective in the national response. The purpose of the paper therefore is to estimate the levels and trends of HIV-related stigma in the country using three Botswana AIDS Impact Surveys (BAIS) I, II and III. It is assumed that any reduction in HIV/AIDS-related stigma and discrimination is a result of the anti-stigma interventions that the Government of Botswana has embarked on.

2. Methodology

2.1 Data

Data for this paper were drawn from the Botswana AIDS Impact Surveys (BAIS) conducted in 2001, 2004 and 2008. The main objectives of the BAIS were to provide information to: assess whether programs are operating as intended; assess performance of intervention programs; assess whether people are changing their sexual behavior; establish the proportion of people in need of care due to HIV infection; establish the proportion of people who are at risk of HIV infection; assess the impact of the pandemic at household level; and provide information on issues related to the impact of HIV/AIDS on households and communities (Republic of Botswana, 2002a).

All the three surveys have asked the same questions that can be used to assess the level and trends in HIVAIDS-relates stigma and discriminatory attitudes. In this paper, the following

three questions were used to assess HIV/AIDS-related stigma and discrimination: i) If a member of your family became sick with HIV/AIDS, would you be willing to care for him or her in your household? ii) If a teacher has HIV/AIDS but is not sick, should s/he be allowed to continue teaching in school? iii) If you knew that shopkeeper or food seller had HIV/AIDS, would you buy vegetables from them? These questions were asked in the three surveys in the same way that makes them comparable.
Respondents who did not complete the individual questionnaire were excluded from the present analysis. The analysis was also restricted to those aged 10-64 years.

2.2 Measurement of variables

2.2.1 Response variables

Stigma is often rooted in social attitudes and it is in this context that trends and levels of HIV-related stigma and discrimination are investigated using variables assumed to measure social attitudes. Participants who did not respond in the affirmative to any of the below three questions were considered to harbor discriminatory attitudes towards people living with HIV/AIDS. The following three response variables were used in this study as measures of stigma and discriminatory attitudes towards people with HIV/AIDS:

2.2.1.1 Unwillingness to care for a family member with HIV/AIDS

Respondents were asked: "If a member of your family became sick with HIV/AIDS, would you be willing to care for him or her in your household?" This indicator is a dummy variable that equals one for respondents who said "no" or zero if it was "yes".

2.2.1.2 Should not allow a teacher with HIV/AIDS to teach

Respondents were asked: "If a teacher has HIV/AIDS but is not sick, should s/he be allowed to continue teaching in school?" This binary variable was coded in such a manner that the response "no" equals one or zero if it was "yes".

2.2.1.3. Would not buy vegetables from a shopkeeper with HIV/AIDS

Respondents were asked: "If you knew that a shopkeeper or a food-seller had HIV/AIDS, would you buy vegetables from them?" This variable was a dummy variable that equals one for respondents who stated "no" or zero if it was "yes".

2.2.2 Control variables

Control variables used for this study included age (10-19, 20-29, 30-39, 40-49, 50-59 and 60-64 years), current marital status (married (married plus living together), once married (divorced, separated, widowed) and never married), and the highest level of education attained (no education, primary (non-formal plus primary), secondary and higher).

2.2.3 Statistical analysis

The proportions of the people expressing discriminatory attitudes toward people living with HIV/AIDS were calculated using percentages. Cross tabulations were used to present the proportions of males and females with discriminatory attitudes toward people living with HIV/AIDS. Graphs were used to examine levels and trends in the proportions of people with discriminatory attitudes. Because comparison of percentages between the three surveys may not be reliable because of differences in the age structures in the three sample populations, direct standardization procedure was used to eliminate the compositional effects or confounding. Standardization involved taking the 2001 population in 10-year age groups from 10 to 64 years as a standard and applying to it the specific proportions expressing discriminatory attitude for the populations being compared. This produced the number of expected population expressing discriminatory attitudes which was compared with the actual number of people expressing discriminatory attitudes in the standard population. The ratio of expected divided by observed gave the standardized proportion. The standardized proportions were used to examine the levels and trends in the population expressing discriminatory attitudes toward people living with HIV/AIDS.

3. Results

The results are presented in the form of tables and figures as shown below. The results indicated that although the percentage of people expressing discriminatory attitudes toward people living HIV/AIDS remains high, it has been declining over the past several years. Figures I to III show trends in the percentage of people expressing discriminatory attitudes toward people living with HIV and AIDS, classified by gender.

Figure I shows that men tended to discriminate a shopkeeper who sells vegetables more than other people living with HIV and AIDS. Men were less discriminating when it came to their family members who were living with HIV and AIDS. However, over time these discriminatory attitudes appear to be declining, which may suggest that anti-stigma and discrimiation interventions that the Government of Botswana has embarked on are producing the desired outcomes.

Figure II portrays that females compared to their male counterparts were less discriminating against people living with HIV and AIDS. The percentage of females reporting discriminatory attitudes were much lower than those of their male counterparts. In addition, the speed or pace of the decline in the percentage of females expressing discriminatory attitudes against people living with HIV and AIDS is much faster than those of the males over time. It is also evident from this figure that females were less discriminating when their family members were involved compared to those who were considered distant family-wise.

Figure III simply presents the percentage of both males and females combined who discriminate against people living with HIV and AIDS. This figure shows results very similar to what has already been discussed. Overall, discriminatory attitudes toward people living with HIV and AIDS have declined over time. Family members living with HIV and AIDS were less discriminated against compared to other groups of people.

3.1 Levels and trends in percentage of people who reported that they would not care for a family member sick with HIV and AIDS

From Table 1 and Figure 3, the percentage of the population who reported that they would not care for a family member sick with HIV and AIDS decreased from 11.5 percent in 2001 to 7.6 percent in 2004 and finally to 3.6 percent in 2008. Generally, a higher percentage of males were more likely to portray HIV-related stigma and discriminatory attitudes than their female counterparts (see Figures 1 and 2). For example, in 2001, 13.2 percent of males reported that they would not care for a family member sick with HIV and AIDS compared to 10.1 percent of females. The same pattern emerged in the BAIS 2004 and 2008 results (11.8 percent males versus 4.6 percent females in 2004 and 5.3 percent versus 4.3 percent in 2008).

Socio-demographic differentials showed that the proportion of the population who reported that they would not care for a family member sick with HIV and AIDS decreased as age increased, although slightly higher proportions of people aged 50 and above tended to portray higher levels of HIV-related stigma and discrimination. A similar pattern was observed for both males and females.

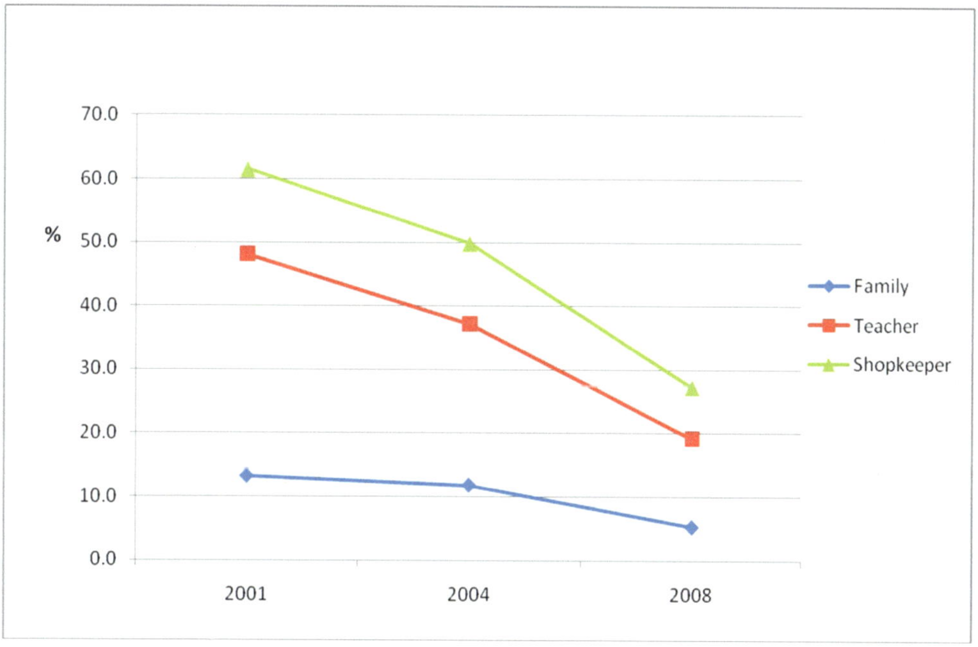

Fig. 1. Levels and trends in the proportion of males who expressed discriminatory attitudes toward people living with HIV and AIDS

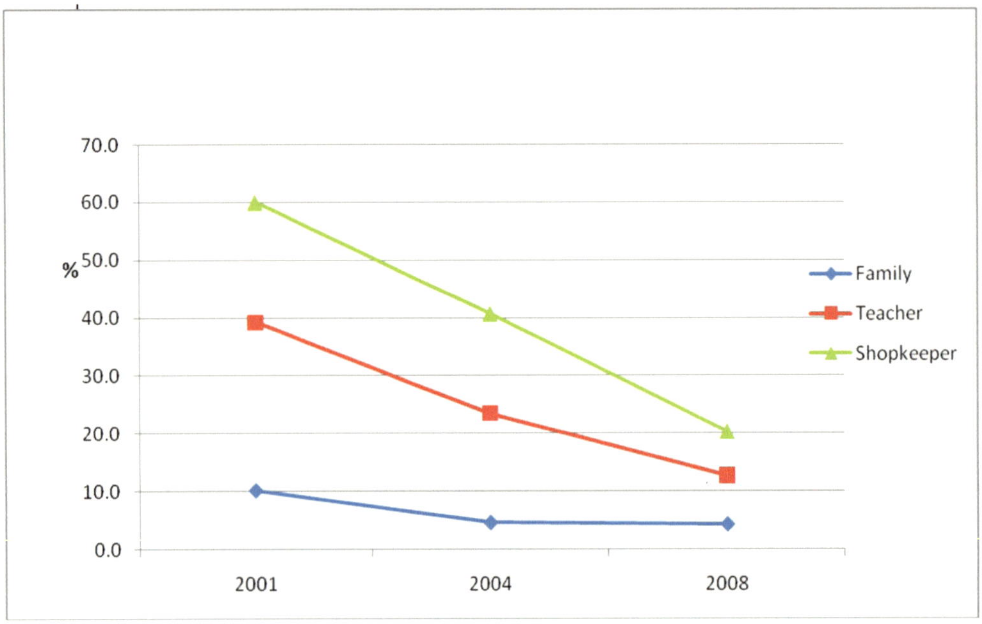

Fig. 2. Levels and trends in the proportion of females who expressed discriminatory attitudes toward people living with HIV and AIDS

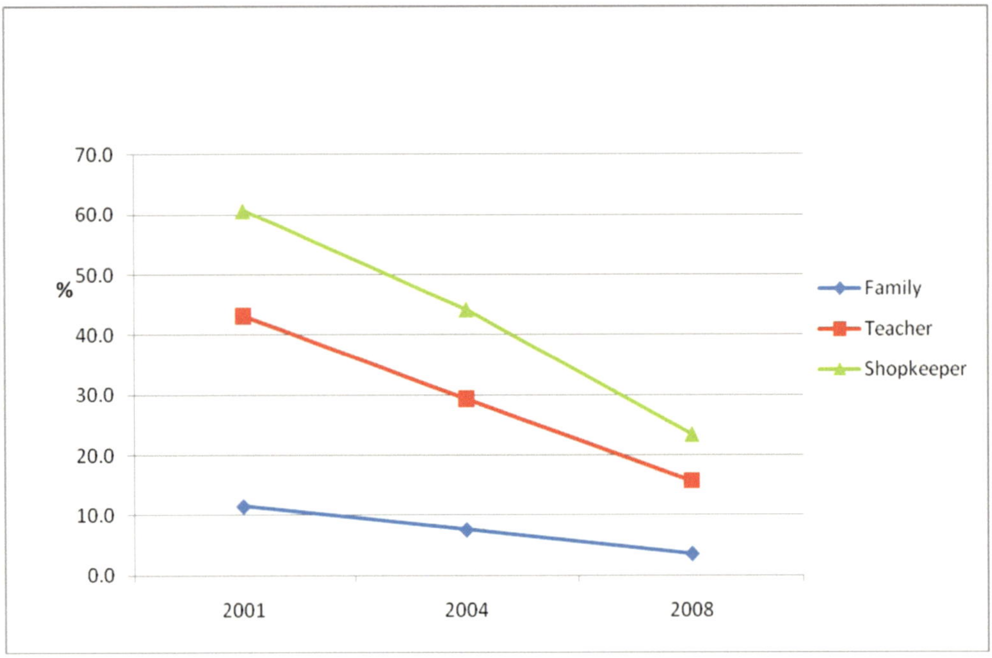

Fig. 3. Levels and trends in the proportion of both males and females who expressed discriminatory attitudes toward people living with HIV and AIDS

Socio-demographic variables	BAIS I			BAIS II			BAIS III		
	Male	Female	Total	Male	Female	Total	Male	Female	Total
Age group									
10-19	22.5	20.5	21.5	19.7	6.3	12.5	8.6	6.7	7.6
20-29	11.0	6.8	8.7	9.0	3.6	5.3	5.1	2.1	3.5
30-39	5.8	2.0	3.5	8.8	3.2	5.6	2.3	1.8	2.0
40-49	5.5	4.3	4.8	2.3	3.3	2.8	1.7	1.5	1.6
50-59	8.1	4.9	6.3	5.8	4.4	5.0	3.4	1.9	2.5
60-64	3.0	5.1	4.2	10.0	7.4	9.0	2.1	5.1	3.8
Education									
No education	7.6	9.8	8.7	13.5	9.1	11.6	5.8	4.7	5.3
Primary	17.9	13.4	15.4	8.9	4.1	6.1	7.7	4.5	5.9
Secondary	12.0	7.9	9.5	9.1	2.9	4.8	3.8	2.3	2.9
Higher	9.1	3.2	6.4	0.9	1.3	1.1	2.5	2.0	2.2
Marital status									
Married	6.0	4.0	4.8	7.7	4.2	5.8	2.1	1.5	1.8
Once married	14.7	5.3	7.6	4.5	2.2	2.6	4.3	2.7	3.1
Never married	16.5	13.4	14.8	10.2	3.8	6.3	6.6	4.3	5.4
Total %	**13.5**	**9.9**	**11.5**	**8.7**	**3.8**	**5.8**	**4.9**	**3.1**	**3.9**
Adjusted Total %	**13.2**	**10.1**	**11.5**	**11.8**	**4.6**	**7.6**	**5.3**	**4.3**	**3.6**

Table 1. Percentage of the population who reported that they would not care for a family member sick with HIV & AIDS, actual and standardized percentages, by survey and sex, Botswana AIDS Impact Surveys (BAIS) I, II & III

Generally, a higher percentage of people with primary education compared to other educational categories tended to report that they would not care for a family member sick with HIV and AIDS compared to those with other educational achievements. People with post-secondary education overall were less likely to report that they would not care for a family member sick with HIV and AIDS. This pattern also emerged regardless of the sex of the respondent.

With regards to marital status, a higher percentage of never married people reported that they would not care for a family member sick with HIV and AIDS compared to people in other marital categories. Married or living together couples were less likely to report that they would not care for a family member sick with HIV and AIDS.

3.2 Levels and trends in percentage of people who reported that a teacher who has HIV and AIDS but not sick should not be allowed to teach

In 2001, 43.2 percent of people stated that a teacher who has HIV or AIDS but not sick should not be allowed to teach compared to 15.7 percent in 2008 (see Table 2).

Again, a higher percentage of males were more likely to portray HIV-related stigma and discriminatory attitudes than their female counterparts (Figures 1 and 2). Overall, 48.1 percent of males indicated that a teacher who has HIV or AIDS but not sick should not be allowed to teach compared to 39.2 percent of females in 2001. These percentages were recorded as 37.2 and 23.5 percent respectively in 2004 and 19.2 and 12.7 percent respectively in 2008.

Socio-demographic variables	BAIS I			BAIS II			BAIS III		
	Male	Female	Total	Male	Female	Total	Male	Female	Total
Age group									
10-19	59.1	48.8	53.7	52.0	26.4	38.6	28.8	20.6	24.6
20-29	40.5	27.9	33.5	27.4	15.4	19.2	11.8	7.3	9.4
30-39	39.8	29.6	33.7	26.9	19.2	22.5	11.6	5.4	8.1
40-49	39.7	43.5	41.8	31.8	24.0	27.6	14.8	9.6	11.8
50-59	52.1	49.5	50.7	29.0	40.7	35.1	22.8	12.8	17.1
60-64	56.8	51.6	53.9	49.8	52.9	51.3	22.7	30.8	27.1
Education									
No education	66.9	65.0	66.0	55.6	46.0	51.6	31.8	25.8	29.0
Primary	63.5	54.2	58.4	41.6	31.3	35.6	31.0	19.0	24.3
Secondary	37.2	26.8	31.0	21.1	12.0	14.8	11.9	7.0	9.3
Higher	6.8	3.6	5.3	2.5	2.1	2.3	4.0	1.8	2.9
Marital status									
Married	38.5	35.7	36.9	25.9	23.2	24.4	13.4	7.8	10.3
Once married	64.8	44.1	49.3	5.3	29.6	25.5	14.2	13.7	13.9
Never married	52.0	40.5	45.9	39.6	16.8	26.1	20.8	13.7	17.1
Total %	**52.0**	**40.5**	**45.9**	**31.9**	**20.7**	**25.3**	**18.1**	**11.5**	**14.5**
Adjusted Total %	**48.1**	**39.2**	**43.2**	**37.2**	**23.5**	**29.3**	**19.2**	**12.7**	**15.7**

Table 2. Percentage of the population who reported that a teacher who has HIV & AIDS but not sick should not be allowed to teach, actual and standardized percentages, by survey and sex, Botswana AIDS Impact Surveys (BAIS) I, II & III

The proportion of the population who reported that a teacher who has HIV or AIDS but not sick should not be allowed to teach that a teacher who has HIV or AIDS but not sick should not be allowed to teach did not vary significantly by age for both males and females. There is no clear trend that can be discerned from the data in terms of age differentials.

Generally, a higher percentage of people with no or primary education compared to other educational categories tended to report that a teacher who has HIV or AIDS but not sick should not be allowed to teach compared to those with higher educational achievement (see Table 2). People with tertiary education were less likely to report that a teacher who has HIV or AIDS but not sick should not be allowed to teach. This pattern also emerged regardless of the sex of the respondent.

With regards to marital status, a higher percentage of never married people reported that a teacher who has HIV or AIDS but not sick should not be allowed to teach compared to people in other marital categories. Married or living together couples were less likely to state that they would not care for a family member sick with HIV and AIDS.

3.3 Levels and trends in percentage of people who reported that they would not buy vegetables from shopkeeper who had HIV and AIDS

Overall, the percentage of people indicating discriminatory attitudes toward a shopkeeper who has HIV or AIDS has been decreasing over time (Figures 1 to 3). About 60.7 percent of people in 2001 compared to 23.5 percent in 2008 indicated that they would not buy vegetables from a shopkeeper who had HIV or AIDS (see Table 3).

The majority of people who stated that they would not buy vegetables from a shopkeeper who had HIV or AIDS were predominantly males.

The percentage of the population that reported that they would not buy vegetables from an HIV positive shopkeeper varied in an unclear direction in terms of ages for both males and females. It would appear that young people generally stated that they would not buy vegetables from a shopkeeper who had HIV or AIDS.

A higher percentage of people with no education and those with primary education compared to other educational categories tended to report that they would not buy vegetables from a shopkeeper who had HIV or AIDS compared to those with higher educational achievement. People with tertiary education were less likely to report that they would not buy vegetables from a shopkeeper who had HIV or AIDS. This pattern also emerged regardless of the sex of the respondent.

With regards to marital status, a higher percentage of never married people reported that they would not buy vegetables from a shopkeeper who had HIV or AIDS compared to those people in other marital categories. Married couples were less likely to state that they would not buy vegetables from a shopkeeper who had HIV or AIDS.

4. Discussion

The purpose of the paper was to estimate the levels and trends of HIV-related stigma in Botswana using three Botswana AIDS Impact Surveys (BAIS) I, II and III. The study shows that HIV/AIDS-related discriminatory attitudes among Batswana are declining. HIV/AIDS-related discrimination is much lower when an HIV infected person is a family member of the respondent. The study results showed that people who were more likely to report that a teacher who has HIV or AIDS but not sick should not be allowed to teach were males, those who had primary education, and the never married. The results showed that people who were more likely to report that a teacher who has HIV or AIDS but not sick should not be allowed to teach were males, those who had primary education, and the never married. The study also showed that people who were more likely to report that they would not buy vegetables from a shopkeeper who had HIV or AIDS were males, those who had no or primary education, and the never married.

It is evident from the results that in the past, most Batswana discriminated against people living with HIV and AIDS. Letamo (2003) found that close to two-thirds of people in 2001 expressed discriminatory attitudes toward people living with HIV and AIDS and the majority of these people were males. This percentage dropped to 44.3% in 2004 and later in 2008 to 23.5%. The reductions in the proportion of people who discriminate against those living with HIV/AIDS are believed to be due to government efforts to reduce stigma and discrimination. The consistent declining trends in discriminatory attitudes towards people living with HIV and AIDS may be suggestive of the fact that the Government of Botswana initiatives in fighting stigma and discrimination associated with HIV and AIDS are starting to produce desired results.

A consistent finding emerging out of the data is that people tend to express accepting attitudes toward people living with HIV and AIDS if they are family members but more discriminating if they are unrelated to them. Like it was earlier stated in Letamo (2003), the more tolerant attitude to care for a family member who is living with HIV/AIDS probably reflect the government intervention of promoting community home-based care programmes. The concept of community home-based care was introduced in 1992 to reduce the relieve public hospitals of the burden of caring for increasing number of AIDS patients. Community home-based care is a programme desired to ensure that family members of people living with HIV and AIDS actively participate in the care of their members. In other words, one can conclude that community home-based care indirectly promotes tolerant attitudes towards people living with HIV and AIDS.

Another emerging observation from the results is that females rather than males have more tolerant attitudes toward people living with HIV and AIDS. The more tolerant attitudes toward people living with HIV and AIDS of females may reflect the current set-up where a disproportionate number of women provide care to all members of the family. Community home-based care is almost exclusively shouldered by women (Population Reference Bureau, n.d.).

5. Conclusions

This study found that although HIV/AIDS-related discrimination has been decreasing over the years, there are still those who harbour these negative attitudes toward people living with HIV and AIDS. Unattended to, these negative attitudes may hamper utilization of various HIV/AIDS care services. It is evident that government efforts or interventions to address HIV/AIDS-related stigma and discrimination are producing desirable outcomes, even though there is room for improvement. Current anti-stigma interventions need to be strengthened in order to uproot HIV/AIDS-related stigma and discrimination completely. It is also important to conduct further studies to understand why people stigmatise and discriminate against those living with HIV or have AIDS.

6. Acknowledgement

The author would like to express his sincere gratitude to the comments made by colleagues during the presentation of the draft manuscript to the STARND Consortium members before it was submitted for consideration of publication as a book chapter. The comments made were invaluable and helped to improve the current manuscript. The author would also like to express his heartfelt gratitude to Central Statistics Office in the Ministry of Finance and Development Planning for granting him permission to use the BAIS data.

Socio-demographic variables	BAIS I			BAIS II			BAIS III		
	Male	Female	Total	Male	Female	Total	Male	Female	Total
Age group									
10-19	71.4	66.1	68.6	55.2	44.3	49.3	36.9	32.0	34.4
20-29	54.6	52.3	53.3	46.4	34.7	38.4	21.6	13.1	17.0
30-39	54.7	53.4	53.9	46.4	34.3	39.4	17.0	10.2	13.2
40-49	58.3	62.1	60.5	50.2	41.1	45.3	21.9	15.8	18.4
50-59	59.6	71.8	66.5	44.3	54.2	49.9	28.9	20.8	24.1
60-64	61.5	63.4	62.6	43.8	66.0	52.6	37.9	32.5	34.9
Education									
No education	72.6	77.6	75.0	72.8	59.1	66.8	40.4	30.6	35.8
Primary	75.5	70.1	72.6	60.5	50.0	54.4	39.0	26.2	31.9
Secondary	52.1	51.9	52.0	34.6	29.6	31.1	19.6	15.3	17.2
Higher	28.8	27.6	28.3	14.4	10.5	12.7	10.3	6.5	8.4
Marital status									
Married	53.4	58.7	56.5	42.1	39.3	40.6	19.4	13.9	16.3
Once married	66.0	63.9	64.5	22.5	39.0	36.4	25.9	20.3	21.6
Never married	65.2	60.2	62.6	55.7	36.6	44.3	29.6	21.8	25.6
Total %	**61.9**	**59.9**	**60.8**	**48.1**	**38.0**	**42.1**	**25.7**	**18.7**	**22.0**
Adjusted Total %	**61.5**	**60.0**	**60.7**	**49.8**	**40.7**	**44.3**	**27.2**	**20.3**	**23.5**

Table 3. Percentage of the population who reported that they would not buy vegetables from a shopkeeper who had HIV & AIDS, actual and standardized percentages, by survey and sex, Botswana AIDS Impact Surveys (BAIS) I, II & III

7. References

Avert (n.d.) *HIV and AIDS stigma and discrimination*. http://www.avert.org/hiv-aids-stigma.htm: Accessed on the 11/03/2011.

Letamo, G. (2003). Prevalence of, and Factors Associated with, HIV/AIDS-related Stigma and Discriminatory Attitudes in Botswana, *Journal of Health, Population and Nutrition*, 21(4): 347-357.

Parker, R., Aggleton, P., Attawell, K., Pulerwitz, J. & Brown, L. (2002). *HIV/AIDS-related Stigma and Discrimination: A Conceptual Framework and an Agenda for Action*. Horizons Progam and Population Council.

Population Reference Bureau (n.d.). *Rooting out AIDS-related stigma and discrimination.* http://www.prb.org/Template.cfm?Sectio...RelatedStgma_and_Discrimination.htm, Accessed on 11/03/2011.

Republic of Botswana (2002a). *Botswana AIDS Impact Survey 2001.* Central Statistics Office. Gaborone, Botswana

Republic of Botswana (2002b). *Botswana National Strategic Framework for HIV/AIDS 2003-2009.* National AIDS Coordinating Agency. Gaborone, Botswana

Tabengwa, M., Menyatso, T., Dabutha, S., Awuah, M., Stegline, C. (2001). *Human rights, gender and HIV/AIDS: analysis of the existing legal system and its shortcomings;* In Republic of Botswana: report of the First National Conference on Gender and HIV/AIDS, 21-23 June., Gaborone: Ministry of Labour and Home Affairs: 35-42.

UNAIDS (2007). *Reducing HIV Stigma and Discrimination: a critical part of national AIDS programmes.* Geneva: Joint United Nations Programme on HIV/AIDS.

USAID (2006). *Can We Measure HIV/AIDS-Related Stigma and Discrimination? Current Knowledge about Quantifying Stigma in Developing Countries.* USAID.

13

The Impact of HIV/AIDS on the Health Transition Among Under-Five Children in Africa

Michel Garenne
Institut Pasteur, Epidémiologie des Maladies Emergentes, Paris,
Institut de Recherche pour le Développement (IRD),
France

1. Introduction

Child survival improved dramatically throughout the world over the past century. Measured as the under-five death rate (the probability of dying before reaching the fifth birthday), child mortality declined from values as high as 300 to 600 per 1000 live births to values as low as 5 to 10 per 1000 in most advanced countries, sometimes even lower, and values around or below 100 per 1000 in most developing countries. [Stolnitz, 1955 & 1965; United Nations, 1982; Ahmad et al., 2000] In industrialized countries this mortality decline was associated firstly with the development of hygiene, clean water supply, sanitation, improved nutrition, and more recently with major advances in preventive and curative medicine. [Szreter, 2003] In developing countries of Africa and Asia, child mortality decline seems more associated with preventive and curative medicine, and less so with hygiene and nutrition, although these have also improved in most cases. [Preston, 1980; Feachem and Jamison, 1991, Ahmad et al., 2000; Jamison et al., 2006]

Beyond regular improvements associated with economic development, social change and modern medicine, reversals in the health transition might occur as a result of external shocks, such as emerging diseases. When a new very lethal disease appears, it may cause an increase in child mortality, despite a decline in mortality from other causes of death. Since 1980, the most important of these emerging diseases is HIV/AIDS, and the continent the most hardly hit by HIV is sub-Saharan Africa. [Newell et al., 2004; UNAIDS, 2010; Jamison et al., 2006] In addition to emerging infectious diseases, other heath threats could also contribute to increasing mortality, for instance various pollutions or exposure to health hazards which may cause cancer, and behavioural changes such as smoking, substance abuse and obesity, although these are more likely to affect adults than under-five children.

Sub-Saharan Africa is very heterogeneous in terms of level of income, level of education, hygiene and sanitation, as well as culturally. Some countries are already quite advanced and modern (e.g. countries in the Southern cone), whereas others lag behind, with low income, low education, low hygiene and poor public health (e.g. Sahelian countries). The effects of an external shock such as an emerging disease are therefore likely to differ among these countries, partly because the spread of the disease might differ, partly because the response to it might differ, and partly because baseline values also differ. Trends in under-five mortality are also determined by other dynamics, and are often related with political stability (or crises) and with economic growth (or recessions), and with the local development of public health, so that the whole picture might appear confusing at first glance.

HIV stroke Africa in the mid-1970's, and spread rapidly throughout the continent, and extensively in Eastern and Southern Africa, with some pockets in West and Central Africa. [Buve et al., 2002; UNAIDS, 2010] By the mid-1990's HIV prevalence was already high in about half of African countries and increasing rapidly, with values ranging from 5% to 15%, well beyond the 1% threshold considered necessary for a rapid spread in the general population. By the mid-2000's the epidemics had stabilized, and HIV prevalence was declining in most countries. Data on HIV prevalence deal primarily with adults aged 15-49 years, and often ignore the children. However, mother to child transmission of HIV is common, either before birth, during delivery or after delivery through breastfeeding, so that a significant proportion of newborns are infected with the virus, and likely to die shortly afterwards. Until recently, HIV infection to children born to HIV positive mothers was common and resulted in high mortality. Since then, efforts were made to limit the mother to child transmission by various means, and to treat infected children with newly available drugs.

The dynamics of HIV epidemics in Africa vary widely, with some countries heavily infected (as in Southern Africa) and some other hardly touched by the disease (as in Sahelian West Africa). As a result, the net effect of HIV/AIDS on child mortality is likely to be contrasted, depending on the country.

Several studies have tried to estimate the net effect of HIV/AIDS on child mortality in Africa. [Houweling et al. 2006; Korenromp et al., 2004, Mahy, 2003]. Adetunji [2000] provided an overview by comparing point estimates of under-five mortality in the late 1980's and early 1990's with the late 1990's, using published estimates from Demographic and Health Surveys (DHS). He showed an increase in mortality in countries with high HIV seroprevalence, but a decline in others. He found that in Africa HIV mortality accounted from 13% to 61% of under-five mortality depending on the country. Newell et al. [2004] conducted a similar exercise by using parameters of survival after HIV infection drawn from empirical evidence, and concluded that by year 2002 some 10% of deaths of children were caused by HIV/AIDS. Zaba et al. [2003] compared several countries, and found that HIV/AIDS could account from 10% of deaths of under-five children (in Malawi) to 60% (in Botswana). Walker et al. [2002] found 7.7% of under-five children due to HIV in 1999 in 39 African countries, with a range from 0.4% to 42% (in Botswana). Several authors have reproduced the figures recently issued by UNAIDS, and quote a value of 4.4% of under-five deaths due to HIV/AIDS in Africa [Black et al., 2010; Stanecki et al., 2010].

The aim of this paper is to provide a synthesis on the probable impact of HIV/AIDS on child mortality trends in Africa, in a broad historical context since 1950. We will stop in year 2005, the time when HIV/AIDS mortality was the highest among children. The situation changed after this date with respect to mother to child transmission and treatment with anti-retroviral therapy. Furthermore, data were lacking after 2005 for many of countries selected for the study. We will focus on long term trends, and on the heterogeneity between countries, summarized in large areas or groups of countries. This study is an extension of earlier work which presented a full scale reconstruction of under-five mortality trends in countries of sub-Saharan Africa since 1950. [Garenne, 1996; Garenne & Gakusi, 2004 & 2006a]

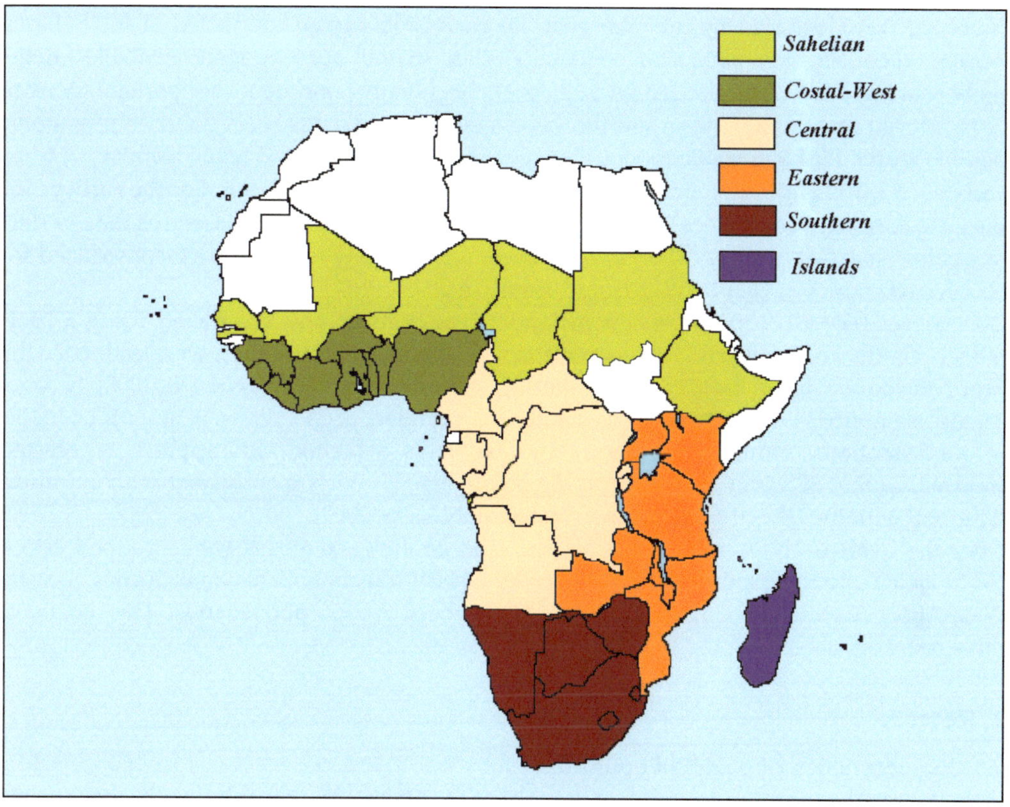

Fig. 1. Sub-Saharan African countries with DHS surveys, by large area

2. Data

Data on under-five mortality were drawn from the maternity histories recorded in Demographic and Health Surveys (DHS). These surveys provide data that allow one to compute age specific death rates by period, and therefore the under-five death rate by calendar year. All 38 countries for which data were available were kept for the final analysis, covering most of continental sub-Saharan Africa, and several islands (see Figure 1). Data on HIV seroprevalence among pregnant women were taken primarily from the UNAIDS database. [UNAIDS, 2008] When necessary, they were completed with data from DHS surveys in a few countries. Data on Gross Domestic Product (GDP) were drawn from the data base built by Angus Maddison and colleagues in its latest edition [2010]. These income data are given in Purchasing Power Parity (PPP), and in constant 1990 dollars.[1]

3. Methods

The method for reconstructing under-five mortality trends has been explained in details in other documents [Garenne & Gakusi, 2004]. In brief, age specific death rates are computed

[1]'Purchasing Power Parity' corrects for the value of a common basket of goods across countries. 'Constant value' of the dollar corrects for inflation overtime.

from maternity histories, by calendar year, for each DHS survey conducted in sub-Saharan Africa, unless access to data was restricted. When several surveys were available for the same country, they were merged by adding events (deaths) and exposure periods (person-years at risk) for the same year and the same age groups. Trends were fitted on monotonic periods with a Linear-Logistic model. Changes in trends were tested using standard T-tests, and only those changes significant at $P< 0.05$ were kept for final analysis. For the early years, the DHS data were sometimes supplemented with other sources, such as census data or data from other sample surveys. All together, under-five mortality trends were reconstructed for all selected countries, year by year from 1950 up to 2005.

Estimating HIV/AIDS mortality among under-five children was completed using a basic model. Firstly, trends in HIV seroprevalence among pregnant women were estimated by year and country using the UNAIDS database, in its latest edition [UNAIDS, 2008]. Second, a standard mother to child transmission rate was assumed, at 25%, consistent with UNAIDS recommendations. Third, a standard AIDS mortality schedule was applied to infected children, so that 60% were assumed to die before age 5, which is consistent with empirical data, and with the UNAIDS recommendations. [UNAIDS, 2002]

Once the database was constructed by year and country, countries were grouped into 6 major areas, selected for their different profiles of HIV infection: Sahelian countries, Coastal West-Africa, Central Africa, Eastern Africa, Southern Africa, and Islands. The details of these countries are shown in Figure 1.

4. Results

4.1 Characteristics of selected countries

Out of the 51 countries counted in sub-Saharan Africa, 38 countries with appropriate mortality data were kept for the final analysis. (Table 1) They account for most of the population of sub-Saharan Africa, and only tiny countries were excluded. The six areas

Large area	Percent Population	HIV prevalence (percent)	GDP-PPP (1990 $)	Number of countries Total	in DHS sample
Sahelian	25.2	1.5	775	11	7
Coastal West	27.4	3.1	1117	10	8
Central	15.1	3.8	633	9	8
Eastern	19.7	7.9	819	6	6
Southern	9.7	17.4	3284	6	6
Islands	3.0	0.3	1497	9	3
Total	100.0	5.1	1119	51	38

Sources: Population from United Population Division; HIV prevalence among adults 15-49 from UNAIDS, 2010 Global Report; GDP-PPP from Maddison (2010)

Table 1. Main characteristics of sub-Saharan African countries

selected were all well covered: 7 out of 11 countries in Sahelian Africa, 8 out of 10 countries in Coastal West Africa, 8 out of 9 countries in Central Africa, all countries in Eastern and Southern Africa. Many tiny islands were excluded, but the largest (Madagascar) accounts already by itself for 95% of the population of this group. Islands have a very low prevalence of HIV, followed by the other groups in the order presented in Table 1. Average seroprevalence ranged from 1.5% in the Sahelian group to 17.4% in the Southern group, a major difference in terms of potential impact on child mortality. Note that if the Southern group is the wealthiest and the Sahelian group among the poorest, there is no linear relationship between income and HIV prevalence. For instance the Eastern group has almost the same income level as the Sahelian group, but five times more HIV, whereas the Islands group is the second wealthiest, but has the lowest HIV prevalence.

4.2 Basic calculations and order of magnitude

To illustrate the rationale of the calculations, one could firstly present aggregate values. According to the UNAIDS database, some 5.1% of adults of both sexes were infected by year 2005 in sub-Saharan Africa. This corresponds to about 6.1% women aged 15-49 infected, and to about 7.3% pregnant women infected. The coefficients used for deriving these numbers were taken from the African DHS surveys with data on HIV seroprevalence, found in 20 countries. The differences are due to higher infection rates among young women compared with young men, and to higher infection rates at the peak of fertility (around age 30 years) compared with younger and older women. Among the babies delivered by these women, some 1.8% will become infected, and 60% of them will die before age 5, so that AIDS mortality will be about 11 per 1000 live births. Compared with an average under-five mortality of 123 per 1000 in year 2005, this leads to an estimate of about 9% of deaths of under-five children attributable to HIV/AIDS. Of course, this is a rough estimate for the whole continent; however it provides an order of magnitude for the effect of HIV/AIDS on overall mortality levels. Since there is a strong interaction between level of mortality and HIV prevalence (the countries the most affected by HIV are also those with the lowest mortality), the formal calculations by country are likely to be somewhat different (see below).

4.3 Overview of mortality trends by area

The mortality decline has been steady for the continent as a whole since 1950. (Table 2, Figure 2) For this group of 38 countries, the under-five death rate was estimated at 346 per 1000 in 1950, 229 per 1000 in 1970, 166 per 1000 in 1990, and 123 per 1000 in 2005. The pace of mortality decline averaged -2.1 per cent per year from 1950 to 1970, somewhat less (-1.6 per cent per year) from 1970 to 1990, and -2.0 per cent per year from 1990 to 2005, the period where HIV spread and hit these countries the hardest. Overall, HIV/AIDS did not change radically the speed of the mortality decline, which remained at an average level between 1990 and 2005. This decline was even somewhat faster than between 1970 and 1990, a period of turmoil for many countries, and of long lasting economic recession. [see Garenne & Gakusi, 2006b, Gakusi & Garenne, 2007 for more details on the impact of political and economic crises]

Mortality levels and trends differed quite significantly among the six groups of countries. Firstly, the levels at baseline differed: countries from the Southern and the Islands groups had much lower levels of mortality in 1950 as well as in 1970. By 1990 the situation was different, since Madagascar underwent a major rise in mortality for about 13 years for reasons other than HIV/AIDS. By 1990, Southern Africa had from far the lowest mortality, but this favourable trend reversed dramatically because of HIV, so that mortality in 2005 was much higher than in 1990, with an average rate of increase of +2.5 per cent per year.

This is the only case of serious reversal for the six groups considered. In contrast, the Islands groups continued with a fast decline, and by 2005 had almost recovered on trends that prevailed before 1970. This group had virtually no HIV/AIDS over the 1990-2005 period.

	Under-five mortality Per 1000 live births				HIV mortality		Mortality decline, Average per year		
Large area	1950	1970	1990	2005	2005	Relative impact %	1950-1970	1970-1990	1990-2005
Sahelian	372	273	195	124	8	6.3	-0.015	-0.017	-0.031
Coastal West	349	231	189	149	9	5.7	-0.021	-0.010	-0.016
Central	348	229	154	133	9	7.0	-0.021	-0.020	-0.010
Eastern	367	222	165	105	21	20.0	-0.025	-0.015	-0.030
Southern	250	143	58	85	52	60.8	-0.028	-0.045	+0.025
Islands	283	188	157	77	1	0.7	-0.021	-0.009	-0.048
Total	346	229	166	123	15	12.3	-0.021	-0.016	-0.020

Source: Author's calculations from DHS surveys

Table 2. Effect of HIV on under-five mortality, 38 countries in sub-Saharan Africa

For the other groups, mortality trends were favourable, and apparently not correlated with HIV prevalence. Over the 1990-2005 period, the Sahelian group and the Eastern group had a fast mortality decline (-3.1 and -3.0 percent per year respectively), despite slower mortality decline in the previous period (-1.7 and -1.5 percent per year respectively between 1970 and 1990). The Coastal-West and the Central groups did not perform as well, although they also had a regular decline (-1.0 and -2.0 percent per year respectively).

In conclusion, the HIV/AIDS epidemic had only a minor impact on under-five mortality trends, except in the Southern Africa region where it led to a strong reversal in mortality trends. This area accounts only for 10% of the total population, so that its contribution to trends in the sub-continent remains small.

The fact that mortality trends remained favourable over the 1990-2005 period, and in fact went faster than in the previous period (1970-1990), except in the Central and Southern groups, is due to other phenomenon: increase in the ratio of physicians per capita, large scale public health programs, in particular EPI vaccination, treatment of diarrhoeal diseases and of acute respiratory infections, prevention and treatment of malaria and of malnutrition. These important actions overcame the effect of HIV/AIDS in many countries.

4.4 Discounting for HIV/AIDS mortality

If one subtracts the estimated HIV/AIDS mortality from the observed mortality, one finds a declining trend that is even faster (Figure 2). Without HIV/AIDS, under-five mortality would have been about 108 per 1000 live births in 2005, and the pace of mortality decline in the 1990-2005 period would have been –2.2%, basically as fast as during the favourable years 1950-1970 during which income per capita increased steadily by about the same absolute value (+2% a year). This gives a measure of the progresses that were achieved in these recent years once the effect of HIV/AIDS is discounted. Note that this later period (1990-2005) is also associated with a rise in income per capita, again by about +2% a year, whereas the 1970-1990 was associated with a recession of about -1% per year in GDP-PPP.

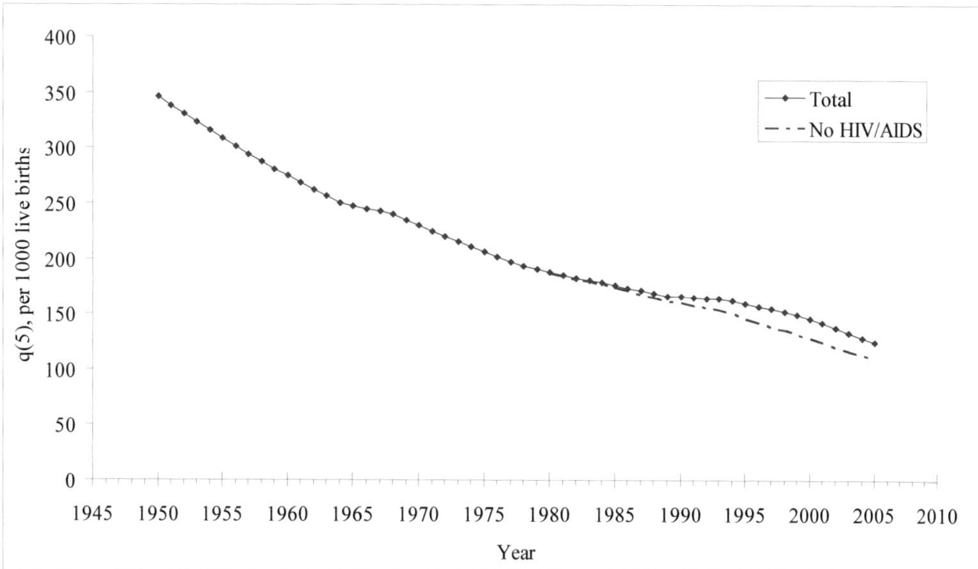

Fig. 2. Trends, with and without HIV/AIDS, 38 countries in sub-Saharan Africa

4.5 Contribution of HIV to mortality levels

Even if HIV/AIDS did not change much the overall trends in mortality, its contribution to mortality levels is still noticeable. According to our calculations, HIV/AIDS mortality accounted for about 12% of total under-five mortality in 2005. This is somewhat higher than our raw estimate presented above (9%), and due to the interaction between mortality level and HIV prevalence. Indeed, the contribution of HIV/AIDS is the largest (61%) in the Southern group, which had the lowest mortality at baseline, because of high HIV mortality combined with low non-HIV mortality. It is also significant (20%) in the Eastern group, for the same reason: higher HIV mortality combined with lower than average non-HIV mortality. Elsewhere the contribution of HIV is smaller (less than 10% in Sahelian, Coastal-West and Central groups), and negligible in the Islands group.

5. Discussion

Under-five mortality decline continued after 1990, despite the HIV/AIDS epidemic. This is due to a balance between very positive effects, associated with continuous improvements in public health and medicine and in income per capita, despite the negative effects of HIV. Even if this decline is not fast enough to meet the Millenium Development Goal 4, which implies an average annual decline -4.4 per cent per year, sub-Saharan Africa appears still on the right tracks. Note that a -2.2% annual mortality decline compares with the path of European countries between 1880 and 1939, at similar mortality levels, as in Sweden (-2.6% per year) or in England and Wales (-2.7% per year) [data from Human Life Table Database, 2008].

Some of our mortality figures may be somewhat under-estimated, because we neglected the interaction between mother's survival and child survival. When a mother dies, she may leave behind young orphans, who were found repeatedly to be at higher risk of mortality, even when seronegative. Of course, this woman will not be interviewed in a DHS survey, so that we may undercount the mortality of children by selecting out mothers who were still alive at time of survey and whose children were under five year of age. However, when women are in an advanced stage of AIDS, and therefore likely to die shortly, they tend to have lower fertility, so that the bias might be smaller that anticipated.

Our estimates of the contribution of HIV/AIDS to under-five mortality are consistent with some of the early estimates quoted above, but differ from some of the more recent estimates. Most of those are based on the method developed by the UNAIDS / UNGASS group, which is more sophisticated than ours, and takes into account numerous other parameters. Our approach was simpler, and matched basic information about mother to child transmission and AIDS mortality found in case studies. Until the early 2000's these figures were probably correct, since prevention of mother to child transmission and access to HAART (highly active anti-retroviral therapy) took off only in these years. Why the estimates are so different while using similar parameters remains to be further analyzed. The UNAIDS estimates might have been over-optimistic on recent developments of the epidemiology of HIV and its treatment, while ours might be over-pessimistic by assuming that until recently AIDS mortality was quite natural. In particular, some of the estimates quoted by Black et al., [2010], such as the proportion of under-five deaths caused by HIV/AIDS in Botswana, seem abnormally low compared with our estimates, with estimates made by other authors, and with the fast increasing mortality trend seen since 1988.

We tried to check the validity of our estimates on the relative contribution of HIV/AIDS in under-five mortality by comparing with independent sources. In South Africa, under-five mortality was decreasing rapidly before 1992, then it increased from 46 per 1000 in 1993 to 85 per 1000 in 2006. According to previous trends, mortality was expected to be about 25 per 1000 in 2006, which, assuming that all the mortality increase was attributable to HIV, suggests that HIV contributed to some 70% of the total in 2006. Similarly, in Zimbabwe, mortality trends predicted a value of 38 per 1000, whereas an under-five mortality of 85 per 1000 was found in 2005, suggesting that 55% of deaths were due to HIV. In Agincourt, a Demographic Surveillance System (DSS) located a rural area of South Africa where causes of death are available, in 2006 HIV/AIDS accounted for 66% of deaths of under-five children, and a similar proportion (64%) was found in nearby hospitals. [updated from Kahn et al. 2007] In Hlabisa, a DSS located in Kwazulu Natal, some 41% of deaths of under-five children were attributed to HIV/AIDS. [Garrib et al., 2006] However, in Manhiça, a DSS located in Mozambique heavily affected by malaria, HIV/AIDS accounted for only 8.3% of the deaths of children age 0-14 years, but possibly more if one considers that deaths attributed to other causes (tuberculosis, malnutrition, diarrhoea, pneumonia) could be also HIV/AIDS deaths. [Sacarlal et al., 2009]

The large differences in HIV prevalence among African countries remain to be explained. African countries differ in many indicators of economic development as well as in many social indicators. We have argued in another paper that sexual behaviour associated with different marriage patterns, in particular with women's mean age at first marriage, and with permissiveness measured by premarital fertility, were key factors of the dynamics of HIV epidemics. [Garenne & Zwang, 2008; Bongaarts, 2007] This in turn explains some of the patterns found in this study. In more advanced countries of Southern Africa, HIV spread much faster because of later marriage and more permissiveness, and had a stronger relative impact because mortality was much lower at baseline. On the other side of the spectrum, in Sahelian countries, marriage was much earlier, permissiveness much less prevalent, and baseline mortality was much higher, so that the relative impact appeared much lower. This combination of various factors linked both to economic development and to the social make up of African societies could explain a great deal of the variations in the contribution of HIV to under-five mortality levels and trends.

We presented available data by large groups of countries, based on geographical clustering. Of course, these groupings are masking differences by country, and even within countries differences between urban and rural areas, and between provinces or districts. It is beyond the scope of this paper to detail more these differences. As examples of such local patterns, let us remind that in Cote d'Ivoire, and in particular in Abidjan its capital city, under-five mortality increased markedly as a result of fast spreading of HIV in the 1980's. [Garenne et al., 1996] Likewise, in Kenya and in Uganda, and in particular in the areas bordering Lake Victoria, mortality increased also markedly as a result of rapid spread of HIV in the 1980's. [Timaeus, 1998]

The cold mortality data presented in this paper do not reflect the numerous social and economic costs of the HIV/AIDS epidemic for African families, and largely ignores the fate of the many orphans who lost one or both parents because of this disease. Discussing these issues has been done in other documents. [UN Millennium Project, 2005]

The prospects for future trends in HIV/AIDS mortality are not as grim as they were in 1990. Since then, efficient strategies to control mother to child transmission were developed and put in place. Furthermore, HAART treatments became available not only for adults, reducing furthermore the risk of transmission from mother to child, but also for children. The combination of these factors should lead to achieve low AIDS mortality among children. Combined with the progress made for other causes of death, one could hope further improvements in child survival in the years to come. [Ndondoki et al., 2011]

We did not address the issue of adult mortality, simply because available data are much weaker, and no comprehensive reconstruction of trends is yet available. However, some attempts have been made by other authors and by modelists to estimate the impact of HIV/AIDS on adult mortality. [Timaeus, 1998] In turn, adult mortality trends seem to have reversed recently, after a long period of increase, in the most infected countries of Southern Africa, primarily as a consequence of HAART treatments. Here again the prospects for future adult mortality trends appear more favourable than thought at the height of the epidemic in the mid-1990's, before anti-retroviral therapy became available. Further improvements will require a continuous effort in screening and treating the persons who are infected with the HIV virus.

6. Acknowledgements

The study was supported by the French Institute for Research on Development (IRD), and by the Institut Pasteur, Paris.

7. References

Adetunji J. (2000). Trends in under-5 mortality rates and the HIV/AIDS epidemic. *Bulletin of the World Health Organisation*; 78(10):1200-6.

Ahmad OB, Lopez AD, Inoue M. (2000). The decline in child mortality: a reappraisal. *Bulletin of the World Health Organization*, 78(10):1175-1191.

Black RE, Cousens S, Johnson HL, Lawn JE, Rudan I, Bassani DG, Jha P, Campbell H, Walker CF, Cibulskis R, Eisele T, Liu L, Mathers C, and the Child Health Epidemiology Reference Group of WHO and UNICEF. (2010). Global, regional, and national causes of child mortality in 2008: a systematic analysis. *Lancet*; 375:1969e87

Bongaarts J. (2007). Late marriage and the HIV epidemic in sub-Saharan Africa. *Population Studies*, 61(1): 73-83.

Buve A, Bishikwabo-Nsarhaza K, Mutangadura G. (2002). The spread and effect of HIV-1 in sub-Saharan Africa. *Lancet*; 359:2011–2017.

Feachem R, Jamison D., editors. (1991). *Disease and mortality in sub-Saharan Africa,* World Bank / Oxford University Press, New-York, NY, USA.

Gakusi E, Garenne M. (2007). Socio-political and economic context of child survival in Rwanda over the 1950-2000 period. *European Journal of Development Research*; 19(3):412-432.

Garenne M. (1996). Mortality in Sub-Saharan Africa: Trends and Prospects. In: Wolgang Lutz ed.: *The Future Population of the World : what can we assume today?*. Earthscan Publications and IASSA, Laxenburg : 149-169.).

Garenne M, Madison M, Tarantola D, Zanou B, Aka J, Dogoré R. (1996). Mortality impact of AIDS in Abidjan, 1986-1992. *AIDS*, 10:1279-1286.

Garenne M, Gakusi E. (2004) Reconstructing under-five mortality trends in Africa from demographic sample surveys. *DHS Working Papers No* 26. IRD-Macro, Calverton, Maryland, USA. [Available on www.measuredhs.com web site]

Garenne M, Gakusi E. (2006a). Health transitions in sub-Saharan Africa: overview of mortality trends in children under-5-years-olds (1950-2000). *Bulletin of the World Health Organisation;* 84(6): 470-478.

Garenne M, Gakusi E. (2006b) Vulnerability and resilience: determinants of under-five mortality changes in Zambia, *World Development;* 34(10): 1765-1787.

Garenne M, Zwang J. (2008). Premarital fertility and HIV/AIDS in Africa. *African Journal of Reproductive Health*; 12(1): 64-74.

Garrib A, Jaffar S, Knight S, Bradshaw D, Bennish ML. (2006). Rates and causes of child mortality in an area of high HIV prevalence in rural South Africa. *Tropical Medicine and International Health;* 11(12):1841-8.

Human Life Table Database. (2008). University of California at Berkeley, Department of Demography. Available on web site: http://www.mortality.org/

Houweling TAJ, Anton E. Kunst AE, Moser K, Mackenbach JP. (2006). Rising under-5 mortality in Africa: who bears the brunt? *Tropical Medicine & International Health;* 11(8): 1218–1227.

Jamison DT, Feachem RG, Makgoba MW, Bos ER, Baingana FK, Hofman KJ, Rogo KO. 2006. *Diseases and mortality in sub-Saharan Africa*. The World Bank, Washington DC. 2nd edition.

Kahn K, Garenne M, Collison M, Tollman SM. (2007). Mortality trends in a new South Africa: Hard to make a fresh start. *Scandinavian Journal of Public Health;* 35(Suppl 69): 26-34.

Korenromp EL, Arnold F, Williams BG, Nahlen BL, Snow RW. (2004). Monitoring trends in under-5 mortality rates through national birth history surveys. *International Journal of Epidemiology*; 33(6):1293-1301.

Maddison, A. (2010). *Historical Statistics of the World Economy: 1 to 2008 AD.* Paris, France: OECD (Organisation for Economic Cooperation and Development).).

Mahy M. (2003). Measuring child mortality in AIDS-affected countries. United Nations, Population Division. Doc. UN/POP/MORT/2003/15 (paper presented to the workshop on HIV/AIDS and adult mortality in developing countries).

Ndondoki C, Dabis F, Namale L, Becquet R, Ekouevi D, Bosse-Amani C, Arrivé E, Leroy V. (2011). Survie et évolution clinique et biologique des enfants infectés par le VIH traités par les antirétroviraux en Afrique : revue de littérature, 2004–2009. *La Presse Médicale* ; 40(1) (forthcoming)

Newell ML, Brahmbhatt H, Ghys PD. (2004). Child mortality and HIV infection in Africa: a review. *AIDS*;18 Suppl 2:S27-34.

Preston SH. (1980). Causes and consequences of mortality declines in less developed countries during the twentieth century. In: R.A. Easterlin, ed. *Population and Economic Change in Developing Countries.* University of Chicago: 289-353.

Sacarlal J, Nhacolo AQ, Sigaúque B, Nhalungo DA, Abacassamo F, Sacoor CN, Aide P, Machevo S, Nhampossa T, Macete EV, Bassat Q, David C, Bardají A, Letang E, Saúte F, Aponte JJ, Thompson R, Alonso PL. (2009). A 10 year study of the cause of death in children under 15 years in Manhiça, Mozambique. *BMC Public Health*; 9:67.

Stanecki K, Daher J, Stover J, Akwara P, Mahy M. (2010). Under-5 mortality due to HIV: regional levels and 1990-2009 trends. *Sexually Transmitted Infections*; 86 Suppl. 2: ii56-61.

Stolnitz G. (1955). A century of international mortality trends, pt. 1, *Population Studies*, 9(1): 24-55.

Stolnitz GJ. (1965). Recent mortality trends in Latin America, Asia and Africa: review and re-interpretation. *Population Studies* 19(2):117-138.

Szreter S. (2003). The population health approach in historical perspective. *American Journal of Public Health*; 93(3): 421-431.

Timaeus LM. (1998). Impact of the HIV epidemic on mortality in sub-Saharan Africa : evidence from national surveys and censuses. *AIDS*; 12(1): S15-S27.

United Nations, Population Division. (1982). *Levels and trends of mortality since 1950.* UN Population Study No. 74.

UNAIDS Reference group on Estimates, Modelling and Projections. (2002). Improved methods and assumptions for estimation of the HIV/AIDS epidemic and its impact. *AIDS*; 16:W1-W14.

UNAIDS. (2008). UNGASS country reports. United Nations, Geneva.

UNAIDS. (2010). *Report on the global AIDS epidemic.* United Nations, Geneva. UNAIDS/10.11E/JC1958E

UN Millennium Project. (2005). Combating AIDS in the developing world. Task Force on HIV/AIDS, Malaria, Tuberculosis, and access to essential medicines; Working group on HIV/AIDS. Earthcan, London, United Kingdom.

Walker N, Schwartländer B, Bryce J. (Ed). (2002). Meeting international goals in child survival and HIV/AIDS. *The Lancet*, 360(9329): 284 - 289.

Zaba B, Marston M, Floyd S. (2003). The effect of HIV on child mortality trends in sub-Saharan Africa. Paper presented at a Workshop held at the United Nations Population Division, September 2003. UN/POP/MORT/2003/13.

14

HIV/AIDS and the Productivity of Selected Sub-Saharan African Regions

Wilfred I. Ukpere and Lazarus I. Okoroji
[1]*Department of Industrial Psychology & People Management*
University of Johannesburg
[2]*Department of Transport Management, Federal University of Technology Owerri*
[1]*South Africa*
[2]*Nigeria*

1. Introduction

More than 42 million people around the world are currently infected with the Human Immunodeficiency Virus (HIV), which causes the Acquired Immunodeficiency Syndrome (AIDS) (Ojukwu, 2004). Although new cases of HIV/AIDS infections have declined in most developed countries, the virus has spread rapidly through much of the developing world. In some areas of sub-Saharan Africa, one in four adults is infected with the virus (Saloner, 2002). Acquired Immunodeficiency Syndrome (AIDS) comprises a collection of symptoms and infections, which result from specific damage to the immune system as a result of HIV. Latter stages of the condition leave individuals susceptible to opportunistic infections and tumours (Arnett 2001; UNAIDS, 2004).

Most European researchers believe that HIV originated from sub-Saharan Africa. Although this allegation may appear to be libellous, sub-Saharan Africa has become one of the worst affected regions (UNAIDS, 2003). An estimated 38.6 million people currently live with the disease worldwide (Nunn, Baggaley, Melby & Thomas, 2004). According to the joint United Nations Program on HIV/AIDS (UNAIDS, 2006), HIV/AIDS has killed more than 25 million people since it was first recognized in 1981, which makes it one of the most destructive epidemics in recorded history. HIV/AIDS has claimed an estimated 2.4-3.3 million lives, of which more than 570,000 were children in 2005 (WHO, 2006). Almost one third of the deaths accruing to HIV/AIDS, occurred in sub-Saharan Africa. This development has adversely impacted on economic growth and human capital development within this region.

Antiretroviral treatment reduces both mortality and morbidity regarding HIV infection, however, routine access to antiretroviral medication is not available in all countries (WHO, 2003). HIV/AIDS stigma is more severe than that associated with other life-threatening conditions and extends beyond affected individuals, care providers and even volunteers who are involved with caring for people who live with the disease (Salati, 2004).

Evidently, the physical size of a country, its population and its national income level per head, are important determinants of economic potential- a major factor, which differentiates one country from another. A country's potential for economic growth is influenced by its endowment of physical resources (land, minerals and raw materials), in addition to its endowment of human resources (the number of people in a country and their skill level) (Dhar, 1995). However, the latter seems to have been demoted by the scourge of the HIV/AIDS pandemic within regions that are most affected. That HIV/AIDS epidemic has been ravishing the world for the past three decades, is a given fact and, therefore, calls for urgent action both individually and collectively. This paper attempts to ascertain the possibility of a relationship between HIV/AIDS and productivity of worst affected regions pursuant to broadening knowledge regarding HIV/AIDs as it affects the global economy. The following hypothesis is proposed:

- H_{O1}: there is no significant relationship between the productivity of a total population and the productivity of a reduced population owing to the HIV/AIDS epidemic.
- H_{A1}: there is a significant relationship between the productivity of total a population and the productivity of a reduced population owing to the HIV/AIDS epidemic.

2. Diagnoses of HIV/AIDS

Since its inception, several definitions have been developed for epidemiological surveillance such as the Bangui definition and the 1994 expanded World Health Organization AIDS case definition. However, clinical staging of patients was not an intended use for these systems as they are neither sensitive nor specific. In developing countries, the World Health Organization's staging system for HIV infection and disease relied on clinical and laboratory data (UNAIDS, 2004). In 1990, the World Health Organization (WHO) grouped these infections and conditions by introducing a staging for patients infected with HIV-1, which was updated in September 2005 (WHO 2006). Most of these conditions are opportunistic infections that are easily treatable in healthy people.

i. Stage i: HIV infection is asymptomatic and not categorized as AIDS.
ii. Stage ii: includes minor mucocutaneous manifestations and recurrent upper respiratory tract infections.
iii. Stage iii: includes unexplained chronic diaorrhea for longer than a month, severe bacterial infections and pulmonary tuberculosis.
iv. Stage iv: includes toxoplasmosis of the brain, candidacies of the esophagus, trachea, broneli or lungs and Kaposi's Sarcoma, which are all diseases that are indicative of AIDS.

Previously, the Centre for Disease Control and Prevention (CDCP) did not have an official name for the disease, and had often referred to it by other diseases that were associated with it, for example, lymphadenopathy, a disease after which the discoverers of HIV originally named the virus. They also used Kaposi Sarcoma, an opportunistic infection, and named a task force after this, which was set up in 1981. In the general press, the term GRID, which abbreviated Gay-Related Immune Deficiency, was also coined (Goldstein, 1983). However, after determining that AIDS was not confined to the homosexual community, the term GRID became misleading, therefore, AIDS was adopted at a meeting in July 1982 (Altman, 1984). By September 1982, the CDCP began to use the name AIDS to include all HIV positive people with a $CD4^{+}T$ cell count below 200 per μl of blood. However, 14% of all cases in developed countries use either this definition or the pre-1993 CDCP definition.

AIDS diagnosis still applies even if, after treatment, the $CD4^{+}T$ cell count rises to above 200 per μl of blood, and even if other AIDS-defining illnesses are cured (Black, 1986, Nomcebo, 2005). The following criteria should be satisfied before a diagnosis of AIDS can be made:

First and foremost, there should be laboratory evidence of infection with the HIV, which is usually achieved by demonstrating the presence of antibodies, to the virus. In the absence of antibodies a diagnosis may be made by viral isolation or viral antigen detection by means of serological tests (International AIDS Society, 2000). If possible, laboratory evidence of deficient cell mediated immunity should be demonstrated. The following tests should be conducted: total lymphocyte count, T cell subset, delayed hypersensitivity skin testing by using a number of antigens and lymphocyte proliferative studies, which uses various mitogens (Daka & Loha, 2008). In addition, there should be clinical evidence, which is either definitive or presumptive of opportunistic infections, certain cancers or direct central nervous system involvement owing to virus infection of the brain (AVERT, 2009).

3. Pathophysiology

Retroviruses have a unique method of reproducing, which allows the virus to copy its genetic information into a form that can be integrated into the host cells' own genetic code. Each time the host cell divides, viral copies are produced along with more host cells. The HIV attacks and gradually depletes a specialized group of lymphocytes, T helper or T4 cells. T cells normally play a key role in setting the immune system's responses in motion (McMichael, 2000). They send out chemical signals that stimulate production of antibodies and trigger maturation of other types of cells within the immune systems (B cell, macrophages and nerve cells). HIV not only depletes T helper cells, but also prevents remaining cells from functioning properly. B-cells become defective in an ability to produce immunoglobulin in response to appropriate stimuli. Loss of immunity is selective and affects primarily parts of the immune system that are involved in defenses against parasites, viral and fungal organisms, hence people who have AIDS, develop certain unusual life infections (ibid).

Diagrammatic illustration of stages of HIV

Infection

↓

Development of antibodies (seroconversion)

↓

Asymptomatic carrier state

↓

AIDS related complex

(Non-life threatening conditions)

↓

Continuing asymptomatic state -------- recovery ------ continuing illness

↓

AIDS and other life threatening conditions

↓

Death

Source: Ukpere, 2007.

Several common diseases such as tuberculosis, malaria, influenza, measles malnutrition and stress temporarily suppress immune response, but once infection subside immune system returns to normal but in AIDS it does not. Antibodies to HIV form in 1 - 4 months after infection but symptoms may not appear for up to 5 years and beyond in some cases and during these years, a person can transmit the virus to others without knowing.

4. Prevention

Perhaps the most important fact about AIDS is that it is a preventable disease. Ideally, this can be achieved by development of a vaccine, although much effort and money have been directed towards production of a vaccine. However, presently, there is none yet, and, it is unlikely that one will be available within the next five years (National Institute of Allergy and Infections Diseases (NIAID) 2009). In the absence of a vaccine, health education and counselling to create a sense of awareness and to reduce the risk of transmission by employing safe sex practices and other high risk behaviours, should become imperative (Centers for Disease Control & Prevention (CDCP), 2002). Other factors that may prevent the spread of AIDS includes ensuring a supply of safe blood and blood products, no sharing of needles and syringes and deferment of pregnancy among high risk subjects. Surveillance to monitor the size of the problem and how it changes, is an important component of prevention (ibid).

4.1 HIV test

In most developing countries, many people are not aware of their HIV status. Less than 1% of sexually active persons in urban Nigeria have been tested for HIV and this proportion is even lower within rural populations (Akande, 2001). Furthermore, a mere 0.5% of pregnant women who attend urban health facilities are counselled, tested or receive their test results. In fact, this proportion is even lower in rural health facilities. Hence, donor blood and blood products that are used in medicine and medical research, are screened for HIV (Nunn, *et al.*, 2004). A typical HIV test, including the HIV Enzyme Immunoassay (EI) and the Western Blot Assay (WBA), detects HIV antibodies in serum, plasma, oral fluid, dried blood spot and urine of patients. However, the window period (the time between initial infection and the development of detectable antibodies against the infection), can vary. This is why it can take 3-6 months to seroconvert, test and detect other HIV antigens, HIV-RNA, and HIV-DNA (Scripps Research Institute, n.d). In order to detect HIV infection these assays are not officially approved, but are nonetheless routinely used in some countries.

4.2 Transmission

Three main transmission routes of HIV include sexual contact, exposure to infected body fluids or tissues and from mother to child during the prenatal period. It is possible to find HIV in the saliva, tears and urine of individuals but there have not been recorded cases of infection from these secretions (WHO, 2006). Therefore, the risk of infection through saliva, tears and urine is negligible.

4.3 Sexual contact

A majority of HIV infections are acquired through unprotected sexual contact between partners, one of whom has HIV (UNAID, 2004; Ojukwu, 2004). Sexual intercourse is a primary mode of HIV infection worldwide. Sexual transmission occurs with contact between sexual secretions from one partner with the rectal, genital or oral mucous membranes of another. Unprotected receptive sexual acts have a greater risk of transmitting HIV from an infected partner to an uninfected partner through unprotected anal and vaginal intercourse/sex (Nomcebo, 2005). Oral sex is not without its risks as HIV may be transmissible through both assertive and receptive oral sex (HIV InSite, 2003). The WHO (2006) reported that the risk of HIV transmission from exposure to saliva is considerably smaller than the risk from exposure to semen. Contrary to popular belief, one would have to swallow gallons of saliva, for a person to run a significant risk of becoming infected. About 30% of women in ten countries representing 'diverse cultural, geographical and urban/ rural settings', reported that their first sexual experiences were either forced or coerced, which makes sexual violence a key driver of the HIV/AIDS pandemic. Frequent sexual assaults result in physical trauma to the vaginal cavity, which facilitates transmission of HIV. During a sexual act, male/female condoms can reduce the chances of infection with HIV and other STDs, and of course the chances of becoming pregnant (Rutter & Quine, 2002; Nomcebo, 2005). The best evidence, to date, indicates that proper condom use reduces the risk of heterosexual HIV transmission by about 80% over the long-term. The benefit is higher if condoms are used correctly on every occasion. Promoting condom use, however, has often proven controversial and difficult. Several religious groups, particularly the Roman Catholic Church, have opposed the use of condoms on religious grounds and have sometimes perceived condom promotion as an affront to the promotion of marriage, monogamy and sexual morality (BBC News, 2009).

5. Treatment

WHO (2004) reported that there is currently no vaccine or cure for HIV/AIDS. The only known methods of prevention are based on avoiding exposure to the virus and an antiretroviral treatment, which, when taken directly after a highly significant exposure, called post-exposure prophylaxis (PEP), has a demanding four week schedule of dosage. Current treatments for HIV infection consist of highly active antiretroviral therapy (HAART). This has been highly beneficial to several HIV-infected individuals since its introduction in 1996 (UNAIDS, 2009).

In the first decade of the epidemic when no useful conventional treatment was available, a large number of people who have AIDS experimented with alternative therapies (Nomcebo, 2005). The definition of "alternative therapies" in AIDS has changed since then. During that time, the phrase often referred to community-driven treatments, were untested by government or pharmaceutical company research, and which most people hoped would directly suppress the virus or stimulate immunity against it. Despite widespread use of complementary and alternative medicines by people who live with HIV/AIDS, effectiveness of these therapies has not been established (UNAIDS, 2004).

Treatment of AIDS consists of treatment of the HIV infection and complications, which result from the immune deficiency. A number of chemotherapeutic agents such as Zidovudine or AZT, Ribavirin, Suramin, Foscarnet and HPA- 23 have been used as antiviral agents, with limited success. Thus far, only Zidovudine has been approved for use in several countries, since it has been shown to cross the blood brain barrier. However, it is expensive and toxic to bone marrow.

5.1 Economic impact

HIV/AIDS retards economic growth by destroying human capital. According to a UN report, HIV/AIDS epidemics will have devastating consequences in decades to come for virtually every sector of society ranging from households, farms and other economic activities (Nomcebo, 2005). The epidemic is predicted to hinder possibility of achieving UN millennium development goals within most affected regions, particularly sub Saharan Africa (Todaro, 1992).

5.2 Impact on agriculture

Agriculture is one of the most important sectors in several developing countries, particularly when measured by the percentage of people dependent on it for their livelihood. Although the sector may produce only 20% of a country's wealth (measured as a percentage of the gross national product), it might provide a living (survival) for as much as 80% of some developing countries' populations (Agarwal, 2002). Indirectly, it provides a living for other parts of the population, for example, processing workers on sugar estates. The effect of AIDS is debilitating at a family level. As an infected farmer becomes increasingly ill, he and family members who take care of him, spend less and less time working on family crops. The family, therefore, begins to lose income from "un-marketed" or incompletely tended crops, and may even sell off farm implements or household properties as a means to survive (Dhar, 1999).

This cycle is compounded by high costs of health care. Whether the sick person turns to a traditional healer or to health services, he/she will surely spend money. A 1997 study by the Food and Agriculture Organization of the United Nations (FAO) showed that in the mid-west of Cote d' ivories (Ivory Coast), care for male AIDS patients cost, on average, about US$ 300 a year, which is a quarter to a half of the net annual income for most small scale farms (Kaplan, 2000). The time lost by family members should also be taken into account. For instance, repeated absence of another member of the farm to accompany the patient to a healer, also reduces the farm's production. Also, when the most debilitating phases of AIDS coincide with key farming periods such as clearing or sowing, time spent nursing a sick member, certainly has a negative impact on turnover (Answers.com, 2009).

5.3 HIV and business

Some companies in Africa have already felt the impact of HIV on their bottom line. A manager at one sugar processing estate in Kenya counted the cost of HIV infection in a number of ways: absenteeism (8000 days of labour cost owing to sickness between 1995 and 1997 alone); lower productivity (50% drop in the ratio of processed sugar recovered from raw care between 1993 and 1997) and higher overtime costs for workers who are obliged to work longer hours to compensate for the void left by sick colleagues (Booth, 2005).

6. Research methodology

The research methodology encompasses different techniques and procedures that are used to collect and analyze data for research. This is important, since it provides a better view of how the conclusion was made. The methodology covers the population of study, method of data collection and data analysis technique.

6.1 Population of study

The population of study comprises countries that have the highest prevalence of HIV/AIDS epidemic in sub-Saharan Africa. These countries are Botswana, Kenya, Uganda, South Africa and Zimbabwe, and were used to reflect rising trends of the epidemic.

6.2 Method of data collection and analysis

Data for the research was obtained from secondary sources such as textbooks, journal articles and the internet. The data collected was analyzed by use of the T-test, which is used when comparing two population means. The formula for finding significant differences between two independent means is stated as follows:

$$t = \overline{x_1} - \overline{x_2}$$

$$\left(Ns_1^{\,2} + N_2S_2^{\,2}\right)\left(N_1 + N_2\right)$$

$$\sqrt{\left(N_1 + N_2 - 2\right)}\left(N_1N_2\right)$$

Where $\overline{x_1}$ = mean of the first group

$\overline{x_2}$ = means of the second group

N_1 = number of cases in the first group

N_2 =number of cases in the second group

S_1 =standard deviation of the first group

S_2 =standard deviation of the second group

In using this formula, the degree of freedom (d.f) is noted.

At the end, if the value of the critical value is less than the calculated value, the null hypothesis is rejected and the alternative hypothesis is accepted.

6.3 Data presentation and analysis

The essence of this presentation and analysis is to ensure that the collected data is meaningful for decision-making. Therefore, this section is the critical aspect of the research, which provides the background upon which the results and conclusion of the study will rest.

Countries	Total Population (in 000)	Population with HIV/AIDS (in 000)	Population without HIV/AIDS (in 000)
Botswana	1600	300	1300
Kenya	34000	2300	31700
Zimbabwe	12900	2000	10900
South Africa	44900	4700	40200
Uganda	27800	510	27290
Total	12100	9810	111390

Source: Field survey data, 2007.

Table 1.1 Countries that have the highest prevalence of HIV/AIDS

An assumption is proposed that the productivity of these countries is one dollar ($1), in order to show manageable figures. The total population's productivity is then compared with the productivity of the reduced population as a result of the influence of the epidemic. Finally, this is used to represent its effects on the world economy.

Country	Productivity of total population (in 000)	Deviation	Productivity of population without HIV/AIDS	Deviation
Botswana	1,600	22640	1,300	22,940
Kenya	34,000	9,760	31,700	7,460
Zimbabwe	12,900	11,340	10,900	13,340
South Africa	44,900	20,660	40,200	15,960
Uganda	27,800	3,560	27,290	3,050
	n Σp=121,200 101 $\overline{x_1}$= 24,40	n Σd_{x1}=67,960 I=i $\overline{d_{R1}}$=13,592	nx1 ΣP_W=111390 I=i $\overline{X_2}$=22,278	n=i Σd_{X2}=62,750 I=i $\overline{d_{X2}}$=12,550

Table 1.2 Deviation of population with HIV/AIDS productivity and population productivity without HIV/AIDS

$$\text{Standard deviation } \overline{x_1} = \sqrt{13,592} = 116.58$$

$$\text{Standard deviation } \overline{x_2} = \sqrt{12,500} = 111.80$$

$$\text{T} - \text{test} = \overline{x_1} - \overline{x_2}$$

$$\sqrt{\frac{(\text{N1s12} + \text{N}_2\text{S22})}{(\text{N}_1 + \text{N}_2 - 2)} \frac{(\text{N}_1 + \text{N}_2)}{(\text{N}_1 \text{x} \text{N}_2)}}$$

Where, $\overline{X_1}$ is mean of the total population's productivity=24,240
$\overline{X_2}$ is mean of the reduced population's productivity=22,278
N_1 is number of countries in the first group =5
N_2 is the same = 5
S_1= standard deviation of productivity of the total population =116.58
S_2 = standard deviation of the productivity of the reduced= 111.80

$$t = \frac{24,240 - 22,278}{\sqrt{\frac{\left(5(116.58)^2 + 5(118.80)^2\right)}{(5+5-2)} \frac{(5+5)}{(5(5))}}}$$

$$= \frac{1962}{\sqrt{\frac{\left(5(13,590.90) + 5(12,499.29)\right)}{(8)}}}$$

$$= \frac{1962}{\sqrt{\frac{(67,9546 + 62,496.2)}{8}(0.4)}}$$

$$= \frac{1962}{\sqrt{(16,306.34)}(0.4)}$$

$$= \frac{1962}{\sqrt{6522.535}}$$

$$= \frac{1962}{80.76}$$

$$= 24.29$$

Using the degree of freedom: $N_1 + N_2 - 2 = 5+5-2=8$
Therefore, at a level of significance of 0.05, it could be observed that t - critical value is 15.507.

6.4 Decision

Since the calculated value (24.29) > t- critical value (15.507), the null hypothesis is rejected and its alternative is accepted. This implies that there exists a significant relationship between the HIV/AIDS epidemic and productivity of the analysed region.

7. Result and conclusion

From the above analysis, it should be noted that the influence of the HIV/AIDS epidemic on general productivity, cannot be underrated. This could be judged from its influence on the productivity of countries that are most affected by the disease. Some empirical researches have correlated the life expectancies of these countries with their respective GDPs. Therefore, this paper has validated that there is a functional relationship between HIV/AIDS pandemic and a decrease in the productivity of selected affected Sub Saharan African regions.

8. References

Agrawal, A.N. 2002. Indian economy: Problem of development and planning. Pune: Wiley Eastern.

Akande, A. 2001. Risky business: South African youths and HIV prevention. Educational Studies, 27 (3): 237-225.

Altman, L.K. 1994. New U.S. report names virus that may cause AIDS. The New York Times, April 24.

Answers.com, 2009. [Online] Available: http://www.answer.com/topic/c-te-d-ivoire .

Arnett, J.J. 2001. Adolescence and emerging adulthood: a cultural approach. Upper Saddle River: Prentice Hall.

AVERT.org 2009. HIV related Opportunistic infections: Prevention and treatment. http://www.avert.org/hiv-opportunistic-infection.htm.

BBC News 17 March, 2009. [Online] Available: http://news.bbc.co.uk/1/hi/world/africa/7947460.stm.

Black, D. 1986. The plaque years, Chapter 3 part 12.

Booyens, S.W. 1993. Dimension of Nursing Management. Cape Town: Juta.

Booth, K.M. 2004. Local women, global science: fighting AIDS in Kenya. Bloomington: Indiana University Press.

Centers for Disease Control & Prevention, 2002. [Online] Available: http://www.cdc.gov/hiv/resources/factsheet/PDF/cdcprev.pdf

Daka, D. & Loha, E. 2008. Relationship between Total Lymphocyte count (TLC) and CD4 count among people living with HIV, Southern Ethiopia: a retrospective evaluation. [Online] Available: http://www.aidsrestherapy.com/content/5/1/26.

Department of Social Development. 2002. HIV/AIDS case studies in South Africa, vol.1. Pretoria: South Africa.

Dhar, P. K. 1999. Indian economy. New Delhi: Kalyani.

Evian, C., Millier, S., Steinberg, M. 1993. Primary AIDS care. Primary Guide for primary health care personnel in the clinical and supportive care of people with HIV/AIDS. Pretoria: Jacana.

Field survey data, 2007.

Gilbert, L., Seikow, T., Walker, L. 1997. Society, health and diseases. Pretoria: Sigma.

Goldstein, A. 1983. AIDS fears hits Gay populace doctors: more death likely, Miami Herald, June 12.

HIV/AIDS (n.d.) [Online] Available: http://www.wikipedia.org/wiki/HIV/AIDS

HIV InSite, 2003. Risk of HIV infection through receptive oral sex. [Online] Available: http://www.hivinsite.org/InSite?page=pr-rr-05

International AIDS Society 2000. External quality assessment programme for HIV Serological tests in Brazil. Brazil: International AIDS Society.

Kaplan, R.D. 2000. The coming Anarchy: Shattering the dreams of the Post Cold War.

Ojukwu, A. 2004. Kwenu! Our culture, our future. Interview with Dr Chidi Achebe. [Online]Available: http://www.kwenu.com/publications/ojukwu/interview/chidi_achebe.htm.

McMichael, A. 2000. HIV T cell responses to HIV. Current opinion in Immunology 12: 367-369.

National Institute of Allergy and Infections Diseases, 2009. [Online] Available: http://www3naid.nih.gov/topics/HIVAIDS/Understanding/Vaccines/VaccineChallenges.htm

Nomcebo, B. S. 2005. HIV/AIDS knowledge, attitudes and risky sexual behaviours of college students at Nazarene Teacher Training College in Swaziland: A descriptive study. University of the Western Cape: Masters in Human Ecology Thesis.

Nunn, M. Baggaley, R. Melby, J. & Thomas, A. (2004). Drugs alone are not enough: Community-based support for '3 by 5'. Report prepared for Christian AIDS on 15th international AIDS conference.

Rutter, D. & Quine, L. 2002. Changing health behaviour: intervention and research with cognition models. Buckingham: Open University Press.

Salati, F.C. 2004. The knowledge and attitudes of physiotherapists towards patients with HIV/AIDS in the Lusaka province, Zambia. Unpublished Thesis: University of the Western Cape.

Saloner, K.L. 2002. Rising to the challenge: The critical role of social workers in the face of the HIV/AIDS pandemic. Social work/Maatskaplike Work, 38 (2) 154-172.

Soul City Institute. 2004. HIV and AIDS prevention, care and treatment. Pretoria: Jacana.

The Scripps Research Institute, n.d. The Window period in HIV testing- the time between contact and detection. [Online] Available: http://www.squidoo.com/hiv-Window-period

Todaro, M. P. 1992. Economics for a Developing World. London: Longman.

Ukpere, G. 2007. The awareness level of HIV/AIDS amongst female teens in Langa Community: A case study. CPUT: Unpublished research proposal.

UNAIDS, 2003. AIDS epidemic update. [Online] Available: http://www.unaids.org

UNAIDS, 2004. Report on the global AIDS epidemic: 4th global report. Geneva: UNAIDS.

UNAIDS, 2006. Report on the global AIDs epidemic: 5th global report. Geneva: UNAIDS.

UNAIDS, 2009. Uniting the world against AIDS: HIV treatment. [Online] Available: http://www.unaids.org/en/policyAndPractice/HIVTreatment/default.asp.

UN, 2004. New report cites devastating effects of HIV/AIDS [Online] Available: http://www.un.org/News/Press/docs/2004/aids82.doc.htm.

WHO, 2003. Perspective and practices in Antiretroviral Treatment: Access to antiretroviral treatment and care: the experience of the HIV equity initiative, Cange Haiti. [Online] available:

http://www.who.int/hiv/pub/prev_care/en/haiti_e.pdf.
WHO, 2006, Overview of the. [Online] Available: http://www.who.int/hiv/mediacentre/2006_GR_CH02_en.pdf.
WHO, 2004. The World Health Report 2004: Changing history. [Online] Available: http://whqlibdoc.who.int/icd/hq/2004/a85554.pdf.

15

AIDS and Trauma: Adults, Children and Orphans

Rachel Whetten and Kristen Shirey
Center for Health Policy & Inequalities Research
Duke University
USA

1. Introduction

Though HIV/AIDS has become more of a chronically-managed illness in the most well-off of places, it is still a devastating disease that spreads rapidly and silently. Biomedical and behavioral research conducted over the last 25 years has taught us a tremendous amount about HIV: the people it infects, the way it infects and the damage it reaps. While some of this research is headline news, particularly those discoveries that lead us closer to a vaccine or other biomedical prophylaxis like microbicides, and to a lesser extent behavioral research that teaches us about effective prevention efforts, what are infrequently discussed but are no less important are the very substantial effects that trauma has on those infected and affected by HIV. We have found that there are higher rates of past and current trauma in adults infected by HIV than in the general population and subsequently these adults often have higher rates of substance abuse and other high risk activities. In children orphaned and otherwise affected by AIDS, we see they suffer not just the loss of a parent, but also significant emotional wounds that require specific treatments to heal. HIV is more than a virus; it is a disease that exploits already present vulnerabilities like poverty and goes on to wreak havoc on all levels of society. In this chapter, we will talk about trauma and its relationship to HIV in both adults and children. We will use fictitious case studies starting in childhood and moving through adulthood to explicate the complicated life stories, specifically the significant role trauma plays in the lives of people who are affected by HIV.

1.1 Orphans and culture and how AIDS has changed orphanhood

Orphans have been a part of the fabric of all cultures for time immemorial. Parents die at all times of a child's lifespan, from childbirth through the teenage years. AIDS has not created the experience of orphanhood but it has exacerbated the situation in many countries. Today, one hundred and forty-three million children are estimated to have lost one or both parents, fifteen million of these to AIDS (United Nations Children's Fund [UNICEF], 2009). Millions more have been abandoned by their parents. While Africa is most often referenced when discussing the orphan burden with respect to HIV/AIDS, South and Southeast Asian countries are caring for 67.5 million orphans alone (UNICEF, 2009). In both Africa and Asia, high mortality among young parents from conditions such as malaria, tuberculosis, HIV/AIDS, pregnancy complications, injuries, and natural disasters are responsible for the large and increasing number of orphans (World Health Organization [WHO], 2007). Most children in less wealthy nations are orphaned not at birth but at older ages (Norwegian UN Association, 2009; UNICEF, 2009; Zuberi et al., 2005); 36% of all orphans and 29% of double orphans are aged 6-11; almost half of single orphans and nearly two-thirds of double orphans are aged 12-17 (UNICEF, 2006).

Traditionally, cultures all over the world have long had their own unique ways to manage their populations of orphans. Eastern Europe is known for its past history of the institutionalization of children; Western Europe after World War I and II also dealt with orphaning through institutionalization; the United States used institutions and then later foster care became more popular. In many parts of Africa, extended family members are expected to absorb their brother or sister's children into their own families; neighbors or even whole villages tacitly and implicitly agree to care communally for the young members of a household that is suddenly parentless. Even today, many non-governmental organizations (NGOs) and other organizations working to care for orphans and vulnerable children (OVCs) use traditional African village culture as a model and point of reference for setting up care systems all over the world, particularly in Sub-Saharan Africa. Indeed, there have always been ways and means to care for orphans in their own societies, by their own societies.

The difference today is the sheer number of orphans that the HIV pandemic has created, with the most dramatic increases in orphaned children occurring in Sub-Saharan Africa and in Southeast Asia. With the virus killing off men and women of reproductive age the fastest - in some countries up to 40% of the men and women in this age group are infected - the number of children with one or both parents dead has increased exponentially in the last 20 years and has thereby overwhelmed these traditional mechanisms (Ntozi et al., 1999; Nyambehdha et al., 2006; Joint United Nations Programme on HIV and AIDS [UNAIDS] et al., 2004). This orphan epidemic of sorts has has left entire communities with sometimes thousands of children they are unable to clothe, educate or even feed. In some cases children are heading up their own households. HIV/AIDS has made desperate a generation of children who were already vulnerable from poverty. This is a crisis by any definition.

However, before we go too much further into the traumatic experiences that concern children infected and affected by HIV/AIDS, it is also important that we recognize how HIV/AIDS has changed the way we *talk* about orphanhood and orphans, perhaps in a way that does not serve them. According to Helen Meintjes and Sonja Giese at the University of Cape Town, from the time the epidemic first started killing off men and women of reproductive age, the NGO and aid community started referring to children who experienced the death of a parent from the disease as 'AIDS orphans.' This change was significant because typically a child was not labeled an 'orphan' in most parts of the world unless he/she lost both of his/her parents. This is still true today when one is *not* speaking in terms of HIV; the loss of one parent is no less a hardship but a child is not called an orphan. Yet, in the context of HIV/AIDS, losing one parent makes you an orphan according to the international aid community. While the attention and subsequent resources the focus on orphans has brought to countries with the most 'orphans' have no doubt been materially and instrumentally helpful to children who are most certainly in need, it is naïve to believe that focusing on what these children have lost, rather than what they still have - which in *many* situations is another biological parent - has some kind of cultural or at the very least semantic repercussion (Meintjes & Giese, 2008). Further, a child must be identified as an orphan - as someone who has lost something vital and makes him/her the target of aid - in order to receive this aid. How does that affect the recipients, particularly in cultures where the word 'orphan' means more than being without parents: it means you are without care or without love, and is necessarily associated with pity? Does this definition bring to the child its own kind of stigma and therefore *more* suffering instead of less? We do not have answers to these questions, but feel they are, at the very least, important to consider in the context of how we understand and digest the world of 'HIV and orphanhood.' In addition, it is important to note that it is those who have lost both parents who are truly the most vulnerable, and according to the Positive Outcomes For Orphans (POFO) data[1], children who have lost one parent show similar rates of trauma to those who have lost *neither*. We are not the first to point out that we are not the first to point out, that the very thing that makes children *most* vulnerable is not their orphanhood but poverty, to which children, not just orphans, are subject.

Regardless of the language of the international community there is no question that any child who experiences the death of a parent experiences a profound loss.

1.2 Traumatic grief

While the death of a parent at any age is upsetting and painful, even as adults we mourn the loss of a parent in ways specific to the relationship that we do not experience when mourning the death of a friend or even a spouse. For children, the loss of a parent has a particular gravity, by nature definition children do not have the developmental distance from their parents *as their own person* to mourn their passing separate from themselves, since they are by nature dependent on them (Brown et al., 2008). In other words, children are connected to their parents in ways that tie directly to their identification of self; children self-identify through their parents and only learn to separate their identities in their adolescence. So losing a parent during any developmental stage, but particularly for younger children, has a specific weight that is qualitatively different than any other kind of loss one can experience.

All children naturally grieve the loss of their parent(s), and this is very healthy. However, the profound nature of losing a parent, perhaps in the context of other environments that make a child more vulnerable, can bring about a specific kind of grief called 'Childhood Traumatic Grief (CTG)' that researchers and professionals have only in the last decade or so really started to strongly define and parse out from post-traumatic stress disorder (PTSD) or other symptoms of normal grieving following a traumatic experience such as the death of a loved one. The definition of CTG is distinct from depression and PTSD and understood as occurring following a loved one's death and the subsequent natural/normal grieving of the child is interrupted/disturbed by the development of trauma symptoms, which can include intrusive thoughts, intense and prolonged longing for the deceased, and, in school-aged children, inability to concentrate (J. Cohen et al., 2006).

Other research suggests that children who have lost a parent to AIDS face increased burdens related to emotional and psychological well-being. In his Ghanaian study (2009), Doku's findings support the mounting evidence which tells us that children orphaned by AIDS show more problems with their peer relationships when compared to other children their age (Ntozi et al., 1999; Nyambehdha et al., 2006; Cluver et al., 2008). Dowdney explains that

[1] Positive Outcomes For Orphans is a longitudinal research study following orphaned and abandoned children in 5 less wealthy nations funded by the NIH.
http://globalhealth.duke.edu/dghi-fieldwork/open-projects/pofo

that the death of a parent under any circumstances, regardless of the additional burden of a stigmatizing illness, is grounds for increased risk of depression and anxiety. She further suggests that one in five children who experience parental death will "likely develop a psychological disorder" (Dowdney, 2000). Dysphoria and depression are the most widely reported of psychological problems in children following parental death (Dowdney, 2000). Severe depression is a potential issue, but is infrequently found in the literature on childhood bereavement. However, it is important to remember that depression and anxiety are associated with suicidal ideation. The type of despair that can accompany the loss one feels with the death of a parent, when unchecked and unmonitored, particularly in the wake of a stigmatizing illness where there is little to no community supporting that child, is a sobering picture.

There are other behavioral and emotional issues that are potential risks with parental death such as anxiety, temper tantrums, hyperactivity, withdrawal and other kinds of somatizing disorders (stomachaches) but in the case of children orphaned by AIDS, it is difficult to tease out causal variables (AIDS, AIDS orphanhood, orphanhood alone) due to the complexity of challenges when a parent is lost to a stigmatizing illness. There is varying evidence related to whether expected death (long illness preceding death) further complicates or ameliorates the grieving process. Likely there are many mediating and moderating factors, such as the way death is dealt with in the family, the way the illness/death is viewed in the community (stigma), any planning that is done ahead of time, and how much the child is included in these decisions and discussions. Indeed, these are not symptoms unique to children who have been orphaned, but it is necessary to understand the full complexity these children are facing when they lose their parents to HIV/AIDS and why they may be more vulnerable to trauma and traumatic experience.

1.3 HIV-related risk-taking behaviors as it relates to trauma in children

Sexual risk behaviors, and other HIV risk behaviours are of particular concern when discussing the health of OVCs. Studies found orphans to be more sexually active than non-orphans (Kang et al., 2008; Nyamukapa et al., 2008; Palermo & Peterman, 2009; Thurman et al., 2006); and to have higher rates of sexual risk-taking and reported forced sex (Birdthistle et al., 2008). Other research, including pilot study research conducted by these authors, finds orphaned girls more likely to go into sex work and, conversely, sex workers in low and middle income countries (LMICs) to be highly likely to have been orphaned and abandoned children (OAC) (Mangoma et al., 2008). The small, qualitative pilot study was not meant to demonstrate causality but to explore the relationship between OAC and sex work. Qualitative interviews were conducted with 25 female sex workers in Hyderabad, India. Our research team and outreach workers visited 'hot spots' (railway stations and bus stops known as areas where sex workers find customers) and sex workers' homes. While not part of the inclusion criteria for the study, it was notable that 16 of the 25 women (64%) were found to have been either single or double orphans.

Human and animal studies demonstrate that greater stress results in increased propensity for drug and alcohol use (Gordon, 2002). The biological response to early life stress modifies neurodevelopment in permanent ways; these neuroadaptations occur within the same neuronal systems that comprise the drug, sex and risk-taking/gambling reward circuit (Adinoff, 2004; Gordon, 2002). Children who have experienced trauma and chronic stress are more likely to be biologically predisposed to gravitate to drug and alcohol use and risky sexual activity (Adinoff, 2004; Gordon, 2002). Our team's adult HIV studies have demonstrated strong relationships between childhood trauma and adult drug and alcohol use, as well as high-risk sexual activity (Leserman et al., 2005; Mugavero et al., 2007; Pence et al., 2008; K. Whetten et al., 2005). Baseline data from the POFO study indicate ongoing traumatic experiences of OAC (K. Whetten et al., 2011); in the 36 month follow-up, some OAC reported illicit drug use and having been drunk.

1.4 Post-traumatic stress disorder and trauma in children

There is ample evidence associating PTSD with trauma exposure in children, with documented and well-researched examples such as bearing witness to neighborhood or familial violence, war, and/or natural disasters. A plethora of research exists examining the effect of all sorts of traumatic events: following the terrorist attack of September 11th in the United States, post-conflict research in Bosnia-Herzegovnia, Croatia, Cambodia, Algeria and Palestine; victims of both community and personal violence (rape or physical assault); and victims of natural disaster, etc. all documenting rates of PTSD and the effects of traumatic events (Calderoni et al., 2006; Dobricki et al., 2010; Hoven et al., 2005; Klaric et al., 2007; Loncar et al., 2006). However, there are remarkably few articles in the literature examining PTSD among orphans, given the sheer number of orphans and the simple vulnerability of the population. There are some studies that have identified trauma and PTSD as significant factors in the life of a child orphaned by HIV. In her South African study of over 1,000 children ages 10-19, Cluver found that AIDS-orphaned children reported high levels of symptoms of PTSD when controlling for age, migration (moving between homes), household size, and gender. This same study revealed higher levels of other psychological distress among children who were orphaned by AIDS, when compared to children orphaned by other causes and non-orphans. The POFO study also found that in addition to losing 1 or both parents, 98% of the sample of 1,258 children experienced at least 1 more traumatic event and more than half (55%) experienced 4 or more traumatic events. While this study did not diagnose PTSD, the sheer fact of having experienced what have been scientifically proven as potentially traumatic events is ominous, never mind *four* such events.

What may be even more important, particularly as we try to intervene on the behalf of children who have experienced trauma and those who have been diagnosed with PTSD is that children who have already experienced one trauma are at an increased risk of experiencing more traumas. Simply put, trauma begets trauma; this is terrifying because we do know that children who experience trauma and/or have experienced PTSD are more vulnerable in their adult lives to psychological problems like depression and anxiety, as well as an increased risk for contracting HIV and other STDs (K. Whetten et al., 2008; Whitmire et al., 1999) than children who have not experienced trauma/do not have PTSD. A 2009 review of all published psychosocial interventions for children orphaned by or vulnerable from HIV/AIDS, defined psychosocial intervention as including "...psychological therapy, psychosocial support and/or care, medical interventions and social interventions..." with liberal inclusion criteria "..Randomised controlled trials, crossover trials, cluster-randomised trials and factorial trials were eligible for inclusion. If no controlled trials were found, data from well-designed non-randomised intervention studies (such as before and after studies), cohort, and case-control observational studies were considered for inclusion. Studies which included male and female children under the age of 18 years of age, either orphaned due to AIDS (one or more parents died of HIV related-illness or AIDS), or vulnerable children (one or more parents living with HIV or AIDS)…", turned up exactly ZERO tested, evidenced-based interventions available to these children who are in such desperate need and in a clear and present danger (King et al., 2002). In other words, it is documented that there are children in need of help, yet there is little evidence that the 'help' on the ground is based on empirical research.

Currently, these authors are aware of a few pilot studies that are using Judith Cohen's manualized Cognitive-Based Therapy (CBT) to address traumatic grief in children who have been orphaned and early analysis is showing real promise.

2. Joshua – A case study: Father dying of AIDS and the effects of the children to be orphaned

In order to really elucidate the series of challenges and hardships the children who are orphaned by AIDS come to face, we will provide a 'case study' of an orphan and his family: a fictitious orphan who is really a composite of orphans who have been orphaned by AIDS who we have known over the years through our research or intervention work.

Joshua was nine, living in a Sub-Saharan country with his elder sister and two younger brothers. Joshua's father was a farmer and while they were by no means rich, they had two solid meals a day and they were happy. Two years before, Joshua's father fell ill with what everyone told him was malaria. After a few weeks Joshua knew that it wasn't malaria because his father was not getting better. At first his father went to the hospital but after a week the family could no longer afford to pay the doctors, and nor could his mother take the time to bring meals to the hospital, so he was moved home. Though initially he was well enough to do some work, ultimately he became bedridden. Joshua began to notice that their meals were getting smaller and sometimes his mother would not eat at all. One day he overheard his aunties and mother talking about the cost of his father's medication and he understood he would need to work as the man of the household and cease going to school.

HIV/AIDS has infected men and women of reproductive age all over the world, particularly in Sub-Saharan Africa, and these are the breadwinners and caretakers of the household. In households that are managing but live on the margins of poverty, one illness can be the difference between eating and not eating or education and no education for the children of that household. Numerous programs have sought to aid the hardest hit countries and populations by providing life-extending medications, and while these programs have been life saving for many, there are still millions of eligible infected individuals who are unable to access the medications for a plethora of reasons: transportation, inability to leave work or family (lack of time), and concern about stigma. Sometimes parents must sacrifice their children's school fees to pay for these medications. In other cases, children leave school in order to make money to supplement the cost spent on medications. Similar circumstances arise when a family member is hospitalized. Furthermore, it is not unusual for hospitals in less wealthy nations to supply only medical care but not food or drink. As a result, this burden to feed the patient falls to the family which can turn into a full-time job, especially for those families who live far distances from the hospital.

Joshua continued to rise with the sun and to help his mother and sister with the morning chores, but then he would go to the fields to work. Upon returning home he would eat and then sit with his father, who appeared to be losing weight by the day and began to cough often. After several months had passed, in the middle of the night he heard his mother's sobs and then the sobs of the neighboring women. His father had passed on in the night. A funeral followed in two days time and it seemed as though not everyone in the village attended, as was the tradition. He wanted to ask his mother about this, but he was afraid he knew the answer. People were afraid of how his father died.

Stigma is a formidable presence in the lives of children affected by HIV but one that is difficult to measure. Stigma can be witnessed in the form of outright discrimination - not allowing children who are infected or those associated with people infected (like children of infected parents) to play or associate with uninfected children is one of the major ways that children experience stigma. The POFO study sought to measure stigma by asking people employed as caregivers in orphanages and people who took care of children who were not biologically their own if they would hypothetically allow their children to play with a child who was known to be infected by HIV. The research team also asked the participants if they would care for a relative who was sickened by the virus. The results showed that individuals associated with institutions were more accepting of those infected with HIV (willing to care for relatives and/or letting their children play with an infected child) and more knowledgeable about the virus (Messer et al., 2010). Unpublished qualitative data from the same study asked about stigma experienced by both children orphaned by HIV and those who were orphaned by other causes. The participants reported that children orphaned by HIV were sometimes stigmatized and shunned by other children and even their caretakers treated them poorly. A few children reported that they felt that being an orphan 'marked' them either through the simple fact of being parentless or by the poverty that often befell them as a result of losing an adult breadwinner in their family. There have been numerous interventions and attempts at reducing stigma targeted in the areas hardest hit by the epidemic. However, as a global society we have yet to evolve enough to where being HIV+ is not a mark of shame for individuals and/or their families.

Joshua's younger brothers continued to go to school and he continued to work the fields with his mother while his elder sister worked at home and took the vegetables they could afford to sell into town. He missed his father and he had less to time play with his friends. When he did have a little spare time, he had less in common with them because he felt older and more mature than them. He was not sure, but he thought that some of his friend's parents didn't look at him directly anymore, like his friend Michael. His mother used to invite him inside every time he would play football with Michael, but since his father died, she had not invited him in the house. Michael and he used to talk about the other kids in their class a lot. Michael kept him updated on the school gossip, but it just made Joshua sad because he realized while it felt important to be taking care of the family and to be the 'man' of the household, he missed his old life; he missed his friends and he even missed school. He started making up excuses to not play football when Michael came around to spend time with him. It wasn't difficult to come up with reasons to not go, because truthfully there were always more chores, more things to be done for the household – animals to tend to, water to be fetched, children to be bathed. And his mother seemed more tired than usual lately.

Another stress that is not measured or noted much in the literature but is a very real and concerning issue is how children in families affected by AIDS find themselves cut off from their former social networks and from their friends. Most importantly, they are often cut off from their natural emotional outlets for sharing and working through problems with their friends. Whether this is done through sitting down and talking under the acacia tree or on the football field with nine other boys, the outlet is crucial and when these begin to crumble through stigma and through new responsibilities to the family, these children suffer.

Things were different at Joshua's house now. Paul, the seven year old, was getting in trouble in school not infrequently; he was bringing home letters from the teacher detailing his poor behavior during lessons and sometimes discussing fights he instigated with others. When questioned, he claimed he is called names at school and must fight for his honor. At nighttime, both his younger brothers would have nightmares. Sometimes they would call for their father and sometimes for their mother. Beatrice would go to them and hold them and sometimes if they could not be settled she would bring them to mother and show them mother was still with them but she tried not to do this too often because she knew inside mother would not be with them much longer.

Children deal with stress and fear differently and one common way is to 'act out' in school, which a child's attempt to bring attention to themselves in the often unconscious hope an adult will pick up on the underlying problem that they need help with (a sick parent, bullying at school, etc). This acting out is frequently seen as a negative behaviour; being disruptive, not completing assignments, talking back to the teacher, etc.

At first he attributed it to her grieving, to her missing her husband, but he soon noticed that his mother was less able to work the fields and began to take longer and more frequent breaks throughout the day. One day, she left the house very early in the morning, saying she had to take a trip to town – to the clinic - she would be home by nightfall. When she returned her face was very worn and troubled. Not very long after this trip into town, his mother stopped coming to work in the fields. While they did not discuss this change, he knew that the disease that had taken his father was to take away his mother, too. In the coming months, a quiet sadness descended on the household.

It is not uncommon that families do not discuss illness and/or impending death, in spite of its overarching presence. There are a myriad of cultural taboos, in the United States and Europe included, that make discussing difficult subjects like life-threatening illness and death planning difficult or impossible to broach. The inability to discuss and prepare children for such a cataclysmic event has far-reaching repercussions, and NGOs all over the globe have made an effort to break the silence around serious illness and death, particularly for the benefit of the children who are left behind. There are now dozens of 'Memory Book' type projects that seek to help parents and other loved ones create books and other types of media to leave behind for their children. As the child grows without the parent, these books/projects can provide a crucial touchstone, a link to that parent: a positive keepsake containing memories, traditions, and histories that might not have been known had they not been created, and really play an important role in that child's healthy grieving, part of which is having positive memories of the deceased. It is well documented that creating positive memories of the deceased loved one is an important step in the grieving process, particularly for children. In many cases, the children themselves create these books with their sick parent or loved one and the experience in and of itself can be a catalyst for important conversations that may not have been had while the parent was still living (Kilimanjaro Women Against AIDS [KIWAKKUKI], 2005).

Only a few aunts and neighbors came to visit, while others who had previously brought them extra ugali now did not bring them anything. Joshua worked harder and longer in the fields and helped his brothers at night with their homework and tended to his mother as best he could. He desperately tried to maintain a level of normalcy in the home all the while knowing that his mother was slipping away from them, from him. She died in the night, just as his father had. He was 10 and now the man of the household. His sister was 12.

Beatrice, Joshua's sister, tended to her mother as best she could as she suffered her illness. She knew that it was the same sickness that took their father. She knew it was the virus they called AIDS and that was why people shunned them now. She acted as mother to her little brothers, though Joshua now acted as a 'man' of the house, working only in the fields and telling her what to do. Recently, shortly before her mother's death, she had experienced her first blood, so she knew that she was marriageable, though she had not shared this news with brother – partly out of custom, but also out of fear. Tradition demanded she tell her mother of her news, and she did, and she was fairly certain her mother passed this news to her aunt. What this meant for her future was unclear because surely news of the virus in her family was everywhere. Who would want her now? Would she have any choices for marriage? When her mother was still living they would giggle and speculate about the different possibilities for her in the distant future, after she had finished school and maybe even attended university! Beatrice was at the top of her class. School work came easy to her and she knew she possessed an above average intelligence. She often wondered how she could apply this in the future; she loved to argue, she could change minds by virtue of her gift of wordplay and logic. She dreamed of becoming a lawyer, as women did that now in her country. She knew of a few girls who had gone on to university in the city. While her family had been poor and she had no idea how this might happen for her, she knew it was not an impossible dream. Well, it had not been; perhaps there was no place for dreams now perhaps her choices would be made for her.

While the life of the eldest boy child can be directly changed in ways such as dropping out of school to work in the fields or work directly for money/salary, the experience of a girl child with a sick and dying parent is equally life changing but can look quite different. For an older girl, she might also leave school so she can care for younger children, be the caretaker for the sick parent and/or be the primary domestic worker - fetching water or firewood, cooking, buying food at the market, etc. When that parent dies, however, if she does not become the head of household for the remaining children, which is always a dire but very real possibility, she may either marry or go to work.

Early marriage is something that young women and girls face in many parts of the world and the challenges of orphanhood only serve to exacerbate this problem. Already vulnerable and dependent, these young women/girls are, by virtue of being a minor, in an unbalanced power dynamic, and have less power to negotiate their own safety. For example, a young bride whose husband wants sex without a condom - does a 15 year old have the skills to negotiate her own personal value and safety, particularly if there is a cultural belief that supports the idea of her 'obeying' her husband? Sadly, young married women have a higher rate of HIV infection than women of the same age demographic but who are unmarried. Furthermore, young women who are unmarried but in sexual relationships are more likely to become sexually involved with younger men and data show that younger men are more likely to be willing to use condoms (Clark, 2004; Haberland et al., 2005; UNICEF, 2003).

More disturbingly, there are stories out of Africa that males have been seeking out young girls, even infants, who are virgins because they are believed to be safe and free from disease, and that they can in fact 'cure' men of HIV/AIDS by having sex with them.

2.1 Mother dies: Children become double orphans

Joshua continued – The problems began immediately upon his mother's death. First, he had to pay for a proper funeral. Soon after his mother's funeral his mother's sister came to the home and told him to pack his things, as he and his youngest brother were moving to a nearby village where this aunt lived with her husband and children. This came as a complete shock to him because while he knew they were a poor family in terms of wealth, they did have their small plot of land and their home. He expected to inherit this and live here with his siblings. At the very least, the money from the sale of the home and adjoining land was to go to him and his siblings, or so he understood.

One of the biggest legal problems facing families who experience parental/spousal death and orphaning is related to land-grabbing and inheritance loss. Because of poorly enforced or even non-existent laws concerning land and home deeds and property ownership, one repeatedly hears the story of wives and children who expected to continue to live where they did when their loved one(s) was alive only to have relatives claim/take/steal this property for themselves. A lack of will-planning, paper deeds and other 'estate' documentation, and birth certificates as well as a lack of law enforcement related to the above all contribute to orphans/widows losing any property that is left to them by the deceased. For a widowed woman with dependent children, this makes her very vulnerable and often requires her to move in with other relatives or move away from neighbors and friends who might have served as social support during a trying time. For orphans, this can be life-shattering since, as children, their rights are rarely recognized. As a result, they are at the mercy of adult relatives' choices and, in all too many cases, simple greed (Kalanidhi & Coury, 2004; McPherson, n.d.).

Joshua was saddened by the thought of moving from his home and worried that his aunt did not mention his sister and other brother in her announced plans. Joshua yearned for them to never be apart, particularly now – he didn't want to lose anyone else - though he knew he had no say in this matter as he was only a child. Within days he was living in his auntie's house, going to school again, as was his brother, but at a different school. At this new school, the other children did not speak to them and appeared to whisper to one another when the two brothers passed by. They tried to join in games during recess but they were shunned. The teacher looked at them with pity but did nothing. His aunt was kind to him but it was clear her husband resented their presence in his house as extra mouths to feed. He felt funny in the house anyway because he had been a man when his parents were alive and now he was again treated as a child, like he had been demoted, and this felt demeaning – disrespectful, even. Joshua was the one who had run the household following his father's death and his mother's sickness. He was no child! Joshua swore to himself that as soon as he was able, he would run away to the city so he could find a good job. Then he would come back for his brothers and sister if he could find her and they would be together again.

For single orphans whose fathers have died, living with the mother is very common. In the reverse situation, with the mother dead and father living, it is less common that the child live with the remaining parent (UNICEF, 2006). While the data tell us that there are more single orphans with fathers lost than there are double orphans (with both parents lost), when one parent dies of HIV it is likely that the other parent has also been infected and will also die prematurely leaving any children in the family labeled a 'double orphan' (Ainsworth, 2002; UNICEF, 2006). While all children who have been orphaned face hardship and challenges, those who have been double orphaned or abandoned by both parents have a particularly difficult road ahead. There are between 13 and 16 million double orphans in the world today (UNICEF, 2006).

The age of a child at the time of orphaning is significant for what responses both the local/origin community will have in terms of planning for the orphan's future. In the case of those children who have a family member to care for them, the younger they are, the more likely it is that they will be absorbed into another family. Depending on the region of the world, culture and familial circumstance, it is the grandparents, aunts and uncles who are most likely to take on the task of caretaking for the orphaned and/or abandoned children. It is also not unusual for siblings to be split up due to financial hardship of the families who are acting as caregivers - they are limited to how many more children for whom they can care, school fees and costs of uniforms are high, etc.. This can serve as an additional trauma for the orphaned children. After losing their parents, they then lose additional member(s) of the family (United States Agency for International development [USAID] et al., 2002). Research on sibling separation suggests that sibling-orphans who were separated after parental death experienced higher rates of anxiety and depression than those who were not separated from their siblings (Gong et al., 2009).

For children who do not have family to whom to go, there are several possibilities that have been observed. Some children find their way into an institution or orphanage. (While the current 'opinion' in the NGO-aid world is that institutionalization is a last resort and should always remain so, there is evidence to suggest that this is not such a black-and-white situation. Indeed, there is evidence that some institutions, by no means all, do have the ability to provide a child-centered, healthy environment from which a child can grow). The quality and type of institution varies wildly across the worldwide landscape, though it is popularly considered a bad situation for a child to live in an institution of any kind.

Another possibility is for children to enter the work force. There are an estimated 215 million children engaged in what is defined as child labor by the International Labor Organization (ILO) but very little data exists on orphans and child labor. Baseline results from the POFO study show that of the 1258 caregivers who responded for the community based children, of the 1258 caregivers who responded for the children, nearly 22% were engaged in what is defined as child labor - a child under the age of 15 working 28 hours a week. Orphans (and vulnerable children) not attending school were four times more likely to have reported engaging in child labor than those attending school. Moreover, children working more than 28 hours a week were twice as likely to not be attending school than those working less than 28 hours (R.Whetten et al., 2011).

The weeks that followed for Beatrice confirmed her worst fears. Her aunt approached her while she was cooking the family dinner and told her about the man who was to be her husband; the ceremony would take place in four weeks' time. Noting the fear on Beatrice's face, her aunt chided that she should be happy anyone was still willing to take her given the family circumstances (HIV in the family). She would no longer attend school, and university was "clearly out of the question, so don't ever mention it again, as it was difficult enough to get him to agree to have you" is what her aunt told her.

Other consequences of the combination of orphaning and trauma have yet to be seen on a large scale, however there are predictions of nothing short of an alarming societal breakdown in the face of children who, having not been properly cared for, will grow to adulthood and run businesses, ministries, government offices and every other part of the private and civil sector and this is a serious risk to the future of society and the world at large (Barnett & Whiteside, 2002; Bellamy, 2005; Kalanidhi, 2004; Lewis, 2002; Natrass, 2002; UNICEF, 2003). Whether this is a truism or a gross exaggeration remains to be seen. However, at the very least, for children who have experienced the trauma of losing their parent(s) and may have experienced additional traumas, we do know they are at risk for further traumas as they grow up. Trauma begets trauma, and this is a cycle that desperately needs to be broken.

2.2 Exposure to trauma is common in adults, particularly in those living with HIV/AIDS

Many HIV positive adults report having been physically or sexually abused during childhood. A history of childhood trauma is also associated with recurrent exposure to traumatic events in adulthood (Parks et al., 2011). Women who were sexually or physically abused during childhood are 2.5 to 3 times more likely than the general population to experience physical or sexual abuse in adulthood (Parks et al., 2011). Many people living with HIV/AIDS report having experienced some kind of traumatic event in their life, including physical and sexual assault. Poverty , a condition many HIV positive people live with, is another risk factor for numerous kinds of traumatic exposures, from childhood abuse or neglect to sexual and interpersonal violence. (Matzopoulos, 2008). The HIV epidemic has taken hold in the poorest parts of the world, and poverty arguably has been a significant contributor to the spread of the disease. Exposure to violence profoundly impacts emotional and mental health; the connection between trauma, HIV, and poverty becomes inextricably linked, perpetuating HIV transmission and worsening poverty, and mental illness including post-traumatic stress disorder (PTSD), depression, and substance abuse. These factors are transmitted across generations by way of problems including orphanhood, child labor, and childhood trauma.

The cyclical or recurrent nature of exposure to trauma is most striking with respect to sexual assault. In one study of 162 primarily low-income, ethnic minority HIV positive adults, on average 45% (68% of women and 35% of men) reported experiencing a sexual assault at some point in their lifetime (Kalichman et al., 2002). These estimates are dramatically higher than the general population, in which the rates of lifetime forced sex are 6.5% in all adults (10.6% of women and 2.1% of men) (Basile, 2007). History of trauma leads to exposure to even more trauma during the lifespan. For example, people who have been sexually assaulted at least once are likely to experience multiple sexual assaults. 80% of those with a history of sexual assault had been assaulted two or more times, and the mean number of lifetime unwanted sexual events was 9.7. Exposure to even one such traumatic event leaves painful and lasting marks on peoples' lives, so one can imagine the devastating cumulative impact of nine such traumas on every aspect of life, including mental health, behavior, relationships, and work.

Post-traumatic stress disorder is perhaps the most clearly defined and well-known sequela of trauma. A diagnosis of PTSD (American Psychiatric Association, 1995) can be made when an individual has exposure to an event or situation in which s/he experienced a threat of death or grave bodily harm, and that experience was met with feelings of intense fear, helplessness, or horror. In addition to history of exposure to a traumatic event, PTSD is characterized by symptoms in three clusters: intrusive recollection, numbing or avoidance, and hyper-arousal. Symptoms of intrusive recollection include nightmares about the traumatic event and vivid memories of the trauma that may be associated with strong emotional and physical response. A few examples of the numbing or avoidance cluster of symptoms include diminished feelings, activity, or memory of the traumatic event. Hyper-arousal involves having an exaggerated startle response, difficulty sleeping, irritability, impaired concentration, or outbursts of anger. While there are a number of different symptoms associated with PTSD, the impacts of trauma on individuals, families, and communities are far more diverse than what can be conceptualized under the umbrella of this diagnosis. Effects of trauma can manifest in many ways in addition to or instead of PTSD, including depression, substance abuse, exposure to violence as a perpetrator and/or victim, increased health risk behaviors, and physical illness.

Cultural differences in how distress is experienced and expressed may lead to different manifestations of distress in response to trauma exposure (Kira, 2010). There has been much debate over the legitimacy of the PTSD diagnosis across cultures. While it is indeed important to consider cultural context in evaluating the relevance and applicability of Western diagnostic and treatment models, that is not to say that trauma does not profoundly impact people of all different cultural backgrounds. Distress may be expressed with different words or actions, but is still distress. Experiences such as rape or torture cannot be accepted as a normal part of any culture, and we cannot minimize or negate the profound impact of trauma or the importance of working to alleviate such suffering and break the cruel cycle of trauma, poverty, and HIV.

Given the high rate of exposure to traumatic events among people living with HIV/AIDS, it is not surprising that many have a diagnosis of PTSD. Studies have found alarmingly high rates of PTSD among people living with HIV/AIDS ranging from 7% to 54%. In the general population in the US, lifetime prevalence of PTSD is 6.8% (Kessler et al., 2005). In a study of 611 adults living with HIV/AIDS in the southeastern U.S., 7% of respondents were found to have a probable diagnosis of PTSD. A parallel survey conducted in Tanzania of 72 adults revealed that 22% of those surveyed had likely PTSD. Though a number of different traumatic events were reported, particularly notable were high rates of sexual assault in both locations: 36% of participants in the southeastern U.S. and one fourth of Tanzanians in the survey reported history of sexual assault (K. Whetten et al., 2006).

3. A case study: Isaac. Childhood sexual trauma, poverty, and how these circumstances affect HIV risk behaviors

Isaac was raised in a Tanzanian village where his family had a small farm. He was the eldest of four children, and when he turned eight he started to work selling maize in the village. Shortly after he started, he went to an older man's house to see if the man wanted to buy maize, and found that this man was very drunk. The man asked him to come inside, then exposed himself to Isaac. He offered to give Isaac some of his drink, but Isaac said no. Isaac was scared and confused, and asked the man again if he would buy some maize. The man didn't buy any, but told Isaac he would buy maize if he came back the next week. Isaac returned the following week, and the man was again drunk. He exposed himself, and told Isaac that he would only buy maize if Isaac touched his penis. Isaac was scared and did not know what to do. As he slowly approached the man, Isaac told himself that he would touch the man this one time so he could sell the maize, but that he would find a way not to have to go back there. The man did buy maize from Isaac and told him to come back again next week. Isaac didn't want to go back, but he really wanted to sell maize to help his family. He didn't want to tell his parents and worried that they would be upset if he sold less maize than he had the week before. He returned to the man's house every week for the next few years. The man was usually drunk, and would often make Isaac touch his penis. Isaac started taking a few sips of the man's drink and found that it calmed his nerves a bit. Once, the man made Isaac touch his penis with his mouth. Isaac was very ashamed that he did this and thought that if anyone knew what he had been doing with the older man they would be disgusted by him. He had heard stories about men who liked other men, and how they were sinners and were dirty. Isaac thought since the man never touched him back that maybe he wasn't like these men. He started to worry about this a lot and have bad dreams about the man touching him. He had a hard time concentrating when he went to school and when he went to sell maize, he would get very nervous and shaky before going to this man's house.

When he was twelve, Isaac was getting bigger and was able to help his father with farming work. His younger sister started selling maize, and he no longer had to do this. He didn't see the old man again, but still worried a lot about what had happened to him and feared that it may happen to his sister as well. He could not bring himself to say anything to his parents or sister. Isaac's friends were starting to talk about girls, and he wondered if girls would like him after what he had done, even though he had never told anyone. He felt like he was somehow different or dirty, and needed to try hard to cover this up so people wouldn't find out the truth. Isaac started to date girls, and felt like being with them proved that he was in fact a 'real' man. He prided himself on having the prettiest girlfriends in the village, and a few times he even had three or four girlfriends. When he was sixteen, Isaac married a girl named Helen. She moved in with his family, and they both worked on the family plot. During the next year, the family's maize crops started doing poorly, and Isaac started worrying because he had just learned that his wife was pregnant with their first baby. He didn't think they would make enough money on growing and selling maize to get by. Isaac started looking for work on neighboring farms and in the village, but others were having the same difficulties with their crops. There was no work to be found. Some of the other young men in his village were going away to work in a Tanzanite mine a few hours away. He heard that these mining jobs had good pay, and that he could go work for a few months in the mine then come back and support his wife and family for the rest of the year.

Isaac went away to the mine and moved into a boarding house with several other mine workers. They were all young men, most were married, and all were away from their families for the first time in their lives. Mining was difficult work, but Isaac was optimistic that he could make enough money during a few months that he would be able to take good care of his wife and the baby they were expecting. Sometimes, women from the village would come to Isaac's boarding house in the evenings. Most of his roommates would pay to have sex with these women. It was so hard to be away from their families, they said, and nobody at home would ever know. A few of the men did not get together with these women, and the others started talking badly about them, saying that those men preferred the young boys who worked with them in the mines. Isaac started thinking back to what had happened when he was a boy with the older man in his village. He was afraid his roommates would think that of him since he had touched another man. The next time these women came over to the boarding house, Isaac had sex with one of them. He felt guilty, but it took his mind off the loneliness and hardship that filled his life as a miner. When he had a few drinks before the women came over, he was more relaxed and didn't feel so guilty. After all, he was working so hard so that he could be a good husband when he returned, and his wife would never know about what happened here in the mines or in his boarding house. He stayed at the mine for six months, returning home when he learned that his wife had given birth to their first son.

3.1 Trauma and risk of acquiring HIV

Like many people who were sexually abused as children, Isaac became sexually active at a young age and engaged in high-risk sexual behaviors including sexual activity with concurrent partners and hired prostitutes. Traumatic events and PTSD are not only more common in those with HIV, they are also risk factors for contracting HIV. People with history of exposure to trauma are more likely to engage in behaviors that place them at higher risk for developing HIV including unsafe sexual activity and intravenous drug use. In a U.S. study of homeless young adults, physical abuse, neglect, and sexual abuse were correlated with HIV risk behaviors (Melander & Tyler, 2010). The more types of abuse and neglect these young adults had experienced, the more likely they were to engage in HIV risk behaviors. Women prisoners in a U.S. study were surveyed regarding HIV status, traumatic events, PTSD, and sexual risk behaviors, and those with PTSD were 71% more likely to have engaged in prostitution and other high risk sexual behaviors (Hutton et al., 2001). In a longitudinal study of South African women, those who reported a history of intimate partner violence acquired HIV at a significantly higher rate. Forty-five of 123 women who reported more than episode of intimate partner violence acquired HIV, as compared with 83 of 846 who reported one or no incidents of intimate partner violence (Jewkes et al., 2010).

Back at home, Isaac was glad to see Helen and was proud to be a father. The crops were still doing very poorly, and he feared that the money he had made at the mine would not last for the rest of the year as he had hoped. He decided to go back to work at the mine, planning to remain only until his crops started doing better. He would go back to visit his wife, son, and family one weekend every four or five months. It was a difficult and lonely life, but he did feel proud that he was providing for his family, especially when he saw his friends who had stayed in the village and how much they were struggling to get by. He even saw one of his school friends begging on the street. At his boarding house, Isaac continued to have sex occasionally with one of the prostitutes, and over time this became part of his normal routine in his mining life. Several years passed with Isaac working in the mines, he and his wife had two more babies, and his family's maize crop didn't improve very much at all. There was a terrible malaria outbreak one year during which both of his parents and one of his cousins died. With his father gone, Isaac returned home to care for the family's land and look after his family since he was the eldest son.

Isaac was glad to be back with his family and out of the mines, but it was very hard to keep everyone in his family fed. He started growing a few other crops beside maize with a little better luck, but it was still difficult. One day, Isaac learned that his sister-in-law had fallen ill. She had grown very thin and developed a cough. He had seen people at the mine get sick like this, and all of them had to stop working. He heard that many of them died and the disease they had was spreading, but he never knew what it was. Her husband, who was Helen's older brother, had gotten sick like this a few years beforehand; everyone said it was malaria but he thought it was probably the same thing he had seen at the mine and now in his sister-in-law. He worried about what would happen to her children, who had already lost their father. It was so much to think about; his sister-in-law had four children, and Isaac felt like he could barely take care of his own children. He prayed to God to make her better, then tried to put it out of his mind. A few months later, Isaac's sister-in-law died. Two of her children went to stay with other family members, and Isaac and Helen took in her eldest and youngest sons. Isaac sent both boys to school with his own children despite the protests of the eldest son, Joshua, who said he was a man and should stay on the farm and work like the other grown men.

Isaac insisted that Joshua attend school; while he could use Joshua's help on the farm, he felt like it would be dishonoring the family if he didn't keep their orphaned children in school. The boys would already have enough trouble since everyone knew that their parents were dead, and had probably died from the disease that brought so much shame and loss to their villages. Isaac tried to be kind to the boys and treat them as his own, but he found it difficult. The eldest, Joshua, was sullen and did not respect his authority. The younger boy, Paul, often asked about his other two siblings. Isaac didn't like that the brothers and sisters were separated, but he was having a hard enough time feeding them and paying school fees; he knew there was no way he could support the other two siblings. Shortly after she went to stay with her auntie, it was announced that Joshua's younger sister Beatrice was to be married. Even though she was so young, Isaac was happy that there was someone willing to marry her after what had happened to her parents. People whispered to one another about this disease and how it came to those who deserved it. Isaac never talked about it, and nobody in the house ever did either; it was as if their silence would bury the existence of this disease and the pain it had brought to the family.

3.2 Stigma, trauma, and HIV

It has been found that believing the stigma attached to an HIV diagnosis may cause PTSD or increase the severity of PTSD symptoms among individuals living with HIV/AIDS. People with HIV are stigmatized around the world, but where the HIV epidemic has hit the hardest, in sub-Saharan Africa, stigma associated with the disease has been particularly distressing and destructive. In a Nigerian study of 190 HIV-positive patients, 61.6% reported having experienced or witnessed a stigmatizing event, and 27.4% met diagnostic criteria for

PTSD. Of note, 28 of the 52 patients diagnosed with PTSD reported a past history of at least one other traumatic event, which further supports the notion that the effects of trauma exposure during the lifespan are cumulative. Some of the most common stigmatizing events experienced as traumatic in this study included verbal assault, neglect, denial of employment, housing or education due to HIV status, and physical assault because of HIV status (Adewuya, 2009).

In the U.S., HIV-related stigma was heavily focused on gay men during the early years of the epidemic, and the gay community has continued to experience high levels of stigma even as HIV rates have been declining among men and increasing in women, particularly in African-American women. Though to a great extent the face of the HIV epidemic in the U.S. has changed, HIV-related stigma remains pervasive. People living in rural areas experience greater stigma than do those living in urban settings (Heckman et al., 1998; Reif et al., 2006). Those who experience greater stigma have poorer adherence to medications, leading to poorer mental health and medical outcomes in those who have recurrent distressing and traumatic stigmatizing experiences related to their diagnosis of HIV (Logie & Gadalla, 2009). HIV-related stigma is painful for individuals and families. The silence associated with stigma is also a powerful force in perpetuating beliefs about disease and treatment that hinder prevention, testing, and treatment efforts. As stigma also stands in the way of education, employment, and housing opportunities, it contributes to poverty. Stigmatizing events can be *the* traumatic event or part of a perpetual cycle of trauma that permeates the lives of people living with HIV/AIDS.

3.3 Post-traumatic stress disorder and HIV

Arguably, receiving the diagnosis of HIV is traumatic in itself, and can lead to development of depression, PTSD, substance abuse, or to exacerbation of any or all of these conditions. Post-traumatic stress disorder was originally conceptualized as a disorder affecting war veterans after a discrete combat-related traumatic event. The time course associated with PTSD related to HIV diagnosis can be very different, as there are a number of potentially traumatic points throughout the lifespan of a person living with HIV. The initial trauma of disclosure of HIV status is followed by stigma-related traumatic events that are quite commonplace in those living with HIV. Recurrent fear accompanies declines in clinical status such as beginning treatment, discontinuing treatment, developing opportunistic infections, or encountering significant medication-related side effects (Kelly et al., 1998). The future-oriented nature of these fears, i.e. fear of looming death as compared with a response to a past threat of death classically associated with PTSD does pose a challenge diagnostically. While the current diagnostic criteria do not clearly include such fear of death or threat to bodily integrity in the future, mental heath clinicians increasingly agree that living with HIV can be traumatic to an extent that it does cause clinically significant impairment and symptoms consistent with a diagnosis of PTSD (Martin & Kagee, 2011).

Because the time course of HIV is a chronic one punctuated by acute stressors, the development of PTSD related to HIV diagnosis can occur years after the diagnosis was first made (Delahanty, 2004). In a 2008 cross-sectional study of HIV-positive patients attending a public health clinic in South Africa, 54.1% of participants met diagnostic criteria for PTSD during their lifetime, and 40% met criteria for HIV-related PTSD, as described by PTSD symptoms attributed by the patient to receiving the HIV diagnosis and/or living with HIV (Martin & Kagee, 2011). In a South African longitudinal cohort study, 14.8% of patients with recently-diagnosed HIV met diagnostic criteria for PTSD at study baseline, and 26.2% met criteria at 6 month follow-up. One-third of the patients with PTSD identified the diagnosis of HIV as the index trauma causing PTSD (Olley et al., 2005, 2006).

Overall, people with PTSD, whether related to HIV diagnosis, HIV-related stigma, other traumatic experiences, or a combination of these factors, are less likely to adhere to anti-retroviral medications (ARVs). This leads to poorer medical outcomes and higher viral loads, which in turn make them more likely to transmit the virus to others. This taken with the increased HIV risk behaviors in individuals with PTSD, yields a group of people at great risk of infecting other people since they are engaging in high-risk behaviors and, if already HIV-positive, are likely to have higher viral loads. Incomplete adherence is directly related to lifetime traumatic events, and individuals who have experienced more lifetime traumatic events are more likely to be incompletely adherent to ARVs. Similar to the additive effects of multiple traumas on HIV risk behaviors, there is also an additive effect of multiple traumas on ARV adherence. In the CHASE study, overall incomplete adherence was reported in 9.5% of all subjects, 22.4% of subjects who had experienced three categories of trauma, and 34% of those who had experienced five or more categories of trauma (Mugavero et al, 2006).

HIV-positive individuals with PTSD report higher levels of physical pain (Smith et al., 2002) and fatigue (Barroso et al., 2010) than do those without PTSD. Post-traumatic stress disorder impacts physical symptoms, but also appears to directly impact immune function and disease progression in people living with HIV. Kimerling et al. demonstrated a more rapid decline in CD4+/CD8+ cell ratios among women with a history of trauma exposure (Kimerling et al., 1999). Subsequent studies have suggested a more complex relationship between PTSD and HIV disease progression with medication adherence playing the dominant role in CD4 counts and other indicators of immune function and disease progression (Delahanty, 2004).

Isaac started to become very thin. He occasionally wondered if he might be getting the same disease as his brother and sister-in-law, but he dismissed this, telling himself it was because he was working so hard to take care of his family. Isaac and his wife had been skipping meals so that the children would get enough to eat, and even though he heard Helen's stomach growling a lot Issac didn't seem to mind much at all. He started to feel tired and was having a harder time getting his work done on the farm. Joshua noticed that Isaac was slowing down and offered to stay home from school to help him out. The first time that Joshua talked about this to Isaac, he smacked Joshua and told him never to say such foolish things. Isaac was adamant that he could take care of himself, his land, and his family. He also, in the back of his mind, didn't want Joshua, Paul, or his own children to go through what he had experienced as a boy when he was working to sell maize. Over the coming months, Isaac grew even thinner, and fatigue descended over him like a heavy blanket. He sometimes felt like he could barely walk to the door without becoming exhausted. Joshua eventually stopped attending school so he could work on the farm. Isaac said this was temporary, and that as soon as he got better Joshua would go back to school. Joshua knew, and deep down Isaac knew as well, that there would be no return to school. Joshua had been through this with both of his parents and knew what was to come. Isaac started coughing. He started to think more often that he probably had the terrible disease that had taken his brother and sister-in-law as well as some of his friends back at the mine. Even as he grew more certain that he was dying of this disease, Isaac could not bring himself to say it out loud; he wanted to think that he could make it go away if he ignored it.

One day, Paul was accompanied home from school by a man from the village. This man, who was not familiar to Isaac, had heard from Paul's teacher that Isaac was very sick. He wanted to tell Isaac that there was a clinic that could help him and other people with this disease. Isaac did not believe him that there was any help, because everyone he had seen with the disease had died. Isaac was also very ashamed that people in the village knew he was sick, and he didn't want even more people to find out by going to the clinic. He kept getting sicker, though, and when he started coughing blood, at Helen's urging Isaac finally agreed to go to the clinic. Joshua and Helen helped him get to the clinic, a long and tiring walk from the farm. When they arrived, Isaac saw other people waiting who were very thin like him, and also saw some other people who looked well. He recognized one of the ladies working in the clinic from his primary school class. She greeted him, and told him that she also had this disease called HIV. She had been very thin and weak like him but was getting treatment, and with the treatment had gotten much stronger. She told Isaac there was hope for him – and for his family – as there had been for her. He was scared, but did start to feel a little bit of hope.

Isaac had some tests, saw the doctor, and it was confirmed that he had HIV. One of the nurses asked him questions about his history, and one of the things she asked him was if he had ever gone to work in the mines. It seemed that a lot of the young men who had worked in the mines came back with HIV because of how commonplace prostitution had become in mining towns, and this was in fact how the virus had reached a lot of the nearby villages.

Isaac took the prescribed anti-retroviral drugs, and he did start to feel better – less tired, and his cough was easing up. Since his first visit to the clinic, though, Isaac had been very troubled about having HIV, about what had happened when he worked in the mines, and also what had happened to him as a boy. As his body grew stronger, his mind grew more distracted by these bad memories. He started to drink a little, remembering how drinking had eased his nerves and sadness when he was in the mines. He did find that this made the bad memories and nightmares quieter, but he also started to have more arguments with Helen. He gradually spent less and less time with his family, and more time drinking by himself. He stopped taking all of his medications.

Substance use disorders are very common in people with PTSD who are HIV-negative. Data on the prevalence of these disorders in HIV-positive people are limited, but substance abuse, like PTSD, is considerably more common in HIV positive individuals than in the general population. Alcohol and drug use are strongly associated with interpersonal violence including sexual assault and intimate partner violence (Boles & Miotto, 2003; Najavits et al., 1998). The relationship between substance abuse, HIV, and trauma is a complex one; substance use increases the risk of exposure to traumatic events that may lead to PTSD or worsen existing symptoms.

Helen urged him to take his medicine, but as he drank more he felt even more depressed and hopeless. One night he drank so much that he passed out in the field next to his house. Joshua found him there in the morning and helped him back into the house. Isaac stayed in bed, and over the next day developed a high fever and bad cough. Helen called the doctor, and even though he gave Isaac medicine, he told Helen that Isaac might not survive. His body was weak from drinking so much, and since he had stopped taking ARVs the HIV had again taken hold on his immune system. Isaac died the following night.

The relationship between HIV and depression is better characterized than that of HIV and trauma. Depression is very common among HIV-positive individuals, with prevalence rates in the U.S. of 35-36% (Pence et al., 2007; Zierler et al., 2000). Among Rwandan women exposed to trauma during the 1994 genocide, 81% of the respondents who were HIV-positive endorsed clinically significant depressive symptoms (M.H. Cohen et al., 2009). Individuals with HIV who have a diagnosis of PTSD also have worsening of CD4 count that appears to be independent of adherence, suggesting a detrimental effect of PTSD on immune function and disease progression. People with co-morbid depression in addition to PTSD have lower CD4 counts than those with less severe or no depressive symptoms (Sledjeski, 2005).

3.4 Treatment for PTSD and other sequelae of trauma in people living with HIV/AIDS

Isaac and Joshua's family was entangled in a web of poverty, trauma, and HIV, and unfortunately suffered a tremendous amount of loss as a result. Isaac did start ARVs and had a chance at surviving for many years. He was haunted by the traumas in his past, however, and as is unfortunately all too common, this stood in the way of him adhering to treatment. Though remarkably effective, anti-retroviral drugs can only go so far in tackling the HIV epidemic. As HIV medication regimens are improving and becoming accessible to more people with HIV, people are living with HIV for many years. It is therefore crucially important to address trauma in people living with HIV. Targeting interventions for people living with HIV/AIDS who have experienced significant trauma and suffer from psychiatric sequelae including PTSD, co-morbid depression, and substance abuse can alleviate great suffering, decrease HIV transmission, reduce risk of future trauma exposure and HIV risk behaviors, improve ARV adherence, and improve overall health outcomes.

The picture of trauma in people with HIV can appear bleak, and it certainly is complex, but effective and feasible treatments are available for adults and children alike. Cognitive-behavioral interventions (CBI), for example, have effectively been used for people living with HIV/AIDS and have been shown to improve symptoms of depression, anxiety, anger, and stress (Crepaz et al., 2008). CBIs are simple interventions that are readily implemented in primary care or specialized HIV care settings. Further, these interventions can have a beneficial effect on improving immune function as evidenced by CD4 count (Crepaz et al., 2008). Similar treatment interventions have been modified to target ARV adherence, and have been found to be effective in improving adherence in addition to improving depressive symptoms (Safren et al., 2009). Most CBIs have been implemented in the U.S. and other wealthy nations; however, a few studies of CBI in less wealthy nations have yielded promising results. For example, in Thailand, a study of a culturally adapted CBI demonstrated improvement in general health and mental health (Li et al., 2010). Integrating behavioral interventions with HIV care for HIV- positive individuals with co-morbid mental health and substance use disorders significantly reduces psychiatric symptoms and improves medication adherence (K. Whetten et al., 2006). More difficult to quantify are the effects of such interventions on families and communities. Given the profound effects of trauma on mental health, HIV risk behaviors, and medication adherence and the cyclical effect of trauma that begets more trauma, mental illness, and HIV transmission, it is crucial to focus efforts on trauma prevention and care around the world. Effective treatments and interventions for trauma are available, and more widespread understanding of and attention to the grave effects of trauma can go far in improving the lives of people living with HIV, their families, and their communities.

4. Conclusion

While this narrative and illustrative case studies are meant to drive home the reality of many children and adults in the world today, it would be wrong for these authors to suggest that the suffering highlighted here begins and ends with orphanhood, traumatic experience or even AIDS. Poverty has always been the root cause of child labor, child marriage, children dropping out of school to care for ill parents and/or to work to pay for life-saving medications, prostitution, and of families on the edge of hunger and starvation. HIV/AIDS has served as a fierce and highly effective catalyst for pushing people on the precarious fence of poverty right over the edge. HIV/AIDS serves a lens from which we can see the essence of inequalities all over the world. Children who are raised in poverty often become impoverished adults themselves, and HIV/AIDS is a powerful servant on the side of poverty in this cruel cycle. Compounding the forces of trauma and the fallout from traumatic experiences adds that much more vulnerability and challenge to an already desperate situation that is entrenched in poverty. As we have detailed, individuals who have experienced trauma are at a higher risk for experiencing depression later in life, and are also more likely to experience more trauma, contributing to an already heavy emotional and spiritual burden as they enter adulthood. It behooves us as a global society to recognize the reality of traumatic illness and unresolved grief and to make room so those affected can find some help and maybe some peace. This is not only for the benefit for the individual, but for the benefit of society at large. A world of people with unresolved trauma is not a healthy environment for building a global economy, for political diplomacy, for solving public health problems. We owe it to those who have been hurt, but also to ourselves and our own children to have the opportunity to create a healthy and well-functioning global society, one where people aren't constantly looking over their shoulders out of fear, or terrified that everyday will be their last. We owe this to ourselves and to each other. The Lancet Global Mental Health working group recently published a series of articles addressing the issues and challenges of global mental health care provision. In their words: " Change in public health only comes about if three core elements are present: a knowledge base, strategies to implement what we know, and the political will to act.,...Now we need political will and solidarity, from the global-health community...... The time to act is now" (Lancet Global Mental Health Working Group et al., 2007) .

5. References

Adewuya, A., Afolabi, M., Ola, B., Ogundele, O., Ajibare, A., Oladipo, B. & Fakande, I. (2009). Post-traumatic stress disorder (PTSD) after stigma related events in HIV infected individuals in Nigeria. *Social Psychiatry and Psychiatric Epidemiology*, Vol.44, No.9, (September 2009), pp. 761-766, ISSN 0933-7954

Adinoff, B. (2004). Neurobiologic processes in drug reward and addiction. *Harvard Review of Psychiatry*, Vol.12, No.6, (2004), pp. 305-320

Ainsworth, M. & Filmer, D. (2002). *Poverty, AIDS and Children's Schooling: A Targeting Dilemma.* Policy Research Working Paper 2885. World Bank, Washington, D.C.

American Psychiatric Association. (1995). *Diagnostic and statistical manual of mental disorders* (4th ed.), Amer Psychiatric Pub Inc, ISBN 9780890424063, Washington, D.C.

Barnett, T. & Whiteside, A. (2002). *AIDS in the Twenty-First Century: Disease and Globalization* (1st ed.), Palgrave Macmillan Ltd., ISBN 978-1403900067, New York, NY

Barroso, J., Hammill, B., Leserman, J., Salahuddin, N., Harmon, J. & Pence, B. (2010) Physiological and psychosocial factors that predict HIV-related fatigue. *AIDS Behav.* Vol.14, No.6, (December 2010), pp.1415-1427, ISSN 1090-7165

Basile, K., Chen, J., Black, M., & Saltzman, L. (2007). Prevalence and characteristics of sexual violence victimization among U.S. adults, 2001-2003. *Violence and Victims*, Vol.22, No.4, (August 2007), pp. 437-448, ISSN 0886-6708

Bellamy, C. (2004). *The State of the World's Children, 2005: Childhood Under Threat.* United Nations Children's Fund, New York, NY

Birdthistle, I., Floyd, S., Machingura, A., Mudziwapasi, N., Gregson, S. & Glynn, J. (2008) From affected to infected? Orphanhood and HIV risk among female adolescents in urban Zimbabwe. *AIDS and Behavior*, Vol.22, No.6, (March 2008), pp.759-766, ISSN 0269-9370

Boles, S., & Miotto, K. (2003). Substance abuse and violence: a review of the literature. *Aggression and Violent Behavior*, Vol.8, No.2, (March-April 2003), pp.155-174

Calderoni, M., Alderman, E., Silver, E. & Bauman, L. (2006). The mental health impact of 9/11 on inner-city high school students 20 miles north of Ground Zero. *Journal of Adolescent Health*, Vol.39, No.1, (July 2006), pp.57-65

Clark, S. (2004). Early Marriage and HIV Risks in Sub-Saharan Africa. *Studies in Family Planning*, Vol.35, No.3, (September 2004), pp. 149-160

Cluver, L., Gardener, D. & Operario, D. (2007). Effects of stigma on the mental health of adolescents orphaned by AIDS. *Journal of Adolescent Health,* Vol.42, No.4, (April 2008), pp.410-417

Cohen, J., Anthony, P. & Mannarino, E. (2006). *Treating Trauma and Traumatic Grief in Children and Adolescents*, Guilford Press, ISBN 978-159353082, New York, NY

Cohen, M., Fabri, M., Cai, X., Shi, Q., Hoover, D., Binagwaho, A., Culhane, M., Mukanyonga, H., Karegeya, D. & Anastos, K. (2009). Prevalence and predictors of posttraumatic stress disorder and depression in HIV-infected and at-risk Rwandan women. *Journal of Womens Health*, Vol.18, No.11, (December 2009), pp.1783-1791

Coid, J., Petruckevitch, A., Feder, G., Chung, W., Richardson, J., & Moorey, S. (2001). Relation between childhood sexual and physical abuse and risk of revictimisation in women: A cross-sectional survey. *Lancet*, Vol.358, No.9280, (August 2001), pp.450-454

Crepaz, N., Passin, W., Herbst, J., Rama, S., Malow, R., Purcell, D. & Wolitski, R. (2008). Meta-analysis of cognitive-behavioral interventions on HIV-positive persons' mental health and immune functioning. *Health Psychology*, Vol.27, No.1, (January 2008), pp.4-14

Delahanty, D., Bogart, L., & Figler, J. (2004). Posttraumatic stress disorder symptoms, salivary cortisol, medication adherence, and CD4 levels in HIV-positive individuals. *AIDS Care*, Vol.16, No.2, (2004), pp.247-260

Dobricki, M., Komproe, I., de Jong, J. & Maercker, A. (2009). Adjustment disorders after severe life-events in four postconflict settings. *Soc Psychiatry Psychiatr Epidemiol.*, Vol.45, No.1, (January 2010), pp.39-46

Doku, P. (2009). Parental HIVAIDS status and death, and childrens psychological wellbeing. *International Journal of Mental Health Systems*, Vol.3, No.1, (November 2009), p.26

Dowdney, L. (2000). Childhood Bereavement following Parental Death. *The Journal of Child Psychology and Psychiatry*, Vol.41, No.7, (October 2000), pp.819-830

Gong, J., Li, X., Fang, X., Zhao, G., Lv, Y., Zhao, J., Lin, X., Zhang, L., Chen, X. & Stanton, B. (2009). Sibling separation and psychological problems of double AIDS orphans in rural China - a comparison analysis. *Child: care, health and development*, Vol.35, No.4, (July 2009), pp.534-541

Gordon, H. (2002). Early environmental stress and biological vulnerability to drug abuse. *Psychoneuroendocrinology*, Vol.27, No.1-2, (Jan/Feb 2002), pp.115-126

Haberland, N., Chong, E., Bracken, H. & Parke, C. (2005). Early Marriage and Adolescent Girls. *YouthNet*, No.15, (August 2005)

Heckman, T., Somlai, A., Peters, J., Walker, J., Otto-Salaj, L., Galdabini, C. & Kelly, J. (1998). Barriers to care among persons living with HIV/AIDS in urban and rural areas. *AIDS Care*, Vol.10, No.3, (June 1998), pp.365–375

Hoven, C., Duarte, C., Lucas, C., Wu, P., Mandell, D., Goodwin, R., Cohen, M., Balaban, V., Woodruff, B., Bin, F., Musa, G., Mei, L., Cantor, P., Aber, J., Cohen, P. & Susser, E. (2005). Psychopathology among New York city public school children 6 months after September 11. *Arch Gen Psychiatry*, Vol.62, No.5, (May 2005), pp.545-552

Kiliminjaro Women Against AIDS, (KIWAKKUKI). (2005). Memory project, Available from: kiwakkuki.org/?page_id=246; kiwakkuki.org/programs/memoryproject.htm

Hutton, H., Treisman, G., Hunt, W., Fishman, M., Kendig, N., Swetz, A., & Lyketsos, C.G. (2001). HIV risk behaviors and their relationship to post-traumatic stress disorder among women prisoners. *Psychiatric Services*, Vol.52, No.4, (April 2001), pp.508-513

Jewkes, R., Dunkle, K., Nduna, M., & Shai, N. (2010). Intimate partner violence, relationship power inequity, and incidence of HIV infection in young women in South Africa: a cohort study. *Lancet*, Vol.376, No.9734, (July 2010), pp.41-48

Kalichman, S., Sikkema, K., DiFonzo, I., Luke, W. & Austin, J. (2002). Emotional adjustment in survivors of sexual assault living with HIV-AIDS. *Journal of Traumatic Stress*, Vol.15, No.4, (August 2002), pp.289-296

Kang, M., Dunbar, M., Laver, S. & Padian, N. (2008). Maternal versus paternal orphans and HIV / STI risk among adolescent girls in Zimbabwe. *AIDS Care*, Vol.20, No.2, (February 2008), pp.214-217

Kelly, B., Raphael, B., Judd, F., Perdices, M., Kernutt, G., Burnett, P., Dunne, M., Burrows, G. (1998). Posttraumatic stress disorder in response to HIV infection. *General Hospital Psychiatry*, Vol.20, No.6, (November 1998), pp.1048-1060

Kessler, R., Berglund, P., Delmer, O., Jin, R., Merikangas, K. & Walters, E. (2005). Lifetime prevalence and age-of-onset distributions of DSM-IV disorders in the National Comorbidity Survey Replication. *Archives of General Psychiatry*, Vol.62, No.6(June 2005), pp.593-602

Kimerling, R., Calhoun, K. , Forehand, R., Armistead, L., Morse, E., Morse, P., Clark, R. & Clark, L. (1999). Traumatic stress in HIV-infected women. *AIDS Education and Prevention*, Vol.11, No.4, (August 1999), pp.321-330

King, E., De Silva, M., Stein, A. & Patel, V. (2002). Interventions for improving the psychosocial well-being of children affected by HIV and AIDS. *Cochrane database Syst Rev*, Vol.15, No.2, (April 2002), CD006733

Kira, I. (2010). Etiology and Treatment of Post-Cumulative Traumatic Stress Disorders in Different Cultures. *Traumatology*, Vol.16, No.4, (May 2010), pp.128-141

Klaric, M., Klarić, B., Stevanović, A., Grković, J. & Jonovska, S. (2007). Psychological consequences of war trauma and postwar social stressors in women in Bosnia and Herzegovina. *Croat Med J.*, Vol.48, No.2, (April 2007), pp.167-176

Lancet Global Mental Health Group. (2007) *Scale up services for mental disorders: a call for action*. September 4, 2007, www.thelancet.com, DOI:10.1016/S0140-6736(07)61242-2

Leserman, J., Whetten, K., Lowe, K., Stangl, D., Swartz, M. & Thielman, N. (2005). How trauma, recent stressful events, and PTSD affect functional health status and health utilization in HIV-infected patients in the south. *Psychosom Med*, Vol.67, No.3, (May-June 2005), pp.500-507

Lewis, S. (2002). United Nations Press Release: *Statement by Steven Lewis, the Secretary-General's UN Envoy on HIV/AIDS in Africa*, July 2002.

Li, L., Lee, S., Jiraphongsa, C., Khumtong, S., Iamsirithaworn, S., Thammawijaya, P. & Rotheram-Borus, M. (2010). Improving the health and mental health of people living with HIV/AIDS: 12-month assessment of a behavioral intervention in Thailand. *Am J Public Health*, Vol.100, No.12, (December 2010), pp.2418-2425

Logie, C. & Gadalla, T.M. Meta-analysis of health and demographic correlates of stigma towards people living with HIV. AIDS Care, Vol.21, No.6, (June 2009), pp.742-753.

Loncar, M., Medved, V., Jovanović, N. & Hotujac, L. (2006). Psychological consequences of rape on women in 1991-1995 war in Croatia and Bosnia and Herzegovina. *Croat Med J.*, Vol.47., No.1, (February 2006), pp.67-75

Mangoma, J., Chimbari, M. & Dhlomo, E. (2008). An enumeration of orphans and anlysis of the problems and wishes of orphans: the case of Kariba, Zimbabwe. *SAHARA Journal*, Vol.5, No.3, (September 2008), pp.120-128

Martin, L. & Kagee, A. (2008). Lifetime and HIV-related PTSD among persons recently diagnosed with HIV. *AIDS Behav.*, Vol.15, No.1, (January 2011), pp. 125-131

Matzopoulos, R., Bowman, B., Butchart, A. & Mercy, J. (2008). The impact of violence on health in low- to middle-income countries. *International Journal of Injury Control and Safety Promotion*, Vol.15, No.4, (December 2008), pp.177-187

McPherson, D. (2006). Property Grabbing and Africa's Orphaned Generation: A Legal Analysis of the Implications of the HIV/AIDS Pandemic for Inheritance by Orphaned Children in Uganda, Kenya, Zambia and Malawi. HIV/AIDS in Africa Project Paper, University of Toronto:
www.law.utoronto.ca/documents/ihrp/HIV_mcpherson.doc

Meintjes, H. & Giese, S. (2006). Spinning the Epidemic: The making of mythologies of orphanhood in the context of AIDS. *Childhood*, Vol.13, No.3, (2006), pp.407-430, ISSN-0907-5682

Melander, L. & Tyler, K. The effect of early maltreatment, victimization, and partner violence on HIV risk behaviour among homeless young adults. *J Adolesc Health*, Vol.47, No.6, (December 2010), pp.575-581.

Messer, L., Pence, B., Whetten, K., Whetten, R., Thielman, N., O'Donnell, K. & Ostermann, J. (2010). Prevalence and predictors of HIV-related stigma among institutional- and community-based caregivers of orphans and vulnerable children living in five less-wealthy countries. *BMC Public Health*, Vol.10, No.504, (August 2010), doi:10.1186/1471-2458-10-504

Mugavero, M., Ostermann, J., Whetten, K., Leserman, J., Swartz, M., Stangl, D. & Thielman, N. (2006). Barriers to antiretroviral adherence: the importance of depression, abuse, and other traumatic events. *AIDS Patient Care STDS*, Vol.20, No.6, (June 2006), pp.418-428

Mugavero, M., Pence, B., Whetten, K., Leserman, J., Swartz, M., Stangl, D. & Thielman, N. (2007). Predictors of AIDS-related morbidity and mortality in a southern U.S. Cohort. *AIDS Patient Care and STDS*, Vol.21, No.9, (October 2007), pp.681-690

Najavits, L., Gastfriend, D., Barber, J., Reif, S., Muenz, L., Blaine, J., Frank, A., Crits-Christoph, P., Thase, M. & Weiss, R. (1998). Cocaine dependence with and without PTSD among subjects in the National Institute on Drug Abuse Collaborative

Cocaine Treatment Study. *American Journal of Psychiatry*, Vol.155, No.2, (February 1998), pp.214-219

Natrass, N. (2002) AIDS and Human Security in Southern Africa. 2002 CSSR Working Paper 18, *AIDS and Society Research Unit, Center for Social Science Research, University of Capetown*, Available from: www.uct.ac.za/depts/cssr

Norwegian UN Association, UNEP/GRID-Arendal, UNU/Global Virtual University, the University College of Hedmark and the INTIS schools. (2009). Human impact map, Available from: globalis.gvu.unu.edu/.

Ntozi, J., Ahimbisibwe F., Odwee J., Ayiga N. & Okurut F. (1999). Orphan care: the role of the extended family in northern Uganda. *The Continuing African HIV/AIDS Epidemic, (*1999), pp.225-236

Nyambehdha, E., Wandibba, S. & Aagaard-Hansen, J. (2003). Changing patterns of orphan care in Kenya due to the HIV epidemic in western Kenya. *Social Science and Medicine*, Vol.5, No.2, (July 2003), pp.301-311

Nyamukapa, C., Gregson, S., Lopman, B., Saito, S., Watts, H., Monasch, R. & Jukes, M. (2007). HIV-associated orphanhood and children's psychosocial distress: theoretical framework tested with data from Zimbabwe. *American Journal of Public Health*, Vol.98, No.1, (January 2008), pp.133-141

Olley, B., Seedat, S. & Stein, D. (2006). Persistence of psychiatric disorders in a cohort of HIV/AIDS patients in South Africa. *J Psychosom Res*, Vol.61, No.4, (October 2006), pp. 479-484

Olley, B., Zeier, M., Seedat, S., & Stein, D. (2005). Post-traumatic stress disorder among recently diagnosed patients with HIV/AIDS in South Africa. *AIDS Care*, Vol.17, No.5, pp.550-557

Palermo, T. & Peterman, A. (2009). Are female orphans at risk for early marriage, early sexual debut, and teen pregnancy? Evidence from sub-Saharan Africa. *Studies in Family Planning*, Vol.40, No.2, (June 2009), pp.101-112

Parks, S., Kim, K., Day, N., Garza, M. & Larkby, C. (2011). Lifetime self-reported victimization among low-income, urban women: the relationship between childhood maltreatment and adult violent victimization. *J Interpers Violence*, Vol.26, No.6, (April 2011), pp.1111-1128. Epub 2010 May 24.

Pence, B., Reif, S., Whetten, K., Leserman, J., Stangl, D., Swartz, M., Thielman, N. & Mugavero, M. (2007). Minorities, the poor, and survivors of abuse: HIV-infected patients in the US Deep South. *South Med J*, Vol.100, No.11, (November 2007), pp.1114–1122

Pence, B., Thielman, N., Whetten, K., Ostermann, J., Kumar, V. & Mugavero, M. (2008). Coping strategies and patterns of alcohol and drug use among HIV-infected patients in the United States Southeast. *AIDS Patient Care STDS*, Vol.22, No.11, (November 2008), pp.869-877

Pharaoh, R. & Schönteich, M. (2003). AIDS, Security and Governance in Southern Africa: Exploring the Impact. *Institute for Security Studies*, Paper No. 65, (January 2003)

Reif, S., Whetten, K. & Raper, J. (2006). Characteristics of HIV-infected adults in the Deep South and their utilization of mental health services: a rural vs.urban comparison. *AIDS Care*, Vol.18, Supp. 1, (2006), pp.S10 –17

Sabbuharo, K. & Coury, D. (2004). *Reaching out to Africa's Orphans: A framework for Public Action*. The World Bank, Washington, D.C.

Safren, S., O'Cleirigh, C., Tan, J., Raminani, S., Reilly, L., Otto, M. & Mayer K. (2009). A randomized controlled trial of cognitive behavioral therapy for adherence and depression (CBT-AD) in HIV-infected individuals. *Health Psychology*, Vol.28, No.1, (January 2009), pp.1-10

Sledjeski, E., Delahanty, D. & Bogart, I. (2005). Incidence and impact of posttraumatic stress disorder and comorbid depression on adherence to HAART and CD4+ counts in people living with HIV. *AIDS Patient Care and STDS*, Vol.19, No.11, (November 2005), pp.728-736

Smith, M., Egert, J., Winkel, G. & Jacobson, J. (2002). The impact of PTSD on pain experience in persons with HIV/AIDS. *Pain*, Vol.98, No.1-2, (July 2002), pp.9-17

Thurman, T., Brown, L., Richter, L., Maharaj, P. & Magnani, R. (2006). Sexual risk behavior among South African adolescents: is orphan status a factor? *AIDS and Behavior*, Vol.10, No.6, (May 2006), pp.627-635

UNAIDS, UNICEF & USAID. (2004). *Children on the Brink 2004: A Joint Report of New Orphan Estimates and a Framework for Action*. (July 2004), UNAIDS, UNICEF and USAID, New York, NY

UNICEF. (2003). *UNICEF and UNAIDS applaud milestone in forging coordinated global response to growing crisis of children orphaned due to AIDS*, Press Release, Available from: www.unaids.org/en/media/unaids/contentassets/dataimport/media/press-releases01/joint_pressrelease_unicef_21oct03_en.pdf

UNICEF. (2006). Africa's Orphaned and Vulnerable Generations: Children Affected by AIDS, Available from: www.unicef.org/publications/index_35645.html

UNICEF. (2009). *State of the Worlds Children*. New York; 2009.

USAID/SCOPE-OVC/FHI. (2002). *Results of the orphans and vulnerable children head of household baseline survey in four districts in Zambia*. Available from: www.fhi.org/en/HIVAIDS/pub/Archive/OVCDocuments/ovczambia.htm

Whetten, K., Ostermann, J., Whetten, R., O'Donnell, K., Thielman, N. & POFO Research Team. (2011). More than the loss of a parent: Traumatic Experiences of Orphaned and Abandoned Children in 5 Less Wealthy Nations. *Journal of Traumatic Stress*, Vol.24, No.2, (April 2011), pp.174-182

Whetten, K., Reif, S., Ostermann, J., Pence, B., Swartz, M., Whetten, R., Conover, C., Bouis, S., Thielman, N. & Eron, J. (2006). Improving health outcomes among individuals with HIV, mental illness, and substance use disorders in the Southeast. *AIDS Care*, Vol.18, Supplement 1, (2006), pp.S18-26

Whetten, K., Reif, S., Napravnik, S., Swartz, M., Thielman, N., Eron, J., Lowe, K. & Soto, T. (2005). Substance abuse and symptoms of mental illness among HIV-positive persons in the Southeast. *South Med J*, Vol.98, No.1, (January 2005), pp.9-14

Whetten, K., Reif, S., Whetten, R., & Murphy-McMillan, L.K. (2008). Trauma, mental health, distrust, and stigma among HIV-positive persons: implications for effective care. *Psychosomatic medicine*, Vol.70, No.5, (June 2008), pp.531-538

Whetten, R., Messer, L. Ostermann, J. Whetten, K. Pence, B. W. Buckner, M. Thielman, N. O'Donnell, K. and the Positive Outcomes for Orphans (POFO) Research Team. Child work and labour among orphaned and abandoned children in five low and middle income countries. *BioMed Central International Health and Human Rights*, Vol.11, No.1, (January 2011), doi:10.1186/1472-698X-11-1

Whitmire, L. Harlow, L., Quina, K. & Morokoff, P. (1999). *Childhood Trauma and HIV: Women at Risk*, Taylor and Francis, ISBN 9780876309476, Ann Arbor, MI

World Health Organization (WHO). (2007). *World Health Report 2007 - A safer future: global public health security in the 21st century*. Geneva, Switzerland

Zierler, S., Cunningham, W., Andersen, R., Shapiro, M., Nakazono, T., Morton, S., Crystal, S., Stein, M., Turner, B., St Clair, P. & Bozzette, S. (2000). Violence victimization after HIV infection in a US probability sample of adult patients in primary care. *Am J Public Health*, Vol.90, No.2, (February 2000), pp.208–215

Zuberi, T., Sibanda, A. & Udjo, E. (2005). *Demography Of South Africa (General Demography of Africa)*, M.E. Sharpe, ISBN 978-0765615633, Armonk, NY

16

Impact of Socio-Medical Factors on the Prevention and Treatment of HIV/AIDS Among Specific Subpopulations

La Fleur F. Small
Wright State University
USA

1. Introduction

The first cases of what would later be known as AIDS were first identified in the United States in June of 1981 (CDC, 1981). Since this recognition of the HIV/AIDS epidemic in the United States, patterns of morbidity and mortality have been altered, sexual practices scrutinized, and healthcare institutions overwhelmed. Today there are an estimated 1.1 million adults and adolescents living with HIV infection (CDC, 2008), and approximately 56,000 new HIV infections are occurring in the U.S. every year (CDC, 2010; Hall et al., 2008). Current HIV incidence rates have been stagnant since 2000 and are considerably lower than the mid 1980's peak of new HIV infections (*see figure 1*). Incident rates during the 1980's reached 130,000. The advent of highly active antiretroviral therapy (HAART) has helped to slow the progression of HIV to AIDS. However, antiretroviral drug resistant HIV-1 has been noted since 1993 (Eshleman et al., 2007). Today it is possible for people to contract a strain of HIV-1 that is resistant to up to three antiretroviral drug classes (Eshleman et al., 2007). Despite stagnant rates of new HIV infections, and modern biomedical convention that indicates equal susceptibility to contraction of HIV, the epidemic still disproportionately impacts specific subpopulations in the United States and some specific groups show increased incidence of HIV when compared to the general population. These groups often experience political and economic subordination, disenfranchisement, and stigmatization.
The most frequently researched of these subpopulations include; persons who are substance abusers (specifically injection drug users), men who have sex with men (MSM), Latino and African American women, older adults (over the age of 50), and adolescents (ages 13-24). What factors contribute to increase prevalence of HIV among these groups? Access and utilization of health services in the early stages of HIV infection can positively impact survival time (Andersen et al., 2000; Bozzette et al., 2003; Montgomery et al., 2002). The use of HAART is credited with declining rates of HIV associated morbidity, hospitalizations and mortality (Bozzette et al., 2003; Montgomery et al., 2002). Interventions for modifying risk behavior and providing current, appropriate health education and medical care have been tested and proven effective in subpopulations. However, in order to develop and fund effective interventions, an understanding of the social determinants of illness within these groups proves advantageous.

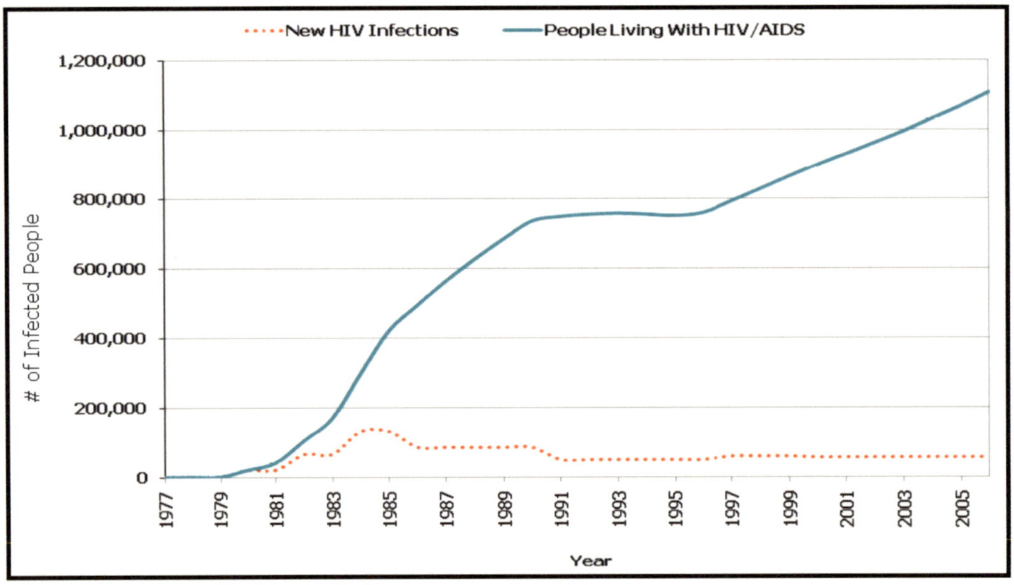

Fig. 1. Estimates of Annual HIV Infection and People Living with HIV/AIDS (1977-2006). (Source: The White House Office of National AIDS Policy, 2010)

This article is a meta-analysis that synthesizes research focusing on the five aforementioned groups. The impetus of this article is to illustrate the unique impact of HIV on each subpopulation by evaluating social factors, social networking, barriers to the receipt of care, unique factors that influence pathogenesis among each group, and to highlight specific interventions developed for each group. Thus, a socio-medical perspective that includes the use of biomedical data, demographic statistics, and an understanding of the individual illness and treatment experience, will be used to analyze increased HIV/AIDS rates amongst these groups.

2. Men Who Have Sex with Men[1] (MSM)

At its onset the HIV epidemic was disproportionately present in the gay community and in resources focused on addressing death and dying (Beckerman & Fontana, 2009). Sexual activity between same sex male partners and intravenous drugs represent some of the most frequent routes of HIV transmission and both groups were highly stigmatized by the general public. In the infancy of HIV/AIDS a strong relationship existed between the stigmatization of persons with same sex orientation and the stigmatization of HIV (Brooks et al., 2005; Edgar et al., 2008). Early in the epidemic, the gay, lesbian, bisexual and transgender (LGBT) community developed its own education campaigns and institutions to reduce HIV in the wake of inaction by government and other institutions (Office of National AIDS Policy, 2010). This coupled with the 1996 introduction of highly active antiretroviral therapy (Beckerman & Fontana, 2009; Brennan et al., 2009; Brennan et al., 2010) changed the perception of HIV as a terminal disease and placed emphasis on adherence to medication,

[1]The term men who have sex with men (MSM) is used in CDC surveillance systems. It indicates behaviors that transmit HIV infections, rather than how individuals self -identify in terms of sexuality.

quality of life and prevention. The demography of HIV/AIDS has changed in the United States, but the majority of newly HIV infections continue to occur among MSM (Benotsch et al., 2002; Brennan et al., 2010). CDC surveillance data indicate that while MSM represent only 2 %[2] of the U.S. population they account for 53% (*n*=28,720) (*see figure 2*)of the newly reported HIV infections (Bachmann et al., 2009; Brennan et al., 2010; CDC, 2008; CDC, 2011;Hall et al., 2008; Office of National AIDS Policy, 2010). Men who have sex with men is one of the only at risk populations that have reported a steady increase in annual numbers of new HIV infections (CDC, 2010; Hall et al., 2008). Diagnoses of HIV in this subpopulation increased 17% from 2005- 2008 (CDC, 2008: CDC, 2010). After initial momentum to decrease HIV/AIDS in the LBGT population, what factors have promoted increase in the rates of infection among MSMs? Emerging factors that may contribute to increased risk for MSMs include "AIDS burnout," (Wolitski et al., 2001) treatment optimism, faulty harm reduction techniques, and sexual risk taking behavior.

AIDS burnout stems from years of exposure to prevention messages and long term efforts to promote safe sex among MSMs and is an independent predictor of unprotected anal intercourse among this group (Wolitski et al., 2001). Often the outdated or overly simplistic safer sex messages ("no glove, no love") have decreased the visibility of HIV prevention messages in some MSM communities (Wolitski et al., 2001). AIDS burnout, coupled with a series of interconnected contextual factors, helps to elucidate the increase in prevalence of HIV among MSMs.

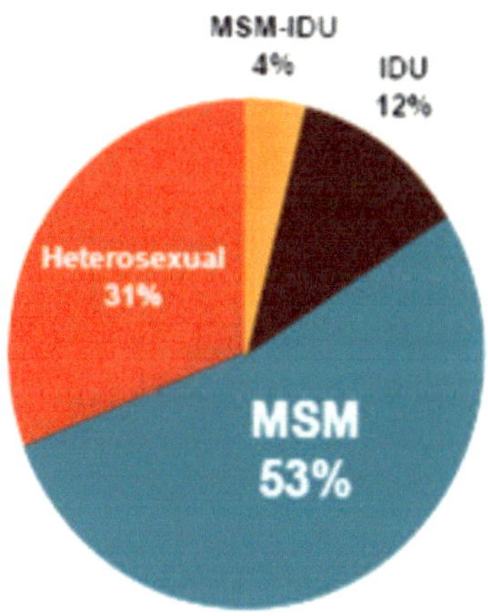

Fig. 2. Estimates of New HIV Infections in the United States, By Transmission Category, 2006. (Sources; CDC, 2010.)

Since the introduction of HAART in 1996, being diagnosed with HIV is perceived as less serious because of the availability of drugs to mitigate the impact of the virus (Bakeman, 2007; Brennan, 2010).This concept defined as treatment optimism is theorized to play a role in increased sexual risk taking behavior among MSMs (Brennan et al., 2009; Brennan et al., 2010). HIV positive MSMs were more likely to report increased treatment optimism than HIV negative MSMs. This belief is grounded in some scientific research that suggests that

[2] The estimate of 2% is based upon the range of 1.4-2.7% in the overall population age 13 and older who engaged in same sex behavior in the last five years.

HIV transmission can be mitigated when infected persons are receiving HAART therapy and has a reduced viral load (Brennan et al., 2010; Quinn et al., 2000). This coupled with the availability of postexposure therapy and viral load monitoring lessens the perceived risk of contracting HIV. However, even if risk is lessened on an individual level, increases in risk taking behavior have implications for population based concern for increased HIV transmission.Yet another social factor that has influenced treatment optimism is diminished public attention. Converse to reports of AIDS burnout, it's believed that in general, media and public attention to HIV/AIDS has decreased since the onset of the epidemic and many no longer view it as a public health emergency. A 2009 Kaiser Family Foundation survey found only 45% of respondents indicated hearing messages highlighting the plight of HIV/AIDS compared to 70% in 2004 (Office of National AIDS Policy, 2010).

In addition to AIDS burnout and treatment optimism, research indicates an increase in sexual risk behavior among MSMs (Benotsch et al., 2002; Blackwell, 2008; Brennan, 2010; Brewer et al., 2006; Parsons, 2005; Van Kesteren, 2007; Wolitski et al., 2001). It is possible that the practice of faulty harm reduction sexual techniques has contributed to the increase of new HIV cases among MSMs. Some of these techniques include HIV positive men positioning themselves as the receptive partner for unprotected anal sex, as a method of strategic positioning designed to reduce sexual risk (Parsons, 2005; Van De Ven et al., 2002). Other risk reduction efforts include serosorting or limiting sexual partners to seroconcordant (similar) HIV status (Barrett et al., 1998; Eaton et al., 2009; Parsons, 2005). Consequently, HIV positive males limit sexual intercourse to other HIV positive males. Conversely, HIV negative males will seek similar partners. Faulty rationalization assumes a skewed perceived susceptibility to contracting HIV, that sexual partners are aware of their HIV status, and/or willing to truthfully disclose this information (Eaton et al., 2009; Parsons, 2005).

Levels of HIV stigma associated with homosexuality reduced as universal susceptibility is encouraged via public health awareness campaigns. UNAIDS defines HIV stigmatizing as a "social process of devaluation that reinforces negative thoughts about a persons living with HIV and AIDS" (Brooks et al., 2005). However, social bias still remains, which in turn creates limited dating outlets (Brooks, 2005). Like other disenfranchised groups, MSMs have few places in which they can meet without fear of social consequences. Several outlets include gay pride cultural events, friendship networks, and sexually charged environments (gay bars, bath houses, and public places) (Bull et al., 2004; Parson, 2005; Van Kersteren, 2007). It is in these sexually charged environments that spontaneous, unexpected and unprotected sex take place. Intentional acts of unprotected sex have become colloquially known as "bare-backing" (Blackwell, 2008; Parsons, 1995). A newly emerging outlet that is of particular interest is the internet. This medium provides a new way of meeting sexual partners without scrutiny (Benotsch et al., 2002; Blackwell et al., 2008; Bull et al., 2004). Description of online sex partner seeking highlights a three stage process that often includes the use of MSM chat rooms, meetings in person, and then ultimately sexual activity (Benotsch et al., 2002; Bull et al., 2004).

2.1 Interventions

Strategies for reducing HIV among MSMs have included; (1) expanded HIV testing so that infected persons can be identified, treated and the risk of transmitting the virus is minimized; (2) individual, small group and community level interventions to reduce risk behaviors ;(3) promotion of condom use ;and the (4) detection and treatment of sexually transmitted diseases (CDC, 2011). Two of the latest prevention strategies include cyberspace educational prevention approaches and Pre-exposure Prophylaxis Initiatives (PrEP). The internet is emerging as an important venue for forming sexual networks among MSMs (Benotsch, et al., 2002). To create effective interventions that are specific to MSMs cyberspace interventions have varying components that include safer sex guidelines, emailing systems for partner notification and psychosocial components designed to increase motivation for behavior change (Benotsch, et al., 2002). Pre-exposure prophylaxis is designed to prevent the acquisition of HIV infection among persons uninfected but exposed to MSMs. Preliminary findings indicate that daily orally administered antiretrovirals may partially reduce HIV among MSMs when provided with regular monitoring of HIV status and ongoing risk reduction adherence counseling (CDC, 2011).The CDC and other U.S Public Health Service (PHS) agencies are developing guidelines for the use of PrEP among MSMs at high risk for HIV.

3. Substance abusers: Injection Drug Users (IDUs)

Transmission of HIV in persons who use illicit drugs remains a major public health challenge. Intravenous (IV) drug use has been a driving force for the spread of HIV/AIDS and contributes substantially to the current HIV burden in the United States (Des Jarlais et al., 1989; Riley, et al., 2010; Rudolph et al., 2010a; Rudolph, et al., 2010b). People who inject drugs are a relatively small share of the U.S. population, but they are disproportionately represented in the HIV epidemic. Of the 16 million drug injection drug users (IDUs) worldwide, an approximately 3 million are HIV infected (Mathers et al. 2008; Vlahov et al., 2010). In the United States there are an estimated 1 million IDUs, yet injection drug use accounts for approximately 16% of new HIV infections (Brady et al., 2008; Hall et al., 2008). Intravenous injection of drugs provides the user with the strongest drug effect with the least cost. Injection into the vein leads to a strong drug reaction (effective crossing of the blood brain barrier) and it's dissolution in liquid prior to injection insures usage of most of the purchased drug, unlike the lost of product associated with smoking or inhaling drugs (Des Jarlais & Seman, 2008). Unfortunately, the injection process also allows a direct route for HIV to enter the human body. While the CDC acknowledged the first cases of HIV among MSMs in 1981, Friedman and colleagues have argued that HIV was present in the IDU New York city population since the mid to late 1970's (2007) (figure 3.1). However infections in this sub-population were ignored due to a hostile legal and sociopolitical environment, influenced by the federal government's "War on Drugs" (Des Jarlais et al., 1989; Des Jarlais et al., 1994; Des Jarlais et al., 2000; Freidman et al., 2007; Santibanez et al., 2006; Stoneburner et al., 1988). This slowed the public health response to the epidemic among IDUs. However, by the mid 1980's the visibility of characteristics of AIDS among IDUs was evident and could no longer be ignored.

Understanding the rates of HIV/AIDS among IDUs proves an arduous task. Drug users tend to be less conspicuous than other high risk groups. Additionally, there is a general lack of advocacy and support groups among persons with substance abuse addiction, often leading to limited information about HIV among this population. Moreover, IDUs represent a heterogeneous group of people whose behavior varies and often impacts seroprevalence. In addition to injection drug use, an IDU may also; (1) be a MSM; (2) or experience high risk heterosexual contact (Santibanez et al., 2006). However, decades of research has highlighted

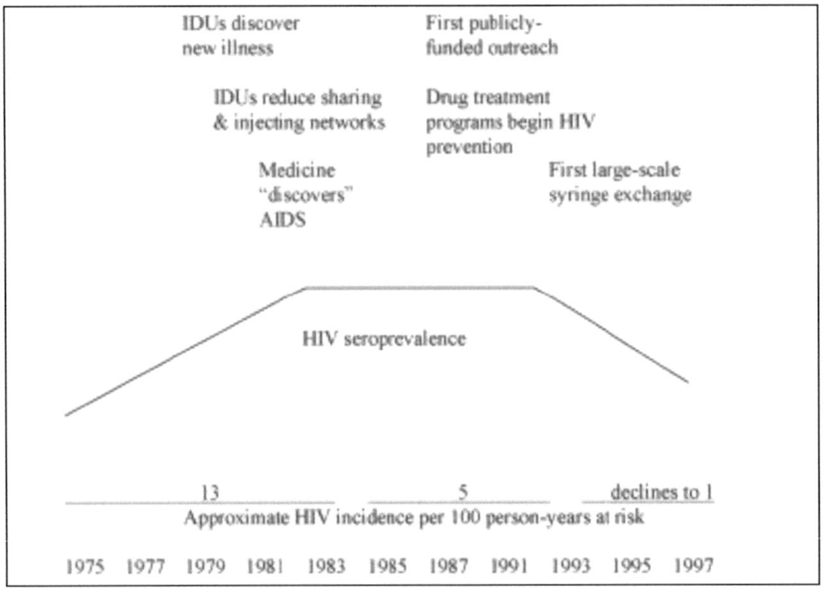

Fig. 3.1. Schematic history of the New York City HIV epidemic among people who inject drugs. (Source; Freidman et al., 2008)

several factors that explain the nexus between IDUs and the transmission of HIV. The first of these factors includes the sharing of used syringes and drug equipment (works) (Friedman et al., 1999; Rudolph et al., 2010).Drug equipment such as; (1) used bottle caps, spoons, or other containers ("cookers"); (2) used pieces of filtering cotton or cigarette filters ("cottons"); and (3) water that was already used to dissolve drugs or clean syringes (Friedman et al., 1999) allows for the transfer of infected bloodproduct from one person to the next. Subsets of IDU's who share works and injection shooting galleries (Des Jarlais & Seman, 2008) ,where one syringe is often rented to numerous clients, or those that participate in backloading[3] or frontloading[4] are particularly more likely to become infected (Des Jarlais & Seman, 2008; Friedman, et al., 1999; Santibanez et al., 2006). IDUs often share works due to restricted access to sterile needles and syringes. For example, mechanisms to limit access to clean syringes can be instituted by state laws that require a prescription to obtain syringes, thereby, outlawing syringe exchange programs (SEPS) in some states. Additionally, law enforcement strategies such as placing police near needle exchange sites and arresting IDUs for drug residue in a used syringe can encourage needle sharing (Des Jarlais & Seman, 2008). However, research indicates that increased access to SEPs exchange has lowered syringe sharing among IDUs, thereby lowering levels of infection among individuals and the larger community, (Riley, et al., 2010; Rotherman-Borus et al., 2010;

[3] Backloading refers to the practice of splitting /sharing drugs, whereby solution of dissolved drugs (and perhaps HIV) is squirted from one person's syringe to another using the back or plunger end of the receiving syringe.

[4] Frontloading refers to the practice of splitting /sharing drugs, whereby solution of dissolved drugs (and perhaps HIV) is squirted from one person's syringe to another. In frontloading, the needle is removed and the drug is transferred through the front of the syringe. Frontloading is less common in the United States because the diabetic syringes commonly used in the US do not have detachable needles.

Rudolph et al., 2010(A); Rudolph et al., 2010(B); Santibanez et al., 2006) and is cost effective and does not lead to increase drug injection or recruit first time injectors (Santibanez et al., 2006).

Lack of available substance abuse treatment programs and HAART is yet another factor that explains the impact of injecting drug use on the HIV/AIDS epidemic. Estimates from the 2007 National Survey on Drug Use and Health (NSDUH) indicate that approximately 7.5 million persons needed treatment for an illicit drug problem and of those needing treatment, about 6.2 million persons did not receive substance abuse treatment (Substance Abuse and Mental Health Services Administration, 2008). Injection drug users experience numerous barriers to treatment. However, a substantial portion of IDUs report an inability to access substance abuse treatment, highlighting a structural barrier to care (Milloy et al., 2009). Pollack and D'Aunno report much IDUs addiction treatment is provided through outpatient treatment centers, however few offer the suggested CDC HIV counseling and testing to their clients (2010), and miss opportunities to diagnose HIV. Additional findings indicate that injection drug itself is a major barrier to HAART initiation (Arasteh & Des Jarlais, 2009; Mehta et al., 2010). Many IDUs do not initiate HAART, or initiate HAART after significant delay (Mehta et al., 2010). Moreover injection drug users have been found to received less HAART and derive less benefit from HAART when received (Arasteh & Des Jarlais, 2009). For IDU's in methadone maintenance programs drug interactions often mean modifications to their HAART regiments (Arasteh & Des Jarlais, 2009). Often physicians are reluctant to prescribe HAART therapy to IDUs because of incomplete adherence, and unstable lifestyles that can promote resistance to antiretroviral therapy (Werb et al., 2010; Wolfe et al., 2010). Greater concerns exists for the possibility that drug -resistant HIV strains could be transmitted to the wider community (Werb et al., 2010).

Sexual transmission of HIV from IDUs to other persons - both other injectors and non-drug user's injection partners has important public health implications (Arasteh & Des Jarlais, 2009; Des Jarlais & Seman, 2008; Meader et al., 2010; Strathdee & Patterson, 2005; Wolfe et al., 2010). IDUs are considered a bridge to spreading HIV to persons through sexual contact and to HIV-infected children. Mothers who reported injection drug use or who had sex with an injection drug user accounted for 51% of cases of mothers documented with HIV (CDC, 2009). In 2006 the CDC revamped universal guidelines requiring HIV testing of all pregnant women without requiring separate written consent allowing early diagnosis of HIV and decreased risk of perinatal transmission from mother to infant (Gaskins, 2010). Early diagnosis and effective antiretroviral therapy has decreased perinatal transmission rates to less than 2% (Gaskin). Nondisclosure of HIV positive status among IDUs may contribute to sexual spread of HIV from IDUs. Significant disincentives and barriers to revealing a HIV positive status may contribute to nondisclosure. Fear of isolation, abandonment, rejection and criminal prosecution[5] may limit disclosure and limit the safety of subsequent sexual activity (Kalichman, 2005). These factors are particularly salient for sex workers infected with HIV. Many IDUs, male and female alike, trade sex for money/or drugs (Friedman et al., 1999). Other factors explaining the impact of injection drug use on sexual transmission highlight that drug use is often concentrated in neighborhoods (Rotheram-Borus et al., 2010), and high rate of injection drug use and risky sexual behavior are often reported among IDUs in low income communities (Wolfe et al., 2010). Des Jarlais & Seman believe

[5] As of 1999 31 states had statues making sexual contact without disclosure a criminal offense and many laws now address exposure (whether or not condoms were involved) not just infection.

that HIV can spread from IDUs to non-injecting sex partners and develop into sustained heterosexual transmission within certain communities (2008). This heterosexual and self-sustained transmission may well explain the high rates of transmission among Black women in the U.S. (*see section 4: Black and Latino women*).

3.1 Interventions

The primary focus of prevention and intervention programs developed for IDUs have been harm reduction strategies and behavioral interventions. Harm reduction is referred to as a set of policies and programs working collaboratively to reduce drug related harm (Friedman, et al., 2007). Harm reduction is based on a strategy that departs from the criminalization of addiction and rather treats addiction as a chronic medical disease. Two of the most popular harm reduction strategies are sterile needle exchange and acquisition programs and opioid agonist therapy (OAT). While both are controversial, these programs have been associated with reductions in and the cessation of injection drug use (Des Jarlais & Seman, 2008; Riley et al., 2010; Rudolph et al.,2010a; Vlahov et al., 2010). Opioid agonist therapies (OAT) were developed to treat opioid dependence, which can involve long lasting physiological and molecular adaptations in the brain. One of the most widely used forms of OAT is methadone maintenance therapy. Methadone blocks the euphoric effects of other opioids and is associated with decreased illicit drug use (Strathdee & Patterson 2005; Vlahov, et al., 2000). Buprenorphine is another popular OAT used among IDUs who are HIV positive. Buprenorphine is safer for use in HIV infected persons receiving HAART because it has fewer drug interactions (Vlahov et al., 2010). Behavioral interventions focus on encouraging IDUs to refrain from risk behaviors (injection drug use, unprotected sex, and sharing drug paraphernalia) that can promote the spread of HIV. These interventions can reduce risk behaviors of IDUs at the level of the individual or social network (Freidman et al., 1999; Santibanez et al., 2006; Vlahov et al., 2010). Drug abuse treatment is the most widely endorsed intervention to reduce HIV-associated risks behaviors among IDUs (Strathdee & Patterson, 2005).

4. Black and Latino women

The HIV/AIDS epidemic rapidly spread and impacted women (Zierler & Kreiger, 1997) and urban communities of color during the period when epidemiological, government and media attention was focused almost solely on the gay population and injection drug users (Weeks et al., 1996). In 1981, six women in the United States were presented with an unexplained underlying cellular immune deficiency. These symptoms were similar to the phenomenon experienced by gay males in the United States that later lead to the official recognition of AIDS. Moreover, research indicates that between 1980 and 1981, 48 women died of AIDS related causes of death (Zierler & Kreiger, 1997). The potential magnitude of the female epidemic continued largely unremarked. Although men continue to represent the majority of new HIV cases, thirty years after the recognition of the disease the proportion of women infected with HIV/AIDS continues to rise.In 1985, women represented 8% of AIDS diagnoses; by 2005 they accounted for 27% (*Figure 4.1*) (CDC, 2007). In 1994, HIV/AIDS represented the third leading cause of death among women (Saul et al., 2000; Weeks et al., 1996;). The route of transmission for an overwhelming majority of new HIV cases among women is through heterosexual contact. The majority of the women infected with the virus are disproportionately women of color; African American and Latino women specifically. While blacks make up only 12% of the U.S. population, they represented nearly half of all people living with HIV in the U.S. in 2006 (46%, or 510,100 total persons). Sixty-four percent of all women living with HIV/AIDS are black. The prevalence rate for black women (1,122 per 100,000) was 18 times the rate for white women (63 per 100,000). Likewise, Hispanics/Latinos account for 15% of the U.S. population, but they accounted for 18% of people living with HIV in 2006 (194,000 total persons). The prevalence rate for Hispanic/Latino women (263 per 100,000) was four times the rate for white women (63 per 100,000) (CDC, 2008; Hall, 2008). An explanation for the disparity in the biological transmission of HIV among women of color is extricable bound to social and economic relations of class, gender, race, and sexuality (Zierler & Kreiger, 1997).

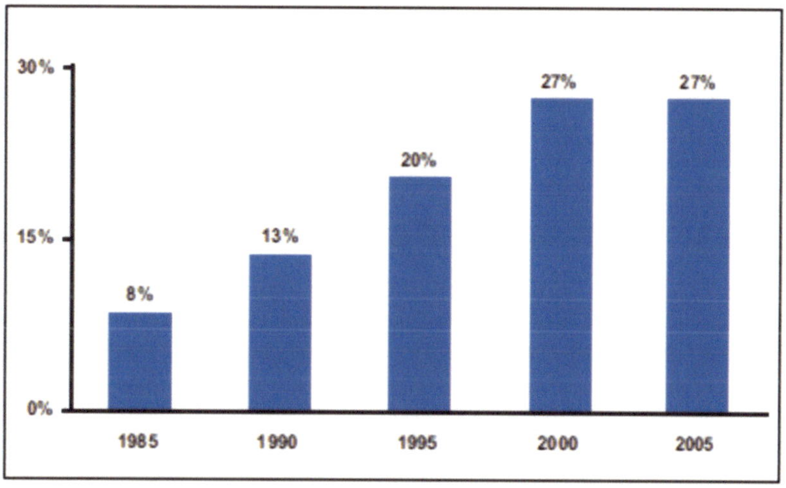

Fig. 4.1. Women as a Proportion of New Diagnosis 1985-2005. (Source; Kaiser Foundation)

There is little difference in opportunistic processes or disease progression in women and men with HIV/AIDS (Gaskins, 2010). However, while heterosexual transmission of the HIV can occur both from males to females and from females to males (Gaskins, 2010), biologically women are more susceptible to contracting the virus (Fasula et al., 2009; Gaskins, 2010; Johnson & Johnstone, 1993; Minkoff et al.,1995;Nichols et al., 2002; Weeks et al,1996; Zierler & Krieger, 1997). There is increased biological efficiency of HIV transmission from the male to female in heterosexual intercourse (Campbell, 1999; Fasula et al., 2009, Minkoff et al, 1995). The proportion of AIDS cases in women attributed to sex with men rose steadily from 15% in 1983 to 38% in 1995 (Minkoff et al., 1995; Zierler &. Krieger, 1997). Today approximately 75%-85% of new HIV infections in women stem from heterosexual contact (Doherty et al, 2009; Fasula et al., 2009) *(figure 4.2)*. Susceptibility to HIV is further increased with the risk of trauma to cervical cells during intercourse (Gaskins, 2010; Nichols et al., 2002), and the presence of sexually transmitted diseases in women (ex. Human Papamoilla Virus (HPV), gonorrhea, Trichomonas vaginalis, chlamydia etc.) and other gynecologic infections,that can facilitate the acquisition of HIV (Gaskins, 2010: Sutton et al., 2009).

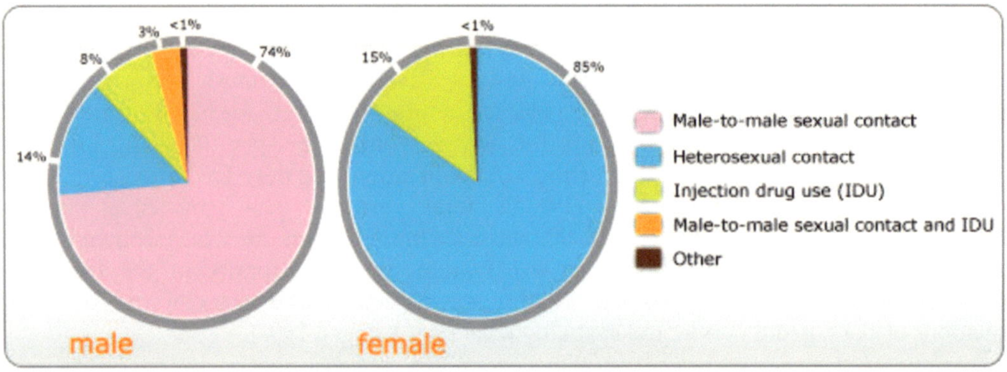

Fig. 4.2. Estimated adult and adolescent new HIV diagnoses in 2009 by transmission route and gender.

Since most infections among women occur through heterosexual sex, their risk is predicated on the risk behaviors of their male partners and gender based-inequality. Abstinence is often not an option for women experiencing domestic violence or victims of sexual violence. Among women living with HIV infection nearly half reported forced sexual experiences (Zierler & Krieger, 1997).The fear of partner violence negatively affects a women's ability to protect themselves sexually (Gonzalez-Guards et al., 2008; Zierler & Krieger, 1997). Even in the absences of partner violence women's economic dependence on men (income, food, housing, child support, etc.) often makes negotiating condom use and safer sex practices difficult (Flaskerud et al, 1996; Gaskins, 2010; Gil, 1995; Saul et al, 2002; Weeks et al, 1996; Zierler & Krieger, 1997). Monogamous relationships can only offer protection if both partners have sex exclusively with each other and do not partake in other HIV/AIDS risk behaviors. Heterosexual intercourse with male partners who are substance abusers (specifically IDUs) helped facilitate the spread of HIV/AIDS amongst women (Campbell, 1999; Minkoff et al, 1995). About 48% of all AIDS cases are in women and are known to be related to IDU in some way (CDC, 2009). Similarly sexual contact with MSMs (who are married or in long term heterosexual relationships) has also heightened the spread of HIV amongst women (Campbell, 1999; .Minkoff et al, 1995).

Black and Latino women experience unique cultural factors that increase their vulnerability to HIV infection. One such issue relates to the high rates of incarceration in these communities and the impact on HIV transmission. Large numbers of incarcerated men creates a gender imbalance in these communities that can fuel HIV transmissions. US Bureau of Justice Statistics indicate that 60% of the 2.3 million incarcerated Americans are Black and Latino (Sabol & West, 2010). Additionally, Black males born in 2001 have 32% chance of going to jail compared to 17% chance for Latino males and 6% for White males. Thus, Black boys are five times and Latino boys nearly three times as likely as white boys to go to jail (Sabol & West, 2010). This trend is influenced greatly by the mandatory drug sentencing policies impacting low income minority communities. Disproportionate incarceration rates among African Americana and Latino men contribute to an imbalance in the ratio of men to women and thereby promote concurrent partnerships (Doherty et al., 2009). Concurrent sexual networks (partnerships overlap temporally) more efficiently promotes the spread of STDs and HIV (Doherty et al., 2009; Margolis et al., 2006). Moreover, incarceration and the "correctional revolving door" further explain the racial disparity in female HIV/AIDS infection rates amongst African American and Latino women versus

White women. While incarcerated inmates are likely to be exposed to and/ or contract HIV, or become exposed to a pleura of risky behaviors which include risky drug use and tattooing practices and consensual and nonconsensual unprotected sexual intercourse (Fullilove, 2008). The HIV/AIDS epidemic is passed to the women in the sexual networks of inmates in these communities as inmates cycle from jails and prisons, back to the general populous, and in many cases return to jails and prisons as recidivist (Fulliove, 2008).

Yet another unique cultural artifact that influences the spread of HIV/AIDS among Black and Latino women are a bipartite of embedded gender inequalities and taboos toward homosexuality and bisexuality. Cultural roles can conflict with behaviors that can decrease the risk of HIV. In Latino communities the gender concept machismo/marianismo implies that household, public, as well as sexual decision making is dominated by men and women have very little power of refusal or negotiation ability (Davila, 2000; Flaskerud et al., 1996; Russell et al., 2000; Saul et al., 2000; Weeks et al, 1996). Moreover, traditional Latino culture emphasizes sexual activity by men and the avoidance of such activity by women (Flaskerud et al., 1996). Therefore Latino women may be especially at high risk of acquiring HIV heterosexually because Latino men are more likely to report multiple sex partners than other racial and ethnic groups (Saul et al., 2000). Within Latino culture, women-initiated sexual decisions, such as condom negotiation may be viewed as a challenge to male authority and trigger male resistance to condom use (Davila, 2000). While the popular image of the Black woman being independent, strong and assertive in their relations with Black men exists (Weeks et al., 1996), Black women face similar cultural restraints. The number of marriageable women far outweighs the number of marriageable men and results in Black women having relatively less power in their sexual relationships (Alleyne & Gaston, 2010; Doherty et al., 2009). Therefore, Black women's risk of contracting HIV increases owning to Black males' engagement in multiple concurrent sexual relationships, and black women's forced willingness to accept man sharing.These factors are further exacerbated by strong cultural beliefs that often stigmatize MSMs in Black and Latino communities. Homosexuality is culturally taboo in Black and Latino communities and is frequently viewed as "a sickness that afflicts only whites" (Bing & Soto, 1991). Consequently men in both minority groups may have great difficulty accepting their sexual orientation (Bing & Soto, 1991) and be secretive about their behavior, and not seek proper treatment for HIV/AIDS (Galanti, 2003). Because men who have sex with men (MSMs) may not identify themselves as homosexual or bisexual because (1); they are on the insertive not receptive end of anal sex (Galanti, 2003; Nichols et al., 2002; Russell et al, 2000); and (2) also engage in sex with women., they place their female partners at great risk. For example, a study showed that 34% of Black men who reported having sex with men also reported having sex with women, while only 6% of the women reported knowledge of having sex with a bisexual male (Brown & Hook, 2006). The confluence of gender inequalities and taboos toward homosexuality and bisexuality, limits opportunities for education, intervention, and treatment of HIV/AIDS, putting women in Black and Latino communities at risk of contracting HIV.

4.1 Interventions

Numerous complexities of race, culture, sexuality, religiosity, socioeconomic status, culture, and power affect HIV/AIDS risks and prevention for Black and Latino women. There exist gaps in the research literature and further gaps in research on gender and sexuality in the sociopolitical context of Black and Latino women (Fitzpatrick et al., 2006; Russell et al., 2000;

Weeks et al., 1996; Zambrana et al., 2004). Moreover, this lack of knowledge limits coalition building, which is critical to HIV/AIDS prevention in women, among women in communities of color (Weeks, et al., 1996). To address these gaps in the research literature, limited enrollment in HIV clinical trials and limited treatment access, in 2003 the Center for Disease Control (CDC) created the Minority HIV/AIDS Research Initiative (Fitzpatrick et al., 2006). This program is designed to provide junior investigators assistance to conduct gap research in communities of color. The rationale for this program highlights the need to; (1) research HIV/AIDS in Black and Latino communities, (2); addressing evident research gaps can only be accomplished by understanding culture-specific nuances ascribed to Blacks and Latinos, and (3); the similarity between researcher and community would remove barriers to conducting effective research (Fitzpatrick et al., 2006). Weeks et al., highlight the need for indigenous female educators and organizers with an understanding of cultural issues to educate women of color about their risk potential (1996). Similarly, these women can also serve as principle investigators and direct research questions to build greater understanding of the social context within which Black and Latino women can make decisions and influence their sexual partners.

5. Older adults

Persons 50 and older comprise approximately 10-15% of all AIDS cases in the U.S. (CDC, 2002; Goodroad, 2003; Inelmen et al., 2005; Jacobs & Kane, 2009; Manfredi, 2002; Ory, et al., 1998; Radda, et al., 2003; Williams & Donnelly, 2002; Zelenetz & Epstein, 1998). However, these numbers may be subject to underreporting bias because they do not include those persons over 50 who are HIV-seropositive but have not developed AIDS (Altschuler et al., 2004; Heckman et al., 2006) or adults diagnosed with AIDS prior to 50 (Altschuler et al., 2004). More recent data indicates that older adults may account for a much higher percentage of people with HIV/AIDS. From 2001-2004 the percentage of all HIV cases in the U.S. for adults age 50 and older increased from 17% to 23% (CDC, 2004; Emlet et al., 2009; Gebo, 2006; Kirk, & Goetz, 2009; Orel et al., 2010). Moreover, the CDC forecasts that by the year 2015 half of all cases of HIV/AIDS will be in persons age 50 and older (Heckman et al., 2006). In creating the definition of "older adult", the CDC assumed a bell-shaped demographic distribution of people with HIV/AIDS infection. Using this approach, a person aged ≥ 50 meets the definition of older adult (CDC, 1992; Luther & Wilkin, 2007 Manfredi, 2002; Orel et al., 2005). The increases in incidence and prevalence of HIV diagnoses within this population are particularly important in lieu of the phenomenon of age transition[6] (UN, 2007). This factor is heightened by the efficacy of Highly Active Antiretroviral Therapy (HAART) rendering HIV/AIDS a chronic disease with declining mortality and fewer AIDS- related opportunistic infections (Manfredi, 2002; Stark, 2006). Consequently, the net effect is a growing, vulnerable, graying HIV-positive population.

Older adults experience specific health challenges (Siegel et al., 1999), HAART treatment issues (Grabar et al., 2006; Nogueras et al., 2006; Silverburg et al., 2007), and social stigma associated with the infection (Emlet, 2006; Goodroad, 2003; Stark, 2006). These health challenges are unique to this subpopulation and create barriers to the receipt of care, and

[6]The age transition refers to a predictable shift from a predominantly younger population when fertility is high to a predominantly older population when fertility is low.

mediate the rising trend of a geriatric HIV positive population. Symptom ambiguity between HIV/AIDS infection and diseases associated with aging (such as diabetes mellitus, decreased renal function, and cardiac disease) often leading to misdiagnosis (Siegel et al., 1999; Zelentz & Epstein, 1998) and delays in diagnosing HIV. Moreover, due to physiologic changes associated with aging, there is a more rapid rate of progression of HIV to AIDS, and increased susceptibility to opportunistic illnesses in older adults (Gebo, 2006; Goodroad, 2003; Mack & Bland, 1999; Manfredi, 2002) (See figure 5). Other health challenges faced by older adults who are diagnosed with HIV include treatment complications due to co-morbidities and polypharmacy (Grabar et al., 2006; Luther & Wilkin, 2007; McLennon, 2003).

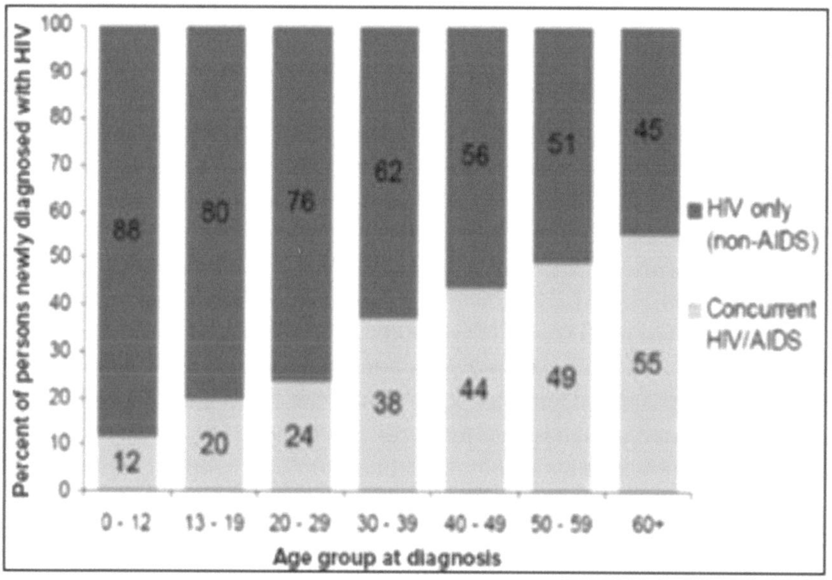

Fig. 5. Concurrent HIV/AIDS among Persons Diagnosed With HIV in 2006, By Age Group in The United States.

In addition to the issues associated with diagnosis of HIV, not too many advances have been made in the provision of effective HAART therapy, amongst older populations. Late diagnosis, impaired immune response, toxicities associated with HAART therapy and lack of knowledge about efficacy of HAART treatment among older adults contribute to high rates of mortality soon after diagnosis (Goetz et al., 2001; Mack & Bland, 1999; Manfredi & Chiodo, 2000; Nokes et al., 2000). Advanced age at seroconversion have always been important prognostic factors in the progression of HIV infection and survival mediated only by the widespread introduction of HAART therapy (Grabar et al., 2006; Manfredi, 2002). However, older patients are often excluded from clinical trials, and studies evaluating efficacy of HAART therapy in older adults are characterized by small numbers and short follow up (Grabar et al., 2006).

Social issues surrounding HIV/AIDS in the older adult are just as important as the biomedical and pharmacotherapeutic aspects. Adults aged ≥50 experience a multidimensional form of HIV-related social stigma. Initially, ageist ideologies among many health care workers contribute to the general lack of understanding and recognition of HIV in the older adult (Goodroad, 2003; Stark, 2006). Research indicates relatively high sexual activity and some risk taking behavior among older adults (Gott, C.M., 2001; Inelman et al., 2005; Jacobs & Thomlison, 2009; Neundorfer et al., 2005; Steinke, 1994). However, ageism and myths concerning elderly populations and infrequent sexual activity, drug use, and other risk taking behavior have made routine screening less common, HIV/AIDS cases more often ignored, and diagnosis of disease delayed (Grabar et al., 2006; Mack & Bland, 1999; Orel et al., 2005). After diagnosis many older adults refrain from disclosing their HIV status to family and friends. Emlet found that older adults were less likely to disclose HIV to relatives, partners, mental health workers, neighbors, and church members than those 20-39 years of age (2006). Limiting the disclosure of HIV status controls the possibility of being stigmatized and facing discrimination (Emlet, 2006; Goodroad, 2003). A latent consequence of such behavior is the forgoing of much needed social support during this health crisis.

5.1 Interventions

Despite being one of the fastest growing segments of the HIV/AIDS caseload, persons age 50 and older have been largely neglected in both education and intervention efforts. While many public health campaigns are designed to target at risk populations and youth in the 13-24 age range, older adults are being ignored in terms of age-specific epidemiology, prevention, intervention and treatment programs (Mack & Ory, 2003; Ory et al., 1998). Hence older adults with HIV/AIDS have been coined in the literature as "the invisible ten percent" and the "hidden population" (Orel et al., 2005). Efforts to understand the rationale behind the unmet need for educational and intervention programs among older adults highlighted the role of state departments of public health in the distribution of current HIV/AIDS health- related information (Orel et al., 2004; Orel et al., 2005). However, findings indicate that only 15 of the 50 state health departments (30%) reported providing HIV/AIDS publications that were specifically intended for older adults (Orel et al., 2004). Successful intervention strategies include embedding and personalizing HIV/AIDS education for older adults with other provided health information. Emlet and colleagues advocate for national collaboration between aging network organizations and AIDS service organizations (ASOs), thereby providing seamless access to services /programs for AIDS and aging service providers (2009). Additionally, the use of HIV peer educators for older adults has been explored by the Senior Intervention Project (SHIP) in south Florida and proven successful not only in education, but also in linking and referring HIV positive patients to care and treatment services (Agate et al., 2003).

6. Adolescents

Adolescents and young adults represent one of the at risk groups for contracting HIV infections in the United States (Belzer et al., 1999). Approximately one quarter of new infections occur among adolescents and young adult (ages 13-29) (CDC, 2008). The definition for adolescence varies depending on the organization and the type of report being produced. The CDC often refers to adolescence between the ages 10-19 and young adults between the ages 20-24 (Wilson et al., 2010). Conversely, the World Health Organization often refers to young people and includes individuals between the ages of 10 to 24 years of age. Due to this variance both adolescents and young adults up till the age of 25 will be discussed in this chapter.

The identification of adolescents with HIV proves difficult because of medicolegal difficulties regarding consent and testing of adolescents, and procurement of this at risk group (Earl, 1993). Historically, these rates of HIV infection have been viewed as a function of adolescent risky sexual and drug use behavior (Di Clemente, 1997; Di Clemente & Wingood, 2000). Initiation of sexual activity often begins in mid adolescences (13-17) (Earl, 1993). Additionally, rates of STD infections are highest for sexually active persons between the ages of 15-24 (Balassone et al., 1993). Findings indicate that a majority of sexually active adolescents do not consistently take precautions to avoid contracting HIV/AIDS and other STDs (Balassone et al., 1993). Adolescence represents a developmental period characterized by risk taking behaviors prefaced on denial, invulnerability, and succumbing to peer influence (Garvie et al., 2009). Yet other risk factors unique to this group, such as, childhood sexual abuse and homelessness contribute to this sub-populations rate of HIV infections. Several studies report incest and sexual abuse survivors may engage in HIV-risky sexual behavior, including sexual compulsivity (Whitmire et al., 1999). In one study, college aged women who reported childhood sexual abuse reported less assertiveness in refusing unwanted sexual activity and less assertiveness about the use of condoms (Whitmire et al., 1999). Many adolescents who experience childhood abuse resort to escapism often becoming homeless runaways (Di Clemente, 1992; National Commission on AIDS, 1994). Consequently, this group may practice survival strategies such as prostitution or pornography that contribute to increased risk for HIV infection (Di Clemente, 1992; Lyon & D' Angelo, 2006; Whitmire et al., 1999). The residential instability of this group of adolescents, dysfunctional family history, lack of perceived life chances, and mental and physical deterioration and may not only contribute to HIV infection, but to rapid progression from HIV to AIDS, compared to their non homeless counterparts (Di Clemente, 1992; Lyon & D' Angelo, 2006; Whitmire et al., 1999). Interesting additional risk factors that influence the contraction of HIV by youths include many of the aforementioned populations in this chapter. These include adolescents who may be; (1) young MSMs; (2) IDUs; (3) racial and ethnic minorities; (4) and heterosexual females; (Kalichman, 2005). The diversity among this group and overlapping needs makes developing effective intervention programs challenging. However, regardless of risk factor experienced adolescents are less likely than adults to adhere to HAART therapy (Belzer, et al., 1999; Lyons & D'Angelo, 2006; Williams et al., 2006). Psychosocial, mental health and substance use problems often make it difficult for youth to adhere to HAART (Garvie et al., 2010).

6.1 Interventions

Adolescents as a group need sensitive and appropriate anticipatory guidance as they transition into adulthood. Adolescents with HIV need considerably more support. Most interventions are designed with an individualistic perspective and are sexual behavior modification interventions, aimed at reducing adolescent vulnerability to HIV by enhancing intrapersonal and interpersonal mediators of preventive behavior (Di Clemente, 1997; Di Clemente & Wingood, 2000). Appropriately tailored interventions addressing; (1) maintaining good physical health; (2) reducing transmission risk behavior and; (3) and promoting and maintaining positive mental health (Kalichman, 2005; Murphy et al., 2000) have been developed. Numerous avenues of dissemination are currently employed in intervention/education efforts and include telephone, internet (Noia et al., 2004) focus group, and individual delivery mechanisms. Current interventions stress the importance of using the parental-child relationship (National commission on AIDS, 1994) and the schools as an intervention setting for risk reduction among adolescents (Di Clemente, 1992; National Commission on AIDS, 1994).

7. Conclusion

In July 2010 the White House Office released a national HIV/AIDS strategy for the United States. The vision for the national HIV/AIDS strategy was stated as follows: "The United States will become a place where new HIV infections are rare and when they do occur, every person, regardless of age, gender, race/ethnicity, sexual orientation, gender identity or socioeconomic circumstances, will have unfettered access to high quality, life extending care, free from stigma and discrimination" (Office of National AIDS Policy, 2010). To this end, the executive branch of government aims to ;(1) reduce the number of people who become infected with HIV, ;(2) increase access to care and optimize health outcomes for people who become infected with HIV; and (3) reduce HIV related disparities. Thirty years after acknowledging the existence of HIV/AIDS, a coordinated government, public health, and community response is needed to achieve a more appropriate response to the HIV epidemic, focusing on interventions and prevention strategies for those most severely impacted by this disease.

8. References

Agate, L.; Mullins, J.; Prudent, E.; & Liberti, T. (2003) Strategies for Researching Retirement Communities and Aging Social Networks: HIV/AIDS Prevention Activities Among Seniors in South Florida. *Journal of Acquired Immune Deficiency Syndromes*, Vol. 33 No. 2, pp S238-S242, ISSN: 1525-4135(print), ISSN; 1077-9450(online).

Alleyne, B.; & Gaston, G. (2010). Gender disparity and HIV risk among young black women in college: A literature review. *Journal of Women and Social Work,* Vol.25, No.2, pp. 135-145, ISSN: 1552-3020

Altschuler, J.; Katz, A.; Tynan, M. (2004). Developing and implementing an HIV/AIDS educational curriculum for older adults. *The Gerontologist*, Vol.44 No.1, pp. 121-126, ISSN: 0016-9013 (print) 1758-5341 (electronic)

Andersen, R.; Bozzette, S.; Shapiro, M.; St. Clair, P.; Morton, S.; Crystal, S.; Goldman, D.; Wenger, N.l; Gifford, A.; Leibowitz, A.; Asch, S.; Berry, S.; Nakazono, T.; Helin, K.; Cunningham, W.; & HCSUS Consortium. (2000). Access of Vulnerable Groups to Antiretroviral Therapy among Persons in Care for HIV Disease in the United States.*Health Services Research,* Vol. *35 No.2, pp.* 389-416, ISSN: 1475-6773 (electronic)

Arasteh, K.; & Des Jarlais, D. (2009). HIV testing and treatment among at-risk drinking injection drug users. *Journal of the International Association of Physicians in AIDS Care (Chicago, Ill.: 2002)*, Vol.8, No.3, pp. 196-201, ISSN: 1557-0886 (print), 1545-1097 (electronic)

Bachmann, L.; Grimley, D.; Chen, H.; Aban, I.; Hu, J.; Zhang, S.; Waithaka, Y.; & Hook III, E. (2009). Risk behaviors in HIV-positive men who have sex with men participating in an intervention in a primary care setting. *International Journal of HIV and AIDS,* Vol.20, pp. 607-612, ISSN: 1179-1373

Bakeman, R.; & Peterson, J. (2007). Do beliefs about HIV treatments affect peer norms and risky sexual behavior among African-American men who have sex with men? *International Journal of STD and AIDS,* Vol.18, pp. 105-108, ISSN: 0956-4624 (print), 1758-1052 (electronic)

Balassone, M.; Baker, S.; Gillmore, M.; Morrison, D.; & Dickstein, D. (1993). Interventions to decrease the risk of HIV/AIDS and other sexually transmitted diseases among high-risk heterosexual adolescents. *Children and Youth Services Review,* Vol.15, pp. 475-488, ISSN: 0190-7409

Barrett, D.;Bolan, G.; & Douglas, J. (1998). Redefining gay male anal intercourse behaviors: Implications for HIV prevention and research. *The Journal of Sex Research,* Vol.35, No.4, pp. 381-389, ISSN: 0022-4499 (print), 1559-8519 (electronic)

Beckerman, A.; & Fontana, L. (2009). Medical treatment for men who have sex with men and are living with HIV/AIDS. *American Journal of Men's Health,* Vol.3, No.4, pp. 319-329, ISSN: 1557-9883 (print), 1557-9891 (electronic)

Belzer, M.; Fuchs, D.; Luftman, G.; & Tucker, D. (1999). Antiretroviral adherence issues among HIV-positive adolescents and young adults. *Journal of Adolescent Health,* Vol.25, pp. 316-319, ISSN: 1054-139X

Benotsch, E.; Kalichman, S.; & Cage, M. (2002). Men who have met sex partners via the internet: Prevalence, predictors, and implications for HIV prevention.*Archives of Sexual Behavior,* Vol.31, No.2, pp. 177-183, ISSN: 0004-0002 (print), 1573-2800 (electronic)

Bing, E.; & Soto, T. (1991). Treatment issues for African-Americans and Hispanics with AIDS. *Psychiatric Medicine,* Vol.9, No.3, pp. 455-467, ISBN: 978-0-7817-8408-5

Blackwell, C. (2008). Men who have sex with men and recruit bareback sex partners on the internet: Implications for STI and HIV prevention and client education. *American Journal of Men's Health,* Vol.2, No.4, pp. 306-313, ISSN: 1557-9883 (print), 1557-9891 (electronic).

Bozzette, S. A.; Berry, S.; Duan, N.; Frankel, M. R.; Leibowitz, A.; Lefkowitz, D.; Emmons, C.; Senterfitt, W.; Berk, M.; Morton, S.; & Shapiro, M. (2003). The care of HIV-infected adults in the United States. *The New England Journal of Medicine,* Vol.*339 No.26,* pp.1897-1904, ISSN: 0028-4793 (print) 1533-4406 (electronic).

Brady, J.; Friedman, S.; Cooper, H., (2008). Risk-based prevalence of infection drug users in the U.S. and in large U.S. metropolitan areas from 1992-2002. *Journal of Urban Health, Bulletin of the New York Academy of Medicine* Vol., 85, pp 323-351. ISSN: 1099-3460 (print version), ISSN: 1468-2869 (electronic version).

Brennan, D.; Welles, S.; Miner, M.; Ross, M.; Mayer, K.; & Rosser, B. (2009). Development of a treatment optimism scale for HIV-positive gay and bisexual men. *AIDS Care,* Vol.21, No.9, pp. 1090-1097, ISSN: 0954-0121 (print), 1360-0451 (electronic)

Brennan, D.; Welles, S.; Miner, M.; Ross, M.; & Rosser, B. (2010). HIV treatment optimism and unsafe anal intercourse among HIV-positive men who have sex with men: Findings from the positive connections study. *AIDS Education and Prevention,* Vol.22, No.2, pp. 126-137, ISSN: 0899-9546.

Brewer, D.; Golden, M.; & Handsfield, H. (2006). Unsafe sexual behavior and correlates of risk in a probability sample of men who have sex with men in the era of highly active antiretroviral therapy. *Sexually Transmitted Diseases,* Vol.33, No.4, pp. 250-255 ISSN: 0148-5717

Brooks, R.; Etzel, M.; Hinojos, E.; Henry, C.; & Perez, M. (2005). Preventing HIV among latino and African American gay and bisexual men in a context of HIV-related stigma, discrimination, and homophobia: Perspectives of providers. *AIDS Patient Care and STD'S,* Vol.19, pp. 737-744, ISSN: 1087-2914 (print), 1557-7449 (electronic)

Brown, E.; & Van Hook, M. (2006). Risk behavior, perceptions of HIV risk, and risk-reduction behavior among a small group of rural African American women who use drugs. *Journal of the Association of Nurses in AIDS Care,* Vol.17, No.5, pp. 42-50, ISSN: 1055-3290

Bull, S.; McFarlane, M.; Lloyd, L.; & Rietmeijer, C. (2004). The process of seeking sex partners online and implications for STD/HIV prevention. *AIDS Care,* Vol.16, No.8, pp. 1012-1020, ISSN: 0954-0121 (print) 1360-0451 (electronic)

Cambell, C. (1999) Women, families, & HIV/AIDS. *Cambridge University Press.* ISBN: 0-521-56211-2

Center for Disease Control and Prevention (CDC) (1981). *Vol. 30, pp.1981, ISSN:* 1080-6059

Center for Disease Control and Prevention. (1992). 1993 revised classification system for HIV infection and expanded surveillance case definition for AIDS among adolescents and adults. *MMWR Recomm Rep,* Vol.41, pp.1-19, ISSN: 1080-6059

Center for Disease Control and Prevention. (2002). *HIV/AIDS surveillance report: U.S. HIV and AIDS cases reported through December 2001.* Year End edition Vol.13, No. 2, ISSN: 1080-6059

Center for Disease Control and Prevention. (2004). *HIV/AIDS surveillance report, 2004.* Vol.16. Atlanta (GA): US Department of Health and Human Services, ISSN: 1080-6059

Center for Disease Control (CDC) (2008).Prevalence Estimates-United States, 2006. *MMWR.* Vol.57, No.39, pp. 1073-1076, ISSN: 1080-6059

Center for Disease Control and Prevention .(2009). HIV/AIDS surveillance report, 2007. Vol. 19, pp.1-63, *ISSN:* 1080-6059

Center for Disease Control (CDC) (2010). HIV in the United States: An Overview. ISSN: 1080-6059

Center for Disease Control (CDC) (2011). Interim Guidance: Preexposure Prophylaxis for the Prevention of HIV Infection IN Men who Have Sex With Men. MMWR. Vol. 60, No.3, ISSN: 1080-6059

Davila, Y. (2000). Hispanic women and AIDS: Gendered risk factors and clinical implications. *Issues in Mental Health Nursing,* Vol.21, pp. 635-646, ISSN: 0161-2840 (print), 1096-4673 (electronic).

Des Jarlais, D.; Freidman, S.; Novick, D.; Sotheran, J.; Thomas, P.; Yancovitz, S.;Mildvan, D.; Weber,J.; Kreek, M.; Maslansky, R.; Bartelme,S.; Spira, T.; Marmor, M.(1989). HIV-1 infection among intravenous drug users in Manhattan from 1977 through 1987. *Journal of American Medical Association,* Vol.261, No.7, pp 1008-1012. ISSN: 0098-7484 (print version), ISSN: 1538-3598(electronic version).

Des Jarlais, D.; Freidman, S.; Sotheran, J.; Wentson, J.; Marmor, M.; Yancovitz, S.; Frank, B.; Beatrice, S.; Mildvan, D. (1994). Continuity and change within an HIV epidemic: Injection drug users in New York City, 1984 through 1992. *Journal of American*

Medical Association, Vol. 217, No. 2, pp 121-127. ISSN: 0098-7484 (print version), ISSN: 1538-3598(electronic version).

Des Jarlais, D.; Marmor, M.; Freidman, P.;Titus, S.; Aviles, E.; Deren, S.;Torian, L.; Glebatis, D.; Murrill, C.; Monterroso, E.; Freidman, S. (2000). HIV incidence among injection drug users in New York City, 1992-1997: Evidence for a declining epidemic. *American Journal of Public Health*, Vol. 9, No.3, pp 352-359. ISSN: 00900036.

Des Jarlais, D.; & Semaan, S. (2008). HIV prevention for injection drug users: The first 25 years and counting. *Psychosomatic Medicine*, Vol. 70, pp. 606-611. ISSN: 0033-3174 (print) 1534-7796 (electronic)

Di Clemente, R. (1992). *Adolescents and AIDS: A Generation in Jeopardy*. Sage Publishers, Newbury Park.ISBN:0-8039-4181-1

Di Clemente, R. (1997). Looking forward: future directions for prevention of HIV among adolescents. In; Sherr, L., ed. *AIDS and Adolescents*. Reading, Berkshire, United Kingdom: Harwood Academic Publishers. 189-199, ISBN: 90-5702-038-6

Di Clemente, R. & Wingood, G. (2000). Expanding the scope of HIV prevention for adolescents: Beyond individual-level interventions, Journal of Adolescent Health, Vol. 26, pp 377-378, ISSN: 1054-139X.

Doherty, I.; Schoenbach,V.; Adimora, A. (2009).Sexual mixing patterns and heterosexual HIV transmission among African Americans in the southeastern United States, *Journal of Acquired Immunodeficiency Syndrome*, Vol. 52. No.1, pp114-120, ISSN: 1525-4135(print), ISSN; 1077-9450(online).

Earl, D. (1993). How to recognize adolescents at risk for HIV infection. *Journal of the Tennessee Medical Association*, Vol.86, No.5, pp. 191-194, ISSN: 1088-6222

Eaton, L.; West, T.; Kenny, D.; & Kalichman, S. (2009). HIV transmission risk among HIV seroconcordant and serodiscordant couples: Dyadic processes of partner selection. *AIDS and Behavior*, Vol. 13, No. 2, pp. 185-195. ISSN: 1090-7165 (print) 1573-3254 (electronic)

Edgar, T.; Noar, S.; Freimuth, V. (2008). Communication perspectives on HIV/AIDS for the 21st century. ISBN: 0805858261

Emlet, C. (2006). A comparison of HIV stigma and disclosure patterns between older and younger adults living with HIV/AIDS. *AIDS Patient Care and STDs*, Vol.*20, No.* 5, pp. 350-358, ISSN: 1087-2914 (monthly) 1557-7449 (electronic)

Emlet, C.; Gerkin, A.; & Orel, N. (2009). The graying of HIV/AIDS: Preparedness and needs of the aging network in a changing epidemic. *Journal of Gerontological Social Work*, Vol.52, No.8, pp. 803-814, ISSN: 0163-4372 (print), 1540-4048 (electronic)

Eshleman, S.; Husnik, M.; Hudelson, S.; Donnell, D.; Huang, Y.; Huang, W.; Hart, S.; Jackson, B.; Coates, T.; Chesney, M.; & Koblin, B. (2007). Antiretroviral drug resistance, HIV-1 tropism, and HIV-1 subtype among men who have sex with men with recent HIV-1 infection. *AIDS*, Vol.21, pp. 1165-1174, ISSN: 0269-9370 (print), 1473-5571 (electronic)

Fasula, A.; Miller, K.; & Sutton, M.Y. (2009). An early warning sign: sexually transmissible infections among young African American women and the need for preemptive, combination HIV prevention. *International Journal of Sexual Health*, Vol.6, pp. 261-263, ISSN: 1931-7611 (print) 1931-762X (electronic)

Fitzpatrick, L.; Sutton, M.; Greenberg, A. (2006). Toward eliminating health disparities in HIV/AIDS: The importance of the minority investigator in addressing scientific gaps in Black and Latino communities. *Journal of the National Medical Association,* Vol. 98, No.12, 1906-1911. ISSN: 0027-9684

Flaskerud, J.; Uman, G.; Lara, R.; Romero, L.; & Taka, K. (1996). Sexual practices, attitudes, and knowledge related to HIV transmission in low income Los Angeles Hispanic women. *The Journal of Sex Research,* Vol.33, No.4, pp. 343-353, ISSN: 0022-4499 (print), 1559-8519 (electronic)

Freidman, S.; Curtis, R.; Neaigus, A.; Jose, B.; Des Jarlais, D. (1999). *Social Networks, Drug Injector's Lives and HIV/AIDS.* Kluwer Academic/Plenum Publishers, NY. ISBN: 0-306-46079-3.

Freidman, S.; Jong, W.; Rossi, D.; Touze, G.; Rockwell, R.; Des Jarlais, D.; Elovich, R. (2007). Harm reduction theory: User's culture, micro social indigenous harm reduction, and the self organization and outside-organizing of user's groups. *International Journal of Drug Policy,* Vol. 18, pp 107-117. ISSN: 0955-3959.

Fullilove, R. (2008). Sociocultural factors influencing the transmission of HIV/AIDS in the United States: AIDS and the nation's prisons. In *Comprehensive Textbook of AIDS Psychiatry.* R. Cohen & J. Gorman (Eds.) *Oxford University Press. NY,* ISBN: 13: 978-0-19-530435-0

Galanti, G. (2003). The Hispanic family and male-female relationships: An overview. *Journal of Transcultural Nursing,* Vol.14, pp. 180-185, ISSN: 1043-6596 (print), 1552-7832 (electronic)

Garvie, P.; Lawford, J.; Flynn, P.; Gaur, A.; Belzer, M.; Sherry, G.; & Hu, C. (2009). Development of a directly observed therapy adherence intervention for adolescents with human immunodeficiency virus-1: Application of focus group methodology to inform design, feasibility, and acceptability. *Journal of Adolescent Health,* Vol.44, pp. 124-132, ISSN: 1054-139X

Garvie, P.; Wilkins, M.; & Young, J. (2010). Medication adherence in adolescents with behaviorally- acquired HIV: Evidence for using a multimethod assessment protocol. *Journal of Adolescent Health,* Vol.47, pp. 504-511, ISSN: 1054-139X

Gaskins, S. (2010). HIV infection in women. In. J.D Durham and F. R. Lashley (eds.) In The person with HIV/AIDS, nursing perspectives. *Springer Publishing Company,* pp.437-459. ISBN: 978-0-8261-2138-7

Gebo, K. (2006). HIV and aging: Implications for patient management. *Drugs Aging,* Vol. *23,* No.11, pp 897-913, ISSN: 1170-229X

Gil, V. (1995). The new female condom: Attitudes and opinions of low-income Puerto Rican women at risk for HIV/AIDS. *Qualitative Health Research,* Vol.5, pp. 178-203, ISSN: 1049-7323 (print), 1552-7557 (electronic)

Goetz, M.; Boscardin W.; Wiley, D.; & Alkasspooles S. (2001). Decreased recovery of CD4 lymphocytes in older HIV-infected patients beginning highly active antiretroviral therapy. *AIDS,* Vol.*15,* pp.1576-1579, ISSN: 0269-9370

González-Guarda, R.; Peragallo, N.; Urrutia, M.; Vasquez, E.; & Mitrani, V. (2008). HIV risks, substance abuse, and intimate partner violence among Hispanic women and their intimate partners. *Journal of the Association of Nurses in AIDS Care,* Vol.19, No.4, pp. 252-266, ISSN: 1055-3290

Goodroad, B.K. (2003). HIV and AIDS in people older than 50. *Journal of Gerontological Nursing*, Vol.*29*, No.4, pp.18-24, ISSN: 0098-9134 (print) 1938-243X (electronic)

Gott, C. (2001). Sexual activity and risk-taking in later Life. *Health and Social Care in the Community, Vol. 9* No.2, pp. 72-78, ISSN: 1365-2524 (electronic)

Grabar, S.; Weiss, L.; & Costagliola, D. (2006). HIV infection in older patients in the HAART era.*Journal of Antimicrobial Chemotherapy,* Vol.*57,* pp. 4-7, ISSN: 0305-7453 (print) 1460-2091 (electronic)

Hall, H.; Song, R.; Rhodes, P.; Prejean, J.; An, Q.; Lee, L.; Karon, J; Brookmeyer, R.; Kaplan, E.; McKenna, M.; & Janssen, R. (2008). Estimates of HIV Incidence in the United States. *JAMA*, Vol.300, No.5, pp. 520-529, ISSN: 0098-7484 (print) 1538-3598 (electronic)

Heckman, T.; Barcikowski, R.; Ogles, B.; Suhr, J.; Carlson, B.; Holroyd, K.; & Garske, J. (2006). A telephone-delivered coping improvement group intervention for middle aged and older adults living with HIV/AIDS. *Annals of Behavioral Medicine*, Vol. *32 No.*1, pp. 27-38, ISSN: 0883-6612 (print) 1532-4796 (electronic)

Inelmen, E.; Gasparini G.; & Enzi, G. (2005). HIV/AIDS in older adults: A case report and literature Review. *Journal of American Geriatrics Society,* Vol.*60 no.*9, pp. 26-30, ISSN: 1532-5415 (electronic)

Jacobs, R.; & Kane, M. (2009). Theory-Based policy development for HIV prevention in racial/ethnic minority midlife and older women. *Journal of Women and Aging,* Vol.21, pp. 19-32, ISSN: 0895-2841 (print), 1540-7322 (electronic)

Jacobs, R.; & Thomlison, B. (2009). Self-Silencing and age as risk factors for sexually acquired HIV in midlife and older women. *Journal of Aging and Health,* Vol.21, No.1, pp. 102-128, ISSN: 0898-2643 (print), 1552-6887 (electronic)

Johnson, M.; & Johnstone, F. (1993). HIV infection in women. *Longman Group UK Limited.* ISBN: 0-443-04885-1

Kalichman, S. (2005). *Positive Prevention: Reducing HIV Transmission among People Living with HIV/AIDS.* New York NY, Kluwer Academic/Plenum Publishers, ISBN: 0-306-48699-7.

Kirk, J.; & Goetz, M. (2009). Human immunodeficiency virus in an aging population, a complication of success. *Journal of American Geriatrics Society,* Vol.57, No.11, pp. 2129-2138, ISSN: 1532-5415 (electronic)

Lyon, M. & D'Angelo, L. (2006). *Teenagers, HIV, and AIDS*. Praeger, Westport Connecticut. ISBN: 0-275-98892-9.

Luther, V; & Wilkins, A. (2007). HIV infection in older adults. *Clinical Geriatric Medicine,* Vol. *23*, pp. 567-583, ISSN: 0749-0690

Mack, K; & Bland, S. (1999). HIV testing behaviors and attitudes regarding HIV/AIDS of adults aged 50-64. *The Gerontologist, Vol. 39*, No.6, pp. 687-694, ISSN: 0016-9013 (print) 1758-5341 (electronic)

Mack, K. & Ory, M. (2003). AIDS and older Americans at the end of the twentieth century. *Journal of Acquired Immune Deficiency Syndromes.* Vol.*33 No.*S21, pp S68-S75., ISSN: 1525-4135(print), ISSN; 1077-9450(online).

Manfredi R., Chiodo R. (2000). A case control study of virological and immunological effects of highly active antiretroviral therapy in HIV-infected patients with advanced age. *AIDS,* Vol. 14, pp. 1475-1477, ISSN: 0269-9370 (print) 1473-5571 (electronic)

Manfredi, R. (2002). HIV disease and advanced age: An increasing therapeutic challenge. *Drugs and Aging*. Vol.*19, No.*9, pp. 647-669, ISSN: 1170-229X (print) 1179-1969 (electronic)

Margolis, A.; MacGowan, R.; Grinstead, O.; Sosman, J.; Kashif, I.; Flanigan, Timothy P.; & The Project START Study Group.

(2006). Unprotected sex with multiple partners: Implications for HIV prevention among young men with a history of incarceration. *Sexually Transmitted Diseases*, 33(3), pp. 175-180. ISSN: 0148-5717

Mathers, B.; Degenhardt, L.; Phillips, B.; Wiessing, L.; Hickman, M.; Strathdee, S.; Wodak, A.; Panda, S.; Tyndall, M.; Toufik, A.; & Mattick, R. (2008). Global epidemiology of injection drug use and HIV among people who inject drugs: A systematic review. *Lancet,* Vol. 372, pp. 1733-1745. ISSN: 0140-6736 (print) 1474-547X (electronic)

McLennon, S.; Smith, R.; & Orrick, J. (2003). Recognizing and preventing drug interactions in older adults with HIV. *Journal of Gerontological Nursing, Vol. 29, No.* 2, pp. 5-12, ISSN: 0098-9134 (print) 1938-243X (electronic)

Meader, N.; Li, R.; Des Jarlais, D.; Pilling, S. (2010). Psychosocial interventions for reducing injection and sexual risk behavior for preventing HIV in drug users. *Cochrane Database of Systematic Reviews*, Issue 1. Art No.:CD007192. ISSN: 1469-493X

Mehta, S.; Kirk, G.; Astemborski, J.; Galai, N.; & Celentano, D. (2010). Temporal trends in highly active antiretroviral therapy initiation among injection drug users in Baltimore, Maryland, 1996-2008. *Clinical infectious diseases: an official publication of the Infectious Diseases Society of America*, Vol.50, No.12, pp. 1664-1671. ISSN: 1058-4838 (print) 1537-6591 (electronic)

Milloy, M.; Kerr, T.; Zhang, R.; Tyndall, M.; Montaner, J.; & Wood, E. (2010). Inability to access addiction treatment and risk of HIV infection among injection drug users recruited from a supervised injection facility (dagger). *American Journal of Public Health*, Vol.32, No.3, pp. 342-349, ISSN: 0090-0036 (print), 1541-0048 (electronic)

Minkoff, H.; DeHovitz, J.; & Duerr, A. (1995). HIV infection in women. *Raven Press*. ISBN: 0-7817-0236-4

Montgomery, J.; Gillespie, B.; Gentry, A.; Mokotoff, E.; Crane, L.; & James, S. (2002). Does access to health care impact survival time after diagnosis of AIDS*? AIDS Patients Care and STDs,* Vol.*16 No.2,* pp.223-231, ISSN: 1087-2914 (print) 1557-7449 (electronic)

Murphy, D.; Moscicki, B.; Vermund, S.; & Muenz, L. (2000). Psychological distress among HIV+ adolescents in the REACH study: Effects of life stress, social support, and coping. *Journal of Adolescent Health,* Vol.27, pp. 391-398, ISSN: 1054-139X

National commission on AIDS (1994). Preventing HIV/AIDS in adolescents. *The Journal of School Health,* Vol. 64, No.1, and pp. 39-51, ISSN: 0022-4391(print), ISSN: 1746-1561(online).

Nichols, J.; Speer, D.; Watson, B.; Watson, M.; Vergon, T.; Vallee, C.; & Meah, J. (2002). Aging with HIV psychological, social, and health issues. *Academic Press. Tampa, Florida*. ISBN: 0-12-518051-9

Nogueras, M.; Navarro, G.; Anton, E.; Sala, M.; Cervantes, M.; Amengual, M.; & Segura, F. (2006). Epidemiological and clinical features, response to HAART, and survival in

HIV-infected patients diagnosed at the age of 60 or more. *BMC Infectious Diseases, Vol. 6*, pp. 159-169, ISSN: 1471-2334

Nokes, K.; Holzemer, W.; Corless, I.; Bakken, S.; Brown, M.; Powell-Cope, G.M.; Inouye, J.; Turner, J. (2000). Health related quality of life in persons younger and older than 50 who are living with HIV/AIDS. *Research on Aging, Vol. 22*, No.3, pp. 290-310, ISSN: 0164-0275 (print) 1552-7573 (electronic)

Noia, J.; Schinke, S.; Pena, J.; & Schwinn, T. (2004). Evaluation of a brief computer-mediated intervention to reduce HIV risk among early adolescent females. *Journal of Adolescent Health*, Vol.35, pp. 62-64, ISSN: 1054-139X

Nuendofer, M.; Harris, P.; Britton, P.; & Lynch, D. (2005). HIV-risk factors for midlife and older women. *The Gerontologist, Vol. 45*, No.5, pp. 617-625, ISSN: 0016-9013 (print) 1758-5341 (electronic)

Office of National AIDS Policy. (2010). National HIV/AIIDS strategy for the United States. *The White House, United States*, pp. 1-45.

Orel, N.; Spence, M.; & Steele, J. (2005). Getting the message out to older adults: Effective HIV health education risk reduction publications. *The Journal of Applied Gerontology*, Vol. *24, No.*5, pp. 490-508, ISSN: 0733-4648 (print) 1552-4523 (electronic)

Orel, N.; Stelle, C.; Watson, W.; & Bunner, B. (2010). No one is immune, a community education partnership addressing HIV/AIDS and older adults. *Journal of Applied Gerontology*, Vol.29, No.3, pp. 352-370, ISSN: 0733-4648 (print) 1552-4523 (electronic)

Ory, M.; Zablotsky, D.; & Crystal, S. (1998). HIV/AIDS and aging: identifying a prevention research and care agenda. *Research on Aging*, Vol. *20*, No.6, pp.637-652, ISSN: 0164-0275 (print) 1552-7573 (electronic)

Parsons, J. (2005). HIV-Positive gay and bisexual men. In: S.C. Kalichman (eds.) Positive prevention reducing HIV transmission among people living with HIV/AIDS. *Kluwer Academic/ Plenum Publishers*, pp. 99-133. ISBN: 0-306-48699-7

Quinn, T.; Waver, M.; Sewankambo, N.; Serwada, D.; Li, C.; Wabwire Mangen, F.; Meehan, M,; Lutalo, T.; Gray, R.; Rakai Project Study Group. (2000). Viral load and heterosexual transmission of Human Immunodeficiency virus type. New England Journal of Medicine, Vol. 342, No.13, pp 921-929, 0028-4793 (print), ISSN 1533-4406 (electronic).

Radda, K., Schensul, J., Disch, W., Levy, J., Reyes, C. (2003). Assessing human immunodeficiency virus (HIV) risk among older urban adults: A model for community-based research partnership. *Family and Community Health*, Vol. *26*, No.3, pp. 203-213, ISSN: 0160-6379 (print), 1550-5057 (electronic).

Riley, E.; Kral, A.; Stopka, T.; Garfein, R.; Reuckhaus, P.; & Bluthenthal, R. (2010). Access to sterile syringes through SanFrancisco pharmacies and the association with HIV risk behavior among injection drug users. *Journal of urban health: bulletin of the New York Academy of Medicine*, Vol.87, No.4, pp. 534-542. ISSN: 1099-3460 (print) 1468-2869 (electronic)

Rotheram-Borus, M.; Rhodes, F.; Desmond, K.; & Weiss, R. (2010). Reducing HIV risks among active injection drug and crack users: the safety counts program. *AIDS and behavior*, Vol.14, No.3, pp. 658-668, ISSN: 1090-7165 (print), 1573-3254 (electronic)

Rudolph, A.; Crawford, N.; Moped, D.; Benjamin, E.; Stern, R.; & Fuller, C.; (2010a). Comparison of injection drug users accessing syringes from pharmacies, syringe exchange programs, and other syringe sources to inform targeted HIV prevention and intervention strategies. *Journal of the American Pharmacists Association: JAPhA*, Vol.50, No.2, pp. 140-147. ISSN: 1086-5802

Rudolph, A.; Standish, K.; Amesty, S.; Crawford, N.; Stern, R.; Badillo, W. (2010b). A community-based approach to linking injection drug users with needed services through pharmacies: an evaluation of a pilot intervention in New York City. *AIDS Education and Prevention: Official Publication of the International Society for AIDS Education*, Vol.22, No.3, pp. 238-251. ISSN: 1943-2755

Russell, L.; Alexander, M.; & Corbo, K. (2000). *Journal of the Association of Nurses in AIDS Care*, Vol.11, No.3, pp. 70-76, ISSN: 1055-3290

Sabol, W. & West, H. (2010). *Prisoners in 2009.* U.S. Bureau of Justice Statistics. NCJ231675

Santibanez, S.; Garfein, R.; Swartzendruber, A.; Purcell, D.; Paxton, L.; & Greenberg, A. (2006). Update and overview of practical epidemiologic aspects of HIV/AIDS among injection drug users in the United States. *Journal of Urban Health,* Vol. 83, No. 1, pp. 86-100. ISSN: 1099-3460 (print) 1468-2869 (electronic).

Saul, J.; Norris, F.; Bartholow, K.; Dixon, D.; Peters, M.; & Moore, J. (2002). Heterosexual risk for HIV among Puerto Rican women: Does power influence self-protective behavior? *AIDS and Behavior,* Vol.4, No.4, pp. 361-371, ISSN: 1090-7165 (print), 1573-3254 (electronic)

Siegel, K.; Dean, L.; & Schrimshaw, E. (1999). Symptom ambiguity among late-middle -aged and older adults with HIV. *Research on Aging*, Vol.*21,* No.4, pp. 595-618, ISSN: 0164-0275 (print) 1552-7573 (electronic)

Silverberg, M.; Leyde, W.; Horberg, M.; Delorenze, G.; Klein, D.;& Quesenberry, C.; (2007). Older age and response to and tolerability of antiretroviral therapy. *Archives of Internal Medicine, Vol. 167,* pp. 684-691, ISSN: 00039926

Stark, S. (2006). HIV after age 55. *Nursing Clinics of North America,* Vol.*41*, pp. 469-479, ISSN: 0899-5885

Steinke, E. (1994). Knowledge of attitude of older adults about sexuality in Ageing: A comparison of two studies. *Journal of Advanced Nursing,* Vol. *19*, pp. 477-485, ISSN: 0309-2402

Stoneburner, R.; Des Jarlais, D.; Benezra, D.; Gorelkin, L.; Sotheran, J.; Freidman,S.; Schultz, S.; Marmor, M.; Mildvan, D.; Maslansky, R. (1988). A larger spectrum of server HIV-1 related disease in intravenous drug users in New York City. *Science,* Vol. 2, pp 916-919. ISSN: 0036-8075 (print), 1095-9203 (online).

Strathdee, S. & Patterson, T. (2005). HIV-Positive and HCV-Positive Drug Users, pp135-162, In: *Positive Prevention: Reducing HIV Transmission among People Living with HIV/AIDS*, S.C. Kalichman (Ed.) ISBN: 0-306-48699-7.

Substance Abuse and Mental Health Services Administration, *Results from the 2007 National Survey on Drug Use and Health: National Findings* .NSDUH Series H-34, DHHS Publication No. SMA 08-4343) Rockville, MD: Office of Applied Studies, 2008.

Sutton, M.; Jones, R.; Wolitski, R.; Cleveland, J.; Dean, H.; & Fenton, K. (2009). A review of the centers of disease control and prevention's response to the HIV/AIDS crisis among blacks in the United States, 1981-2009. *American Journal of Public Health,* Vol.99, No.S2, pp.S351-S359, ISSN: 0090-0036 (print), 1541-0048 (electronic)

United Nations Population Division. (2007). *World Population Prospectus: The 2006 Revision.* New York: United Nations.

Van De Ven, P.; Kippax, S.; Crawford, J.; Rawstorne, P.; Prestage, G.; Grulish, A.; & Murphy, D. (2002). In a minority of gay men, sexual risk practice indicates strategic positioning for perceived risk reduction rather than unbridled sex. *AIDS Care: Psychological and Sociomedical Aspects of AIDS/HIV,* Vol. 14, No. 4, pp. 471-480. ISSN: 0954-0121 (print), 1360-0451 (electronic)

Van Kesteren, N.; Hospers, H.; & Kok, G. (2007) Sexual risk behavior among HIV-positive men who have sex with men: A literature review. *Patient education and counseling,* Vol. 65, pp. 5-20. ISSN: 0738-3991

Vlahov, D.; Robertson, A.; & Strathdee, S. (2010). Prevention of HIV Infection among Injection Drug Users in Resource-Limited Settings. *Clinical Infectious Diseases,* Vol.50, pp. S114-S121, ISSN: 1058-4838 (print), 1537-6591 (online)

Weeks, M.; Singer, M.; Crier, M.; & Schensul, J. (1996). Gender relations, sexuality, and AIDS risk among African American and Latina women. *Gender Relations, Sexuality, and AIDS Risk,* pp. 338-370. ISBN: 0-13-079427-9

Werb, D.; Mills, E.; Montaner, J.; & Wood, E. (2010). Risk of resistance to highly active anti retroviral therapy among HIV-positive injecting drug users: a meta-analysis. *Lancet Infectious Diseases,* Vol.10, No.7, pp. 464-469, ISSN: 0140-6736 (print) 1474-547X (electronic)

Whitmire, L., Harlow, L., Quina, K., Morokoff, P. (1999). Childhood Trauma and HIV: Women at Risk. Taylor & Francis Group, Ann Arbor, MI. ISBN: 0-87630-947-3.

Williams, E. & Donnelly, J. (2002). Older Americans and AIDS: Some guidelines for prevention. *Social Work,* Vol.*47, No.*2, pp. 105-111, ISSN: 1468-0173 (print) 1741-296X (electronic)

Williams, P.; Storm, D.; Montepiedra, G.; Nichols, S.; Kammerer, B.; Sirois, P.; Farley, J.; & Malee, K. (2006). Predictors of adherence to antiretroviral medications in children and adolescents with HIV infection. *Journal of the American Academy of Pediatrics,* Vol.118, No.6, pp. e1745-e1757, ISSN: 1073-0397

Wilson, C.; Wright, P.; Safrit, J.; & Rudy, B. (2010). Epidemiology of HIV infection and risk in adolescents and youth. *Journal of Acquired Immune Deficiency Syndromes,* Vol. 54, pp. S5-S6. ISSN: 1525-4135 (print) 1077-9450 (electronic)

Wolfe, D.; Carneri, M.; Shepard, D. (2010). Treatment and care for injecting drug users with HIV infection: a review of barriers and ways forward. *Lancet Infectious Diseases,* Vol.376, No.9738, pp. 355-366, ISSN: 0140-6736 (print) 1474-547X (electronic)

Wolitski, R.; Valdiserri, R.; Denning, P.; & Levine, W. (2001). Are we headed for a resurgence of the HIV epidemic among men who have sex with men? *American Journal of Public Health,* Vol. 91, No. 6. ISSN: 0090-0036 (print) 1541-0048 (electronic)

Zambrana, R.; Cornelius, L.; Boykin, S.; & Lopez, D. (2004). Latinas and HIV/AIDS risk factors: Implications for harm reduction strategies. *American Journal of Public Health,* Vol.94, No.7, pp. 1152-1158, ISSN: 0090-0036 (print), 1541-0048 (electronic)

Zelenetz, P.; & Epstein, M. (1998). HIV in the elderly. *AIDS Patient Care and STDs,* Vol.*12,* No.4, pp. 255-262, ISSN: 1087-2914 (print) 1557-7449 (electronic)

Zierler, S.; & Krieger, N. (1997). Reframing women's risk: Social inequalities and HIV infection. *American Journal* of *Public Health,* Vol.18, pp. 401-436, ISSN: 0090-0036 (print), 1541-0048 (electronic)